MW00852007

Out of the Crucible

HOW THE US MILITARY TRANSFORMED COMBAT CASUALTY CARE IN

IRAQ AND AFGHANISTAN

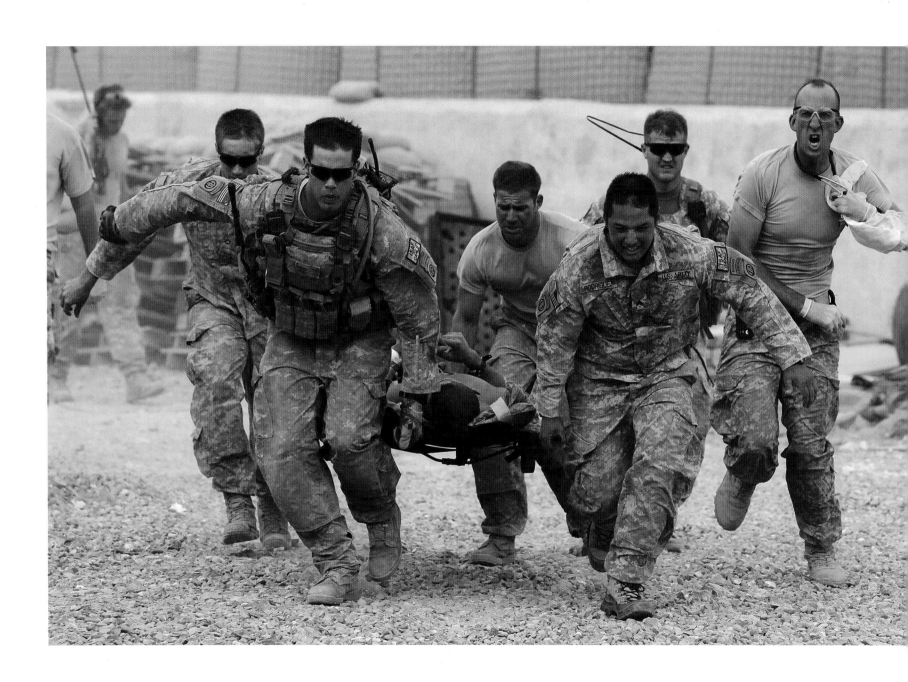

Out of the Crucible

HOW THE US MILITARY TRANSFORMED COMBAT CASUALTY CARE IN IRAQ AND AFGHANISTAN

senior editors

Arthur L. Kellermann, MD, MPH
Professor of Military and Emergency Medicine and Dean, F. Edward Hébert School of Medicine
Uniformed Services University of the Health Sciences

Eric Elster, MD
Captain, MC, US Navy
Professor and Chair, USU-Walter Reed Department of Surgery, F. Edward Hébert School of Medicine
Uniformed Services University of the Health Sciences

associate editors

Charles Babington
Principal, WaVe Communications

Racine Harris, MPH
Program Manager, Defense Health Horizons
Henry M. Jackson Foundation for the Advancement of Military Medicine

BORDEN INSTITUTE

US ARMY MEDICAL DEPARTMENT CENTER AND SCHOOL
HEALTH READINESS CENTER OF EXCELLENCE

Fort Sam Houston, Texas

JOHN H. GARR, MD, MSE, FACEP, Colonel, MC, US Army | *Director & Editor-in-Chief, Borden Institute*

JOAN REDDING | *Senior Production Editor*

VIVIAN MASON | *Volume Editor*

CHRISTINE GAMBOA, MS, MBA | *Creative Director & Production Manager, Fineline Graphics LLC*

The views expressed are those of the authors and do not necessarily represent those of the US Army, the US Department of Defense, or the United States Government. Use of trade or brand names in this publication does not imply endorsement by the Department of Defense. Partial support for this book was provided by Defense Health Horizons, a policy analysis unit at the Uniformed Services University of the Health Sciences.

CERTAIN PARTS OF THIS PUBLICATION PERTAIN TO COPYRIGHT RESTRICTIONS. ALL RIGHTS RESERVED. NO COPYRIGHTED PARTS OF THIS PUBLICATION MAY BE REPRODUCED OR TRANSMITTED IN ANY FORM OR BY ANY MEANS, ELECTRONIC OR MECHANICAL (INCLUDING PHOTOCOPY, RECORDING, OR ANY INFORMATION STORAGE AND RETRIEVAL SYSTEM), WITHOUT PERMISSION IN WRITING FROM THE PUBLISHER OR COPYRIGHT OWNER.

Published by the OFFICE OF THE SURGEON GENERAL

Borden Institute

US Army Medical Department Center and School

Health Readiness Center of Excellence

Fort Sam Houston, Texas

2017

Library of Congress Cataloging-in-Publication Data

Names: Kellermann, Arthur, editor. | Elster, Eric, editor. | Babington, Charles, editor. | Harris, Racine, editor. | Borden Institute (U.S.), issuing body.

Title: Out of the crucible : how the US military transformed combat casualty care in Iraq and Afghanistan / senior editors, Arthur L. Kellermann, Eric Elster ; associate editors, Charles Babington, Racine Harris.

Other titles: Out of the crucible (Kellermann)

Description: Fort Sam Houston, Texas : Borden Institute, 2017. | Includes bibliographical references.

Identifiers: LCCN 2017032811

Subjects: | MESH: Emergency Medical Services | Military Medicine | War-Related Injuries—therapy | War-Related Injuries—rehabilitation | Iraq War, 2003-2011 | Afghan Campaign 2001-

Classification: LCC RC971 | NLM WB 116 | DDC 616.9/8023—dc23 LC record available at https://lccn.loc.gov/2017032811

PRINTED IN THE UNITED STATES OF AMERICA

24, 23, 22, 21, 20, 19, 18, 17   5 4 3 2 1

[*Title Page image*] US Army Soldiers carry a critically wounded American Soldier on a stretcher to an awaiting MEDEVAC helicopter from Charlie Co., Sixth Battalion, 101st Airborne Combat Aviation Brigade, Task Force Shadow, June 24, 2010, near Kandahar, Afghanistan. Photo by Justin Sullivan/Getty Images. Reproduced with permission from: Getty Images.

For sale by the Superintendent of Documents, U.S. Government Publishing Office
Internet: bookstore.gpo.gov   Phone: toll free (866) 512-1800;   DC area (202) 512-1800
Fax: (202) 512-2104 Mail: Stop IDCC, Washington, DC 20402-0001

ISBN 978-0-16-094179-5

contents

Section One: Foundations

Section Two: Innovations

Section Three: Challenges

"Without question, our military medical professionals reflect the amazing light of creativity, compassion, and exquisite care . . . and it's especially brilliant in the darkest moments."

General Daniel B. Allyn

contributors

Hassan Alam, MD
Norman Thompson Professor of Surgery, Section Head of Surgery, Department of Surgery, University of Michigan, Ann Arbor, Michigan; Associate Professor of Surgery, Uniformed Services University of the Health Sciences, Bethesda, Maryland

Daniel B. Allyn, MA
General, US Army; 35th Vice Chief of Staff of the Army; Office of the Vice Chief of Staff, Washington, DC

Romney C. Andersen, MD
Colonel (Retired), Medical Corps, US Army; Chairman Emeritus, Department of Orthopaedics, Walter Reed National Military Medical Center; Professor, Department of Surgery, Uniformed Services University of the Health Sciences and the Walter Reed National Military Medical Center, Bethesda, Maryland

Rocco Armonda, MD
Colonel (Retired), Medical Corps, US Army; Associate Professor of Surgery, Uniformed Services University of the Health Sciences and the Walter Reed National Military Medical Center, Bethesda, Maryland

John H. Armstrong, MD
Affiliate Associate Professor of Surgery, Morsani College of Medicine, University of South Florida Health, Tampa, Florida

Regina C. Armstrong, PhD
Director of the Center for Neuroscience and Regenerative Medicine; Professor of Anatomy, Physiology and Genetics, Uniformed Services University of the Health Sciences, Bethesda, Maryland

Anthony Atala, MD
Director, Wake Forest Institute for Regenerative Medicine, Winston-Salem, North Carolina

David G. Baer, PhD
Deputy Director, Department of Defense Combat Casualty Care Research Program, US Army Medical Research and Materiel Command, Fort Detrick, Maryland

Jeffrey Bailey, MD
Colonel, Medical Corps, US Air Force; Director of Surgery, Walter Reed National Military Medical Center; Professor of Surgery, Department of Surgery, Uniformed Services University of the Health Sciences and the Walter Reed National Military Medical Center, Bethesda, Maryland

Arnaud Belard, MBA
Executive Director, Surgical Critical Care Initiative (SC2i), Henry M. Jackson Foundation for the Advancement of Military Medicine; Department of Surgery, Uniformed Services University of the Health Sciences and the Walter Reed National Military Medical Center, Bethesda, Maryland

Randy Bell, MD
Commander, US Navy; Division of Neurosurgery, Walter Reed National Military Medical Center; Associate Professor of Surgery, Department of Surgery, Uniformed Services University of the Health Sciences and the Walter Reed National Military Medical Center, Bethesda, Maryland

David M. Benedek, MD
Colonel, Medical Corps, US Army; Professor/Deputy Chair, Department of Psychiatry, Associate Director, Center for the Study of Traumatic Stress, Uniformed Services University of the Health Sciences, Bethesda, Maryland

Donald M. Berwick, MD
President Emeritus and Senior Fellow, Institute for Healthcare Improvement, Cambridge, Massachusetts

Kimberlie Biever, AN
Lieutenant Colonel, US Army; Deputy and 66S and 66T Assignment Officer; Army Nurse Corps Branch, Human Resources Command; Office of The Surgeon General Consultant, En Route Critical Care, US Army Human Resources Command, Fort Knox, Kentucky

Raquel Bono, MD
Vice Admiral; Medical Corps, US Navy; Director, Defense Health Agency, Falls Church, Virginia

Chester C. Buckenmaier III, MD
Colonel (Retired), Medical Corps, US Army; Professor of Anesthesiology; Director, Defense & Veterans Center for Integrative Pain Management; Department of Military Emergency Medicine, Uniformed Services University of the Health Sciences, Bethesda, Maryland

Frank K. Butler, MD
Captain (Retired), Medical Corps, US Navy; Chairman, Committee on Tactical Combat Casualty Care; Director, Prehospital Trauma Care, Joint Trauma System, San Antonio, Texas

Leopoldo C. Cancio, MD
Colonel (Retired), Medical Corps, US Army; Medical Officer (General Surgery), US Army Burn Center, Joint Base San Antonio–Fort Sam Houston, Texas

Jeremy W. Cannon, MD
Colonel, Medical Corps, US Air Force Reserves; Clinical Assistant Professor, Division of Traumatology, Surgical Critical Care, and Emergency Surgery, Perelman School of Medicine, University of Pennsylvania, Philadelphia, Pennsylvania

Andrew P. Cap, MD, PhD
Lieutenant Colonel, Medical Corps, US Army; Chief, Blood Research, US Army Institute of Surgical Research, Joint Base San Antonio–Fort Sam Houston, Texas; Associate Professor of Medicine, Uniformed Services University of the Health Sciences; Deputy Hematology-Oncology Consultant to the Surgeon General; Program Director, Clinical Research Fellowship, San Antonio Military Medical Center

Paul K. Carlton Jr, MD
Lieutenant General (Retired), Medical Corps, US Air Force; former US Air Force Surgeon General; Managing Member, PK Concepts, LLC, Melrose, Florida

Marcus H. Colyer, MD
Lieutenant Colonel, Medical Corps, US Army; Opthalmology Residency Program Director, Walter Reed National Military Medical Center and National Capital Consortium; Department of Surgery, Uniformed Services University of the Health Sciences and the Walter Reed National Military Medical Center, Bethesda, Maryland

Rory A. Cooper, PhD
Director and Senior Career Scientist, Human Engineering Research Laboratories, Rehabilitation Research and Development Service, US Department of Veteran Affairs; Distinguished Professor and FISA Foundation–Paralyzed Veterans of America Chair, Department of Rehabilitation Science and Technology, University of Pittsburgh, Pittsburgh, Pennsylvania

Kory Cornum, MD
Brigadier General (Retired), US Air Force; Air Mobility Command Surgeon, Scott Air Force Base, Illinois; formerly, Commander, Keesler Medical Center, Keesler Air Force Base, Mississippi

Rhonda Cornum, MD
Brigadier General (Retired), US Army; formerly, Commander, Landstuhl Regional Medical Center, Landstuhl, Germany; formerly, US Army Forces Command Surgeon, Fort Bragg, North Carolina; formerly, US Army Assistant Surgeon General for Force Projection; formerly, Director, Comprehensive Soldier Fitness

Stephen J. Cozza, MD
Colonel (Retired), Medical Corps, US Army; Professor of Psychiatry, Department of Psychiatry, Uniformed Services University of the Health Sciences; Associate Director, Center for the Study of Traumatic Stress, Bethesda, Maryland

Alicia T. Crowder, PhD
Manager, Neurotrauma Research Portfolio, Department of Defense Combat Casualty Care Research Program, US Army Medical Research and Materiel Command, Fort Detrick, Maryland

Brian Curry, MD
Lieutenant, Medical Corps, US Navy; Staff Neurosurgeon, Department of Surgery, Uniformed Services University of the Health Sciences and the Walter Reed National Military Medical Center, Bethesda, Maryland

Jerri Curtis, MD
Captain (Retired), Medical Corps, US Navy; Executive Director, National Capital Consortium, Designated Institutional Official; Associate Dean, Graduate Medical Education, Uniformed Services University of the Health Sciences, Bethesda, Maryland

Marla J. De Jong, PhD
Colonel, US Air Force; Interim Associate Dean for Research; Director, Faye Glenn Abdellah Center for Military and Federal Health Research; Professor, Daniel K. Inouye Graduate School of Nursing, Uniformed Services University of the Health Sciences, Bethesda, Maryland

Patricia A. Deuster, PhD, MPH
Professor and Director, Consortium for Health and Military Performance—A DoD Center of Excellence, Department of Military and Emergency Medicine, Uniformed Services University of the Health Sciences, Bethesda, Maryland

Guy F. Disney
Lieutenant (Retired), Light Dragoons, British Army; Cheltenham, United Kingdom

Patrick Downes, PsyD

Joseph J. Dubose, MD
Lieutenant Colonel, Medical Corps, US Air Force; Associate Professor of Surgery, Department of Surgery, Uniformed Services University of the Health Sciences and the Walter Reed National Military Medical Center, Bethesda, Maryland; Associate Professor of Surgery, University of California–Davis, Travis Air Force Base, California

Brian J. Eastridge, MD
Colonel, Medical Corps, US Army; Professor, Department of Surgery, University of Texas Health Science Center at San Antonio, San Antonio, Texas

Eric Elster, MD
Captain, Medical Corps, US Navy; Professor and Chair, Department of Surgery, Uniformed Services University of the Health Sciences and the Walter Reed National Military Medical Center, Bethesda, Maryland; Director, Surgical Critical Care Initiative (SC2i), Bethesda, Maryland

Andrew D. Fisher, MPAS, PA-C
Major, US Army; Medical Student, Texas A&M Health Science Center College of Medicine, Bryan, Texas; formerly, Physician Assistant, 75th Ranger Regiment, Fort Benning, Georgia

Arnold Fisher
Honorary Chairman, Intrepid Fallen Heroes Fund, New York, New York

Jonathan Forsberg, MD, PhD
Commander, US Navy; Professor of Surgery, Orthopedics Service, Department of Surgery, Uniformed Services University of the Health Sciences and the Walter Reed National Military Medical Center, Bethesda, Maryland

Louis M. French, PsyD
Deputy Director, National Intrepid Center of Excellence Directorate, Walter Reed National Military Medical Center; Associate Professor, Department of Rehabilitation Medicine, Uniformed Services University of the Health Sciences, Bethesda, Maryland

Gregory D. Gadson, MSIS, MPM
Colonel (Retired), US Army; Entrepreneur and Managing Partner, Patriot Strategies LLC, Alexandria, Virginia; formerly, Commander, US Army Garrison, Fort Belvoir, Virginia; formerly, Director, Army Wounded Warrior Program, Alexandria, Virginia

Patrick Georgoff, MD
General Surgery Resident, Surgical Critical Care Fellow, Department of Surgery, Section of General Surgery, University of Michigan, Ann Arbor, Michigan

James J. Geracci, MD
Colonel, Medical Corps, US Marine Corps; US Army III Corps Command Surgeon, Combined Joint Task Force–Operation Inherent Resolve, Camp Arifjan, Kuwait

Robert K. Gifford, PhD
Senior Project Director, Study to Assess Risk and Resilience in Service Members; Executive Officer, Center for the Study of Traumatic Stress, Department of Psychiatry, Uniformed Services University of the Health Sciences, Bethesda, Maryland

Bruce L. Gillingham, MD
Rear Admiral, Medical Corps, US Navy; Deputy Chief of Health Care Operations, Defense Health Agency, Falls Church, Virginia; previously, Commander, Navy Medicine West, San Diego, California

Colin M. Greene, MD, MPH
Colonel, Medical Corps, US Army; Program Manager, Joint Trauma Analysis and Prevention of Injury in Combat Program, US Army Medical Research and Materiel Command, Fort Detrick, Maryland

Jamie Grimes, MD
Colonel, Medical Corps, US Army; Chair, Neurology Department, Uniformed Services University of the Health Sciences; Chief, Walter Reed National Military Medical Center, Bethesda, Maryland

Racine Harris, MPH
Associate Director, Defense Health Horizons, Uniformed Services University of the Health Sciences; Program Manager II, Henry M. Jackson Foundation for the Advancement of Military Medicine, Bethesda, Maryland

Stephen P. Hetz, MD
Colonel (Retired), Medical Corps, US Army; Staff General Surgeon, William Beaumont Army Medical Center, El Paso, Texas

John B. Holcomb, MD
Colonel (Retired), US Army; Director, Center for Translational Injury Research; Chief, Division of Acute Care Surgery; Professor of Surgery, Vice Chair, Department of Surgery, Jack H. Mayfield, MD, Chair in Surgery, University of Texas Medical School, University of Texas–Houston, Houston, Texas

David B. Hoyt, MD
Executive Director, American College of Surgeons, Chicago, Illinois

Paul E. Hurwitz, MPH
Senior Program Manager, Center for the Study of Traumatic Stress and Study to Assess Risk and Resilience in Service Members, Uniformed Services University of the Health Sciences, Bethesda, Maryland

Bart O. Iddins, MD
Major General, Medical Corps, US Air Force, Commander, 59th Medical Wing, Joint Base San Antonio–Lackland Air Force Base, Texas

Kevin Jackson, OD, MPH
Commander, Medical Service Corps, US Navy; Chief of Staff, F. Edward Hébert School of Medicine; Assistant Professor, Department of Preventive Medicine and Biostatistics, Uniformed Services University of the Health Sciences, Bethesda, Maryland

Donald Jenkins, MD
Colonel (Retired), US Air Force; Vice Chair for Quality, Department of Surgery; Professor, Division of Trauma and Emergency Surgery; Betty and Bob Kelson Distinguished Chair in Burn and Trauma Surgery; Associate Deputy Director, Military Health Institute, University of Texas Health Science Center at San Antonio, San Antonio, Texas

Jay Johannigman, MD
Colonel (Retired), Medical Corps, US Air Force; Director, Division of Trauma and Critical Care, Department of Surgery, University of Cincinnati , Cincinnati, Ohio

Stephen L. Jones, MD
Major General (Retired), Medical Corps, US Army; formerly, Chief, US Army Medical Corps and Commanding General, US Army Medical Department Center and School, Health Readiness Center of Excellence, Fort Sam Houston, Texas

Mary Keller, EdD
President and Chief Executive Officer, Military Child Education
Coalition, Harker Heights, Texas

Arthur L. Kellermann, MD, MPH
Professor of Military and Emergency Medicine and Dean, F. Edward
Hébert School of Medicine, Uniformed Services University of the
Health Sciences, Bethesda, Maryland

Jessica Kensky, BSN, RN

Russ Kotwal, MD, MPH
Colonel (Retired), Medical Corps, US Army; Director of Strategic
Projects, Department of Defense Joint Trauma System, Institute of
Surgical Research, Joint Base San Antonio–Fort Sam Houston, Texas

M. Margaret Knudson, MD
Medical Director, Military Health Systems Strategic Partnership,
American College of Surgeons; Professor of Surgery, University of
California–San Francisco, San Francisco, California

John F. Kragh Jr, MD
Researcher, US Army Institute of Surgical Research, Damage Control
Resuscitation, Joint Base San Antonio–Fort Sam Houston, Texas

Daniel Kral, MSMOT
Colonel, Medical Corps, US Army; Director, Telemedicine and
Advanced Technology Research Center, US Army Medical Research
and Materiel Command, Fort Detrick, Maryland

M. Benjamin Larkin, PharmD
Second Lieutenant, Medical Services Corps, US Army; Medical Student,
Uniformed Services University of the Health Sciences, Bethesda,
Maryland

Brian C. Lein, MD
Major General, Medical Corps, US Army; Commanding General,
US Army Medical Department Center and School, Health Readiness
Center of Excellence, Fort Sam Houston, Texas; formerly, Command-
ing General, US Army Medical Research and Materiel Command, Fort
Detrick, Maryland

Craig Llewellyn, MD, MPH
Colonel (Retired), Medical Corps, US Army; Emeritus Professor of
Military and Emergency Medicine, Uniformed Services University of
the Health Sciences, Bethesda, Maryland

Robert L. Mabry, MD
Colonel, Medical Corps, US Army; Chief, Combat Casualty Care,
Office of The Surgeon General; Defense Health Headquarters,
Falls Church, Virginia

Matthew J. Martin, MD
Colonel, Medical Corps, US Army; Associate Professor, Department of
Surgery, Uniformed Services University of the Health Sciences and the
Walter Reed National Military Medical Center, Bethesda, Maryland;
Trauma Medical Director, Madigan Army Medical Center, Tacoma,
Washington

Sean L. Murphy, MD
Brigadier General, Medical Corps, US Air Force; Command Surgeon,
Air Combat Command, Joint Base Langley–Eustis, Virginia

Clinton K. Murray, MD
Colonel, Medical Corps, US Army; Corps Specific Branch Proponent
Officer and Deputy Corps Chief for the US Army Medical Corps;
formerly, Chief of the Infectious Disease Service at Brooke Army
Medical Center, Fort Sam Houston, Texas

Kelly A. Murray, MD
Colonel, Medical Corps, US Army; Command Surgeon, US Forces
Korea, Yongsan Garrison, South Korea

Francis G. O'Connor, MD, MPH
Colonel (Retired), Medical Corps, US Army; Professor and Chair,
Military and Emergency Medicine; Medical Director, Consortium for
Health and Military Performance (CHAMP), Uniformed Services
University of the Health Sciences, Bethesda, Maryland

Lisa Osborne, PhD
Captain, US Navy; Associate Professor, Navy Senior Service Leader, Uniformed Services University of the Health Sciences, Bethesda, Maryland

Martin G. Ottolini, MD
Colonel (Retired), Medical Corps, US Air Force; Associate Professor of
Pediatrics and Assistant Dean for Research, F. Edward Hébert School
of Medicine, Uniformed Services University of the Health Sciences,
Bethesda, Maryland

Paul F. Pasquina, MD
Colonel (Retired), Medical Corps, US Army; Chief, Department of
Orthopaedics and Rehabilitation, Walter Reed National Military
Medical Center; Professor and Chair, Department of Physical Medicine
and Rehabilitation, Uniformed Services University of the Health
Sciences, Bethesda, Maryland

Jeremy Perkins, MD
Colonel, Medical Corps, US Army; Chief, Hematology-Oncology
Service, Walter Reed National Military Medical Center; Associate
Professor of Medicine, Uniformed Services University of the Health
Sciences, Bethesda, Maryland

Ron Poropatich, MD
Colonel (Retired), Medical Corps, US Army; Executive Director, Center for Military Medicine Research, Health Sciences at the University
of Pittsburgh; Professor of Medicine, Division of Pulmonary, Allergy,
and Critical Care Medicine, University of Pittsburgh; Senior Advisor of
Telemedicine, University of Pittsburgh Medical Center; Faculty Member,
McGowan Institute for Regenerative Medicine, Pittsburgh, Pennsylvania

Benjamin K. Potter, MD
Lieutenant Colonel, Medical Corps, US Army; Vice Chair (Research)
and Professor, Department of Surgery, Uniformed Services University
of the Health Sciences and the Walter Reed National Military Medical
Center, Bethesda, Maryland

Todd E. Rasmussen, MD
Colonel, Medical Corps, US Air Force; Director, Department of
Defense Combat Casualty Care Research Program; Harris B. Shumaker
Jr. Professor of Surgery, Department of Surgery, Uniformed Services
University of the Health Sciences and the Walter Reed National Military
Medical Center, Bethesda, Maryland

Paula Rauch, MD
Director, Marjorie E. Korff PACT (Parenting At a Challenging Time)
Program; Program Director, Family Support and Outreach, Red Sox
Foundation/MGH Home Base Program, Massachusetts General
Hospital, Boston, Massachusetts

Brian V. Reamy, MD
Colonel (Retired), Medical Corps, US Air Force; Professor of Family Medicine, Senior Associate Dean for Academic Affairs, F. Edward Hébert School of Medicine, Uniformed Services University of the Health Sciences, Bethesda, Maryland

Peter Rhee, MD, MPH
Captain (Retired), Medical Corps, US Navy; Senior Vice President and Chief of Acute Care Surgery, Grady Memorial Hospital, Atlanta, Georgia

Charles L. Rice, MD
Captain (Retired), Medical Corps, US Navy Reserve; President (former) and Professor of Surgery, Uniformed Services University of the Health Sciences, Bethesda, Maryland

Karen Richardson, BA
Senior Manager, Communications, Wake Forest Institute for Regenerative Medicine; Department of Urology, Wake Forest University Baptist Medical Center, Winston-Salem, North Carolina

Mark S. Riddle, MD, DRPH
Commander, Medical Corps, US Navy; Director, Bacterial Diarrhea Vaccines Program, Naval Medical Research Center, Silver Spring, Maryland

Daniel R. Robles
Master Sergeant (Retired), US Army; Garden Ridge, Texas

Michael F. Rotondo, MD
Professor, Department of Surgery, University of Rochester; CEO, University of Rochester Faculty Medical Group, Rochester, New York; formerly, Chairman, American College of Surgeons Committee on Trauma

William R. Rowley, MD
Rear Admiral (Retired), Medical Corps, US Navy; Senior Fellow, Institute for Alternative Futures, Alexandria, Virginia

John W. Sanders, MD, MPH
Captain (Retired), Medical Corps, US Navy; Professor of Medicine, Wake Forest University School of Medicine, Winston-Salem, North Carolina

Eric B. Schoomaker, MD, PhD
Lieutenant General (Retired), Medical Corps, US Army; Professor and Vice Chairman of Military and Emergency Medicine, Uniformed Services University of the Health Sciences; formerly, US Army Surgeon General and Commander of the US Army Medical Command, the North Atlantic Regional Medical Command, and Walter Reed Army Medical Center

Martin A. Schreiber, MD
Colonel, Medical Corps, US Army Reserves; Chief, Trauma, Critical Care and Acute Care Surgery, Oregon Health and Science University, Portland, Oregon

C. William Schwab, MD
Founding Chief, Division of Traumatology, Surgical Critical Care and Emergency Surgery and Emeritus Professor of Surgery, Perelman School of Medicine, University of Pennsylvania; Senior Consultant, Penn Medicine, Philadelphia, Pennsylvania

Patrick Sculley, DDS
Major General (Retired), Dental Corps, US Army; formerly, Senior Vice President, Uniformed Services University of the Health Sciences; formerly, Chief of the Dental Corps, US Army

Dale C. Smith, PhD
Professor of Military Medicine & History, Uniformed Services
University of the Health Sciences, Bethesda, Maryland

Bonnie Smoak, MD, PhD
Colonel (Retired), Medical Corps, US Army; Adjunct Associate
Professor, Preventive Medicine and Biometrics, Uniformed Services
University of the Health Sciences, Bethesda, Maryland

Murray B. Stein, MD, MPH
Distinguished Professor of Psychiatry and Family Medicine & Public
Health; Vice Chair for Clinical Research in Psychiatry, University of
California–San Diego, San Diego, California

Richard W. Thomas, MD, DDS
Major General (Retired), Medical Corps, US Army; President and
Professor of Military Medicine, Uniformed Services University of the
Health Sciences, Bethesda, Maryland; formerly, Chief of Health Care
Operations, Defense Health Agency

Jeffrey W. Timby
Deputy Commanding Officer, Tripler Army Medical Center; Former
Deputy Medical Officer of the Marine Corps and Fleet Marine Force
Specialty Leader

Thomas W. Travis, MD, MPH
Lieutenant General (Retired), Medical Corps, US Air Force; formerly,
US Air Force Surgeon General; Senior Vice President for the Southern
Region, Uniformed Services University of the Health Sciences, Bethesda,
Maryland

David R. Tribble, MD, DRPH
Science Director, Infectious Disease Clinical Research Program; Profes-
sor, Department of Preventive Medicine and Biometrics, Uniformed
Services University of the Health Sciences, Bethesda, Maryland

Robert J. Ursano, MD
Colonel (Retired), Medical Corps, US Air Force; Professor and Chair,
Department of Psychiatry, Uniformed Services University of the
Health Sciences; Director, Center for the Study of Traumatic Stress,
Bethesda, Maryland

James C. West, MD
Captain, Medical Corps, US Navy; Assistant Professor of Psychiatry,
Assistant Chair, Department of Psychiatry, Uniformed Services Univer-
sity of the Health Sciences, Bethesda, Maryland

Susan West, BSN
Data Analysis Branch Chief, Joint Trauma System, Data Analysis
Branch, Joint Base San Antonio, San Antonio, Texas

Brian Wilhelm, MS
Sergeant (Retired), US Army, 4th Infantry Division, Fort Carson, Colorado; Adjunct Faculty Member, Lewis University, Romeoville, Illinois

Jonathan Woodson, MD
Professor of Surgery, Boston University School of Medicine, Boston,
Massachusetts; Brigadier General, US Army Ready Reserves; formerly,
Assistant Secretary of Defense for Health Affairs, Washington, DC

Gary H. Wynn, MD
Lieutenant Colonel, Medical Corps, US Army; Associate Professor,
Department of Psychiatry, Uniformed Services University of the Health
Sciences, Bethesda, Maryland

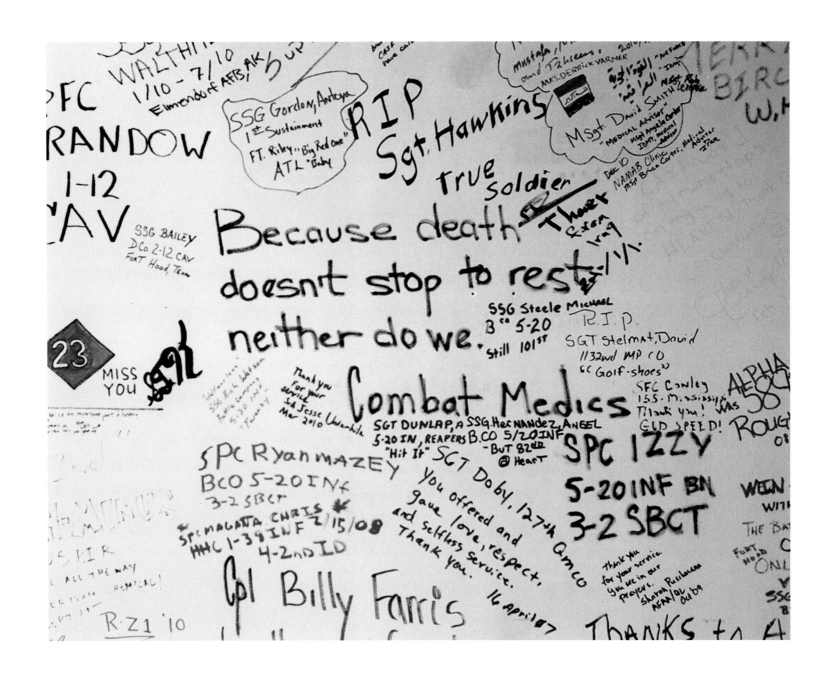

OUT OF THE CRUCIBLE tells one of the most extraordinary stories in the history of American medicine: how our nation's military health system—while working alongside coalition forces fighting two wars on the other side of the world (and simultaneously caring for millions of service members, dependents, and military retirees at home)—completely transformed its approach to combat casualty care.

Few outside our armed forces, and specialists in trauma and emergency care, understand the magnitude of what was done. Fewer still know *how* it was done. We compiled this book to bring these accomplishments to a wider audience, told in the words of those who brought it about.

Typically, medical advances are made incrementally, through painstaking research. This was not feasible in Iraq and Afghanistan or in the skies between these distant lands and the United States. Moreover, few of the innovations were the product of top-down decision making. In every phase of the continuum of care—from the point of injury on the battlefield to rehabilitation and reintegration of wounded warriors into their communities—military innovators challenged existing dogma and pushed the envelope by rapidly devising, implementing, refining, and spreading new techniques and technologies throughout the force. They were able to succeed because the Military Health System was willing to learn from its failures and build on its successes. Through a mix of keen observation and the systematic collection and analysis of data (most notably, creation of the Joint Trauma System), military medicine continually improved.

The results speak for themselves. In the latter years of Operation Enduring Freedom (OEF) and Operation Iraqi Freedom (OIF), America's Military Health System achieved the highest rate of casualty survival in the history of warfare. As a result, thousands of service members who would have died in

[*Opposite*] The contingency aeromedical staging facility walls, formerly located at the Air Force Theater Hospital at Joint Base Balad, Iraq, featured messages from service members and famous people paying tribute to fallen warriors and giving thanks to the staff that worked there. The walls were removed and sent to the National Museum of the US Air Force at Wright-Patterson Air Force Base, Ohio. US Air Force photo by Staff Sergeant Keyonna Fennell.

earlier wars are alive today. Tens of thousands with severe injuries were able to recover substantial function and go on to lead fulfilling lives.

The pace at which this transformation occurred is as astonishing as its scope. It's long been said it takes an average of 17 years for a new discovery to be adopted into medical practice. The US military adopted more than 25 major innovations in care in little more than a decade. Working with a research budget 1/30th the size of the National Institutes of Health, it sponsored high-impact science that answered critical questions and developed products that were rapidly pushed into the field.

In the pages of this book, you'll meet many of the people who brought these changes about. Each chapter is written by subject matter experts who played a key role in the development or adoption of the innovation. In addition, many chapters contain a first-person account written by one or more individuals who personally created, championed, or benefitted from these advances. These include essays by Colonel Kelly A. Murray, a military doctor who earned a Bronze Star for saving her fellow Soldiers during an ambush; Rear Admiral Bruce L. Gillingham, who describes how an enlisted service member in his unit figured out how to prevent wounded warriors from getting dangerously cold during MEDEVAC flights; Colonel (Retired) Greg Gadson, who describes himself as a "former wounded warrior;" and two brave civilians—Jessica Kensky and Patrick Downes—who after being maimed in the Boston Marathon bombings benefitted from rehabilitation care at Walter Reed.

From the founding of our nation to today, Americans have benefitted from advances in military medicine. For example, modern trauma centers and aeromedical emergency medical systems are a direct outgrowth of lessons learned on the battlefields of Korea and Vietnam. Already, innovations developed in Iraq and Afghanistan are being swiftly adopted by civilian emergency and trauma care providers. This cannot happen too soon, because the rise of rampage shootings and terrorist bombings in the United States is quickly blurring the line between civilian and military trauma.

The US military has benefitted from civilian partnerships as well. During OEF and OIF, three professional surgical societies brought many of America's leading surgeons to Landstuhl Regional Medical Center in Germany to work alongside their military counterparts. Today, military surgeons, nurses, and other team members rotate through some of our nation's leading civilian trauma centers to keep their skills sharp.

As impressive as these advances may be, we cannot become complacent. Just as generals and admirals are admonished not to "fight the last war," we must not assume that the next major conflict will unfold like the ones just past. Counterterrorism operations in the vast reaches of sub-Saharan Africa, high-tech warfare in Eastern Europe, or an air-sea battle in the South China Sea will produce radically different challenges than those faced in Iraq and Afghanistan. For this reason, America's Military Health System must retain its capacity to quickly identify emerging health threats and innovate to overcome them.

During OIF, many of the wounded warriors and healthcare providers passing through the aeromedical staging facility at Joint Base Balad on the way to Landstuhl Regional Medical Center in Germany scrawled messages of hope and thanks on the facility's walls. A section was later removed and placed on permanent display at Defense Health Headquarters in Falls Church, Virginia. One note, written in bold letters, stands out: *"Because death doesn't stop to rest, neither do we—Combat Medics."*

The relentless dedication this message conveys has defined American military medicine for 240 years. To be true to this tradition, we must ensure that lessons learned in the crucible of the wars in Iraq and Afghanistan are not forgotten, but instead inspire future military healthcare providers to exceed what is thought possible. This book is dedicated to all who served in Iraq and Afghanistan, and all who worked tirelessly to bring them home.

ARTHUR L. KELLERMANN, MD, MPH
Dean, F. Edward Hébert School of Medicine
Uniformed Services University of the Health Sciences

ERIC ELSTER, MD
Captain, Medical Corps, US Navy
Professor and Chairman, Department of Surgery
Uniformed Services University of the Health Sciences

Bethesda, Maryland
May 2017

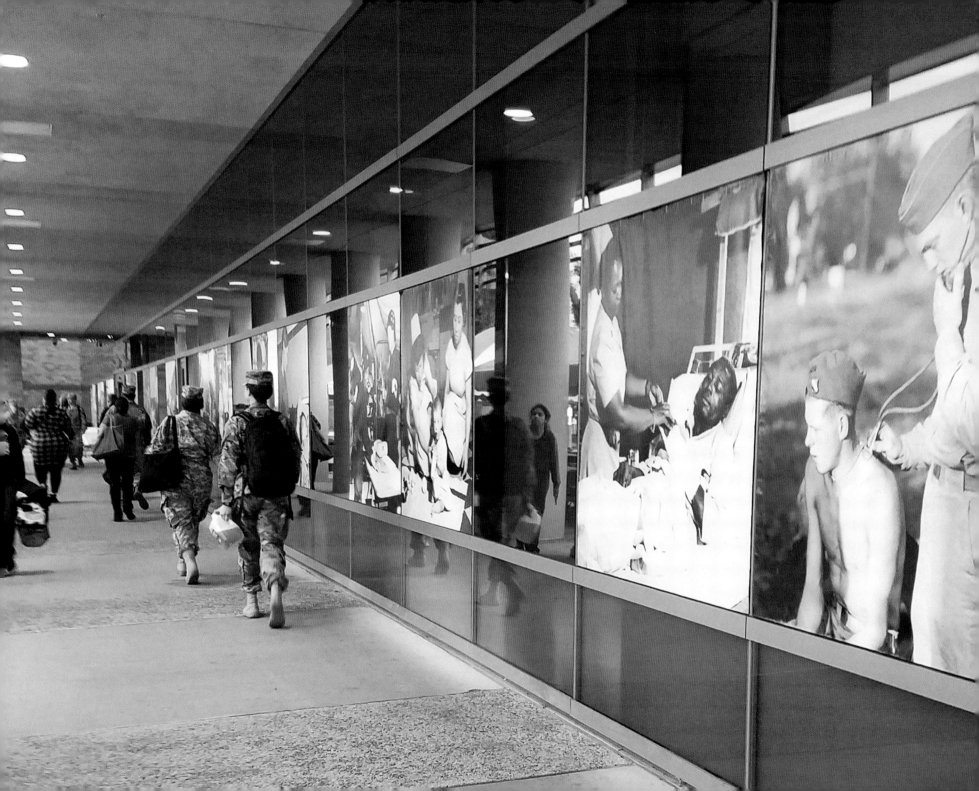

SECTION ONE

Foundations

[*Section One image*] Photos of military medical personnel from World War II through Operation Enduring Freedom are on display along the windows leading to the Garden Entrance of Brooke Army Medical Center, November 4, 2016. The display was provided by the Army Medical Department Museum on Joint Base San Antonio–Fort Sam Houston. US Army photo by Lori Newman/ Released. Reproduced from: https://www.dvidshub.net/image/2986885/bamc-veterans-day-2016.

CHAPTER one

A Soldier's Story

GENERAL DANIEL B. ALLYN

F OR 35 YEARS AS AN INFANTRYMAN, I have experienced firsthand the skill, ingenuity, and passion of our medical professionals across the joint force. I have seen corpsmen, medics, doctors, nurses, and technicians from all services leverage their craft to save lives under the most demanding environments on the face of the earth. More than any other "crucible," war brings out the worst and best of mankind. Without question, our military medical professionals reflect the amazing light of creativity, compassion, and exquisite care . . . and it's especially brilliant in the darkest moments.

This past February, I again saw this truth when I visited two Army Rangers at Walter Reed [National Military Medical Center] shortly after their evacuation from Afghanistan.

Wounded on the objective of a high-value-target, one of the sergeants was shot twice, one bullet passing through his thorax, the other striking his shoulder. Immediately, his fellow Rangers applied buddy aid, and Ranger medics controlled his bleeding and administered freeze-dried plasma, a cutting-edge product developed through the [Food and Drug Administration's] Investigational New Drug Initiative. After a difficult "exfil,"[1] flight medics aboard the MH-47[2] continued to stabilize the Ranger and, using ultrasound in flight, identified another wound causing heavy bleeding. After a tail-to-tail swap,[3] an Air Force flight surgeon inserted two chest tubes and performed a thoracotomy, opening his entire left chest to identify the hemorrhage and surgically correct it.

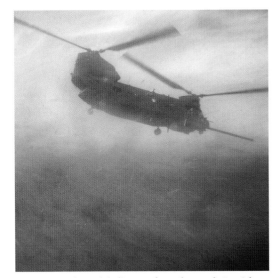

An MH-47 Chinook helicopter from the 160th Special Operations Aviation Regiment takes off during the exfiltration of Army Rangers from the 75th Ranger Regiment during a company live fire training at Camp Roberts, California, January 31, 2014. US Army Photo by Staff Sergeant Teddy Wade/Released. Reproduced from: https://www.dvidshub.net/image/1161150/75th-ranger-regiment-task-force-training.

After four minutes of traumatic arrest, the Ranger regained his breathing and stabilized. He was flown to Bagram [Airfield, Afghanistan], stabilized further, and then transferred directly to Walter Reed, where I had the honor of meeting him as he left the intensive care unit.

This Ranger's story is amazing and one of the thousands our service members have experienced in this long war. There is no military on the face of this earth that matches our level of medical care for its warriors from battlefields to the trauma centers. And as I spoke with this Ranger's father and sister, the thanks I saw in their eyes is the strongest possible tribute to the doctors, nurses, clinicians, and technicians who aided this great young American . . . and proof that Military Medicine changes lives.

So as we share a few moments together this evening,[4] I ask that we keep this Army Ranger's story in the forefront of our minds. Soldiers, Sailors, Airmen, and Marines are the reason we are gathered here today.

To all the military medical professionals in the audience tonight, your efforts each and every day are fundamental to maintaining the readiness, resilience, and battlefield dominance of our joint force. So on behalf of a grateful Army and a grateful nation, thank you for what you do. God Bless you, and Army Strong!

Notes

1. Also known as "exfiltration" or "extraction," "exfil" is a tactical combat term for the process of immediately removing an individual Soldier or unit from a targeted site.
2. The MH-47 Chinook is the primary heavy-lift transport helicopter used by US Army Special Operations personnel. It differs from the more conventional CH-47 Chinook due to features that make it more capable of operating at night and performing missions deep in enemy territory.
3. "Tail-to-tail swap" describes the process of rapidly transferring patients, personnel, or cargo from one rotary-wing aircraft to another. Typically done with rotors turning, it is a loud and chaotic activity.
4. General Allyn's remarks were made at the 2016 "Heroes of Military Medicine" award ceremony in Washington, DC, on May 5, 2016.

CHAPTER two

A Heritage of Innovation

DALE C. SMITH, PHD

I N THE FIRST SEASON OF THE CLASSIC TELEVISION COMEDY M*A*S*H (season 1, episode 17, January 1973), a more experienced surgical commander tells his young protégé, "There are two rules of war. Rule number one is that young men die. Rule number two is that doctors can't change rule number one." In reality, American military doctors have repeatedly and successfully challenged both rules for more than 230 years. Thanks to their efforts, death rates from combat wounds and infectious diseases have fallen to historic lows. The spirit of innovation that produced the innovations described in the subsequent chapters of this book did not spring up overnight. It is based on a long and proud heritage that stretches back to the founding of our republic.

THE REVOLUTIONARY WAR AND THE "COMMAND OF HEALTH"

Within weeks of establishing an army, the Continental Congress authorized a centralized medical support activity, called the "hospital," to care for sick and wounded soldiers above the regimental level. General George Washington provided an enduring example of outstanding command support when he ordered that his troops be inoculated against smallpox while they were isolated in winter encampments. Washington wrote, "Necessity not only authorizes but seems to require the measure, for should the disorder infect the army the natural way, and rage with its usual virulence, we should have more dread from it than from the sword of the enemy."[1] Inoculation broke the back of the epidemic. This was the first time any army in the world was immunized by command order.

THE EARLY 1800S: THE FIRST RESEARCH

After the military setbacks of the War of 1812, our nation's political leaders realized the fledgling republic needed a small standing army for protection. To protect the health of the new force, the Army established a medical department led by Joseph Lovell, the first surgeon general. To understand the health risks his force faced, Dr Lovell began the tradition of reporting cases of disease from all posts, camps, and stations. This practice proved its worth in the Second Seminole War, when members of the Army Medical Department determined the effective dose of quinine to treat troops sickened by malaria by comparing the doses given by different field hospitals to their subsequent outcomes. This was the first time in American history that military doctors applied science to develop a clinical innovation in a war zone. More innovations would follow.

MILITARY-CIVILIAN COOPERATION

The US military's commitment to medical research was cemented by the work of Army surgeon William Beaumont (Figure 2.1), who used an accidentally created gastric fistula to explore the physiology of gastric function. When Beaumont wrote to Washington, DC, for assistance, General Lovell mobilized the nation's best scientific resources to help his subordinate officer with the work. A few years later, when the Philadelphia Naval Hospital opened its doors in the 1830s, surgeon Thomas Harris started a teaching program to prepare young assistant surgeons for their promotion examinations. He persuaded local medical school faculty to help and opened his hospital's wards to assist in educating their medical students.

THE CIVIL WAR AND DEVELOPMENT OF "BATTLEFIELD MEDICINE"

The rapid development of military technology before and during the American Civil War (1861–1865) increased the capacity for both sides to inflict massive casualties. The resulting carnage forced military medicine to advance as well. Within months of Fort Sumter's

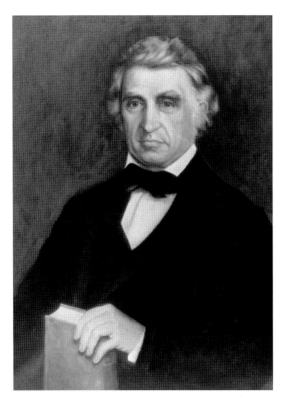

FIGURE 2.1. William Beaumont (November 21, 1785–April 25, 1853). Reproduction of an 1840s painting by Chester Harding. Photograph courtesy of National Library of Medicine, Images from the History of Medicine.

shelling, American military doctors began thinking about how they could better manage battlefield casualties. In 1862, the most forward-thinking member of this group, Major Jonathan Letterman (Figure 2.2), was named medical director of the Army of the Potomac. Over the next two years, he championed a series of innovations, some of which he personally developed and others that he learned from colleagues and rapidly expanded. His system for evacuating and treating casualties worked so well, Letterman is often called the "father of battlefield medicine."

Letterman's first challenge was figuring out how to get large numbers of wounded off the battlefield more quickly than anyone thought possible. He quickly concluded that the teamsters hired for the task were unreliable. Letterman envisioned a group of regular soldiers trained to swiftly evacuate wounded soldiers from the battlefield under the supervision of regular noncommissioned officers and officers. He convinced General George McClellan to approve his plan, and in September 1862, Letterman's first units were partially deployed during the Battle of Antietam. Based on encouraging results, he expanded the system and connected it to a network of field hospitals that delivered necessary treatment as wounded, ill, and injured soldiers were moved behind the lines. He also devised a system to document treatments and outcomes so he could continuously improve care.

Letterman's systematic approach to combat casualty care benefitted patients long after the Civil War. One of his protégés, Dr. Edward Dawson, returned to New York City, where he convinced Bellevue Hospital to establish America's first civilian ambulance service. The trauma and emergency medical service systems widely used today are based on Letterman's pioneering work.

The Army was not the only service branch that advanced military medicine during the Civil War. The US Navy also recognized that casualty care was important to conserving fighting strength. Various Navy surgeons undertook innovations to prepare their crews for the damage of battle. On the *USS Kearsarge*, surgeon J.M. Browne foreshadowed the role of Navy corpsmen when he taught his ship's crew basic skills of treating wounds and bandaging (see Chapter 11). He hoped that they would help him treat shipmates who were injured in battle, but his initial results were disappointing. Following the historic engagement between *USS Kearsarge* and the Confederate commerce raider *Alabama*, Browne lamented that "under the excitement of battle, little reliance could be placed upon their fulfillment of my instructions."[2]

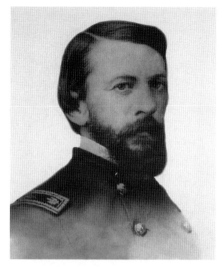

FIGURE 2.2. Major Jonathan Letterman as Medical Director, Army of the Potomac. Photograph courtesy of National Library of Medicine, Images from the History of Medicine.

1865-1904: PROGRESS IN PREVENTIVE MEDICINE

Following the Civil War, Browne became chief of the Navy Bureau of Medicine and Surgery, where he worked to convince line Navy officers that human damage control is as important as ship damage control (see Chapter 15). Browne recognized that without the support of line officers, medical preparedness would not succeed. Another Navy medical officer who understood the value of line support was surgeon Charles Siegfried, who thought the new science of bacteriology could be used to improve health on Navy ships. At the time, bouts of gastrointestinal disease regularly disabled crews for weeks after each port of call. Siegfried knew many Navy mess units (each comprised of 8 to 10 sailors) paid little attention to hygiene as they prepared their food. He envisioned a "consolidated mess," where an entire ship's watch would be fed at once by cooks and helpers trained in proper food-handling techniques. He took the idea to Captain Henry C. Taylor, slated to assume command of the newly commissioned Battleship *Indiana*. Impressed, Taylor offered Siegfried the post of ship's surgeon. Together, they proved that a consolidated mess reduces outbreaks of disease and improves crew morale.

THE DEFEAT OF YELLOW FEVER

In 1901, Major Walter Reed (Figure 2.3) demonstrated that yellow fever is transmitted by a particular species of mosquito instead of direct contact with soiled clothing or bedding (as was widely believed at the time). Reed credited Cuban doctor Carlos Finlay with the original idea that mosquitos are the vector for yellow fever, and thus the key to controlling the disease. Shortly after Reed published his findings, another Army physician, Dr. William Gorgas, put them to good use in Havana and soon thereafter in the Panama Canal Zone.

When Gorgas arrived in Panama, 21,000 of the 26,000 Canal Zone workers had been sick. Fear was high and morale was low. Stories about how the French had suffered death rates of 200 per month before abandoning the project circulated widely. Based on Walter Reed's research, Gorgas believed he could control yellow fever by targeting the mosquitos that transmit it. He proposed fumigating camps, draining the ponds and swamps where mosquitos breed, and extensively using mosquito nets. Initially, the Canal Commission

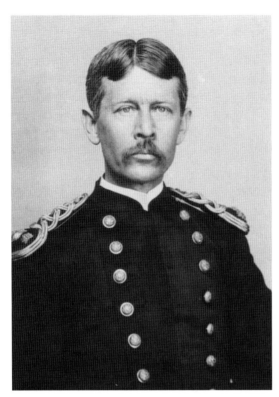

FIGURE 2.3. Walter Reed, MD (September 13, 1851– November 22, 1902). Photograph courtesy of National Library of Medicine, Images from the History of Medicine.

balked over the cost of his interventions, but it relented under pressure from the American public, medical professionals, and ultimately the US president. Once Gorgas' measures were fully implemented, cases of yellow fever dropped dramatically. The Panama Canal was completed in 1914, the same year Gorgas was named the 22nd surgeon general of the US Army.

THE SPANISH-AMERICAN WAR AND THE FIGHT AGAINST TROPICAL DISEASES

In the 1898 Spanish-American War, the United States lost more soldiers to typhoid fever than to combat. This prompted the Army to redouble research on tropical diseases, a commitment it maintains to this day. As a result, Army researchers developed several effective vaccines and prophylactic drugs to protect American service members abroad. Examples include typhoid immunization (1907), and eventually several treatments for malaria, as well as ongoing research to develop a malaria vaccine.

THE 20TH CENTURY: RAPID PROGRESS IN CASUALTY CARE

The 20th century produced numerous breakthroughs in military medicine and surgery, including blood transfusions (World War I), penicillin (World War II), and vascular repair surgery (Korean War). In each case, the crucible of war accelerated the improvement and rapid adoption of medical innovations. During these conflicts, large numbers of civilian healthcare professionals, including several of America's leading academic doctors, were brought into uniform. Once there, they took advantage of the discipline and systematization of military medicine to rapidly advance their research.

World War I

Confronted with massive casualties, World War I military surgeons determined that in some cases, definitive surgery could wait. Building on 19th century experience treating extremity fractures and new data on the spread of germs from contaminated wounds into the bloodstream, military trauma surgeons began to make more informed judgments about when to immediately amputate a badly fractured arm or leg, and when to defer the decision until the patient reached a higher level of care. The 19th century invention of the traction splint by Welsh surgeon Hugh Owen Thomas dramatically improved management of femur fractures. Before the "Thomas splint" was introduced to the battlefield by Robert Jones, mortality was as high as 80 percent. Afterward, it fell to 8 percent.

Surgical specialization grew. Neurosurgeon Harvey Cushing demonstrated that if soldiers with head wounds could be protected from further damage and contamination, it was better to defer treatment to an experienced neurosurgeon rather than have a general surgeon attempt repair. Great leaders of American medicine, including Charles and William Mayo, William H. Welch and George W. Crile, made major contributions to military medicine and surgery during their time on active duty. The bonds they established between military medicine and civilian health systems and specialty societies continue to this day.

World War II

World War II produced numerous advances. The introduction of sulfa and penicillin gave military surgeons weapons to fight otherwise uncontrollable infections. Military doctors also began to recognize the value of physiological monitoring of patients. During the London blitz, recognition of crush injuries from falling masonry and the surgical treatment of hemorrhage taught surgeons to think about massive blood loss and the benefits of blood replacement. Two-stage operations to repair bowel injuries became standard practice, due to well-founded fears of infection and obstruction with a single-stage approach. Dr. Lyman Brewer and colleagues in Auxiliary Surgical Unit No. 2 in Italy developed the concept of positive-pressure respiration therapy to deal with "wet lung syndrome"—a dangerous buildup of fluid in the lungs following chest surgery. Throughout the war, medical personnel refined the system of moving severely injured casualties to higher echelons of care, as Jonathan Letterman first devised in the Civil War.

At the war's end in 1945, 80 American surgeons who had served together in North Africa and the Mediterranean theater met in Rome and founded the Excelsior Surgical Society. They pledged to hold annual meetings to review their wartime experiences and capture the lessons learned. For the next 30 years, the society functioned under the auspices of the American College of Surgeons. Recently, it was reestablished by US military surgeons who served together in Iraq and Afghanistan.

Korea and Vietnam

The technical challenge of treating casualties on remote battlefields, and American's growing biomedical expertise, sparked several major advances during the Korean and Vietnam wars. Korea ushered in the practice of medical evacuation (MEDEVAC) by military helicopter and wider use of the "artificial kidney." After researchers changed World War II policy, injured arteries were successfully repaired using techniques primarily established by Carl W. Hughes. In Vietnam, Norman M. Rich extended vascular surgery to include venous repair, and MEDEVAC helicopters were widely used at the point of wounding. Other advances included improved fluid and electrolyte replacement for burn therapy, postoperative nutritional supplementation, and developments in intensive care.

BRINGING BATTLEFIELD LESSONS HOME

When military doctors returned home from Vietnam, they were appalled that an American's odds of surviving a serious car crash were much worse than a soldier's odds of surviving a severe battlefield injury in the jungles of Southeast Asia. They immediately set about organizing trauma care systems and designating certain hospitals as "trauma centers." Building on the previous civilian work of R. Adams Cowley in Baltimore, they supported the development of civilian helicopter evacuation through the Military Assistance to Safety and Traffic program of 1970 and encouraged building a civilian trauma system on the military model.

Prehospital care was shockingly poor. Until the mid-1960s, hearses often served double-duty as ambulances, and treatment was limited to minimal first aid. Many hospital "emergency rooms" were covered by rotating members of the medical staff who lacked specialized training, or worse yet, by unsupervised interns.

A turning point came in 1966, when the National Academy of Sciences released *Accidental Death and Disability: The Neglected Disease of Modern Society*.[3] This landmark report contrasted the marked improvements in emergency care the military developed in Vietnam with the carnage on America's highways. It galvanized the public. Spurred into action, Congress established the National Highway Traffic Safety Administration (NHTSA). One of NHTSA's first acts was to draft a national curriculum to train "emergency medical technicians." Modern emergency medical services were born.

One advance that helped trauma care systems steadily improve was the creation of comprehensive data registries that documented methods of treatment and the outcomes they produced. The Vietnam Vascular Registry, established by Army surgeon Norman Rich in 1966, was an early example. It served as the prototype for the civilian National Trauma Data Bank, which in turn informed the development of the Department of Defense Trauma Registry used today.

TABLE 2.1. Army Medical Department Advances In Combat Casualty Care.

Reproduced from:
Murray CK, Hitter SR, Jones SL. Army Medical Department at War: lessons learned. *Army Med Dep J.* 2016;Apr–Sep:2.

Data sources:
1. Pruitt BA Jr. The symbiosis of combat casualty care and civilian trauma care: 1914–2007. *J Trauma.* 2008;64:S4-S8.
2. Pruitt BA Jr, Rasmussen TE, Gueller G. The formula for success in military medical research. *J Trauma.* 2015;79:S64–S69.

World War I
Use of intravenous fluids and blood transfusions
Motorized ambulances
Laparotomy for penetrating abdominal wounds
Use of surgical specialists
Effective topical antisepsis: Dakin-Carrel wound irrigation system
Antitetanus serum
Radiologic localization of foreign bodies
Neurosurgical trauma databank
Characterized bacteria and infection rates associated with wounds

World War II
General availability of whole blood and plasma
Formulaic resuscitation of burn patients
Availability of "well trained" surgeons and use of specialty-specific auxiliary surgical groups
Hierarchical organization of trauma care
Use of antibiotics
Use of fixed wing aeromedical evacuation
Identification of "wet lung in war casualties"

Korean War
Fluid resuscitation adequate to correct shock and prevent organ failure
Availability of board-certified surgical specialists
Forward availability of definitive surgery
Use of helicopters for patient transport
Primary repair and vascular grafts for injured vessels
Use of hemodialysis in theater of operations
Identification of high output renal failure
Recognition of seasonal variation in bacteria recovered from battle wounds

Vietnam War

General use of helicopters for patient transport

Monitoring of organ function in theater of operations

Blood gas measurements

Serum chemistries

Portable radiology equipment

Use of mechanical ventilators in theater of operations

Effective topical antimicrobial chemotherapy for burns

Staged intercontinental aeromedical transport of burn patients

Identification of acute respiratory distress syndrome

Establishment of Vietnam Vascular Registry

Operation Desert Shield/Desert Storm

Burn team augmentation of evacuation hospitals to provide theater-wide burn care

Reactivation of intercontinental burn patient transport system

Operations in Iraq and Afghanistan

Development of a military trauma registry

"Low volume" resuscitation fluids (colloids and red blood cells)

Hemostatic agents (systemic and topical)

Use of "damage control" initial surgery

Use of endovascular stents

Common use of external fixators

Improved tourniquets

Computer-assisted design and manufacture of limb prostheses

Pain control

Concussion care

Established clinical practice guidelines for combat casualty care

Identification of coagulopathy in injury

Challenges of treating infections with fungus and multidrug-resistant bacteria

Deployed Electronic Health Record

Reach-back capability with telehealth and programmatic email communication

LEARNING FROM "BLACK HAWK DOWN"

In early October 1993, the 2nd General Hospital (now called Landstuhl Regional Medical Center) in Germany was inundated with casualties from Operation Restore Hope, the Battle of Mogadishu, as memorialized in the book and movie Black Hawk Down.[1] Without the heroic efforts of medics, doctors, and nurses on the front line and subsequently in the operating rooms, intensive care units, and wards of my hospital, our losses would have been higher.

As a brand-new general surgeon assigned to Landstuhl, I was frustrated by the lack of coordinated trauma care, and overwhelmed with the volume and complexity of combat wounded we received from Somalia. The trauma experience in my surgical residency had not prepared me for the severity and intensity of these wounds.

Although the military had developed a robust casualty care process in support of Desert Storm/Desert Shield less than two years earlier, the lessons from those conflicts were quickly forgotten. As a result, we scrambled to adapt when Operation Restore Hope—a humanitarian relief operation to address widespread starvation in Somalia—turned into a combat mission.

After the Battle of Mogadishu, in-depth analyses of the medical lessons learned by military medical visionaries (John Holcomb, Frank Butler, Bob Mabry, John Uhorchak, and many others) led to significant and dramatic improvements in combat casualty care.[2-4]

Fast forward to 2007–2009. I was again stationed at Landstuhl, this time as the facility's commander. The transformation in combat casualty care I observed was remarkable. It clearly led to significant and sustained improvements in survival on the battlefield and during subsequent hospital care.

A partial list of the improvements I observed included widespread adoption of Tactical Combat Casualty Care, aggressive use of tourniquets, deployment of new-generation clot-promoting dressings, Critical Care Air Transport Teams (CCATTs), and the development of the Joint Trauma System. The casualty care skills of military providers were enhanced through the establishment of American College of Surgeons (ACS) Committee on Trauma-designated trauma centers in military hospitals, the ACS Visiting Surgeon Program, and regular analysis of data from a seamless trauma registry (the Joint Trauma Registry), fully wedded to the military's electronic medical record. Each of these components, and many others, were integral parts of the military health system's casualty care program.

Our responsibility—now, and in the years ahead—is to retain the lessons we have learned and ensure that the systems and programs we worked so hard to establish are ready when needed. This is why the military health system focuses so intensely on continuous improvement, evidence-driven practice, requirements-driven research, communication, and both individual and team-based training. These activities must be sustained through appropriate resourcing and firmly codified into doctrine and policy at the Department of Defense level.

We cannot assume that future conflicts will afford us the luxury of a months-long buildup and just-in-time training. The only way we can assure we will be ready to swiftly and effectively respond is if the military health system continually keeps its edge by maintaining high-performing teams of trauma-trained military health professionals at every level—from our front line combat medics, corpsmen, and MEDEVAC personnel to our forward surgical teams, critical care nurses, CCATTs, trauma surgeons, orthopedists, and rehabilitation specialists. These teams must be ready to deploy, at a moment's notice, anywhere in the world to protect the health of our forces, conduct humanitarian assistance missions, and if needed, provide state-of-the-art care to our wounded, ill, and injured.

Major General Brian C. Lein
Commander, Army Medical Department Center and School
Health Readiness Center of Excellence, San Antonio, Texas

Notes

1. Bowden M. *Black Hawk Down: A Story of Modern War*. New York, NY: Signet Books, 1999.
2. Mabry RL, Holcomb JB, MD, Baker AM, et al. United States Army Rangers in Somalia: an analysis of combat casualties on an urban battlefield. *J Trauma*. 2000;49:515–529.
3. Butler FK Jr, Hagmann J, Butler EG. Tactical combat casualty care in special operations. *Mil Med*. 1996;161(Suppl):3–16.
4. Eastridge BJ, Jenkins D, Flaherty S, Schiller S. Holcomb JB. Trauma system development in a theater of war: experiences from Operation Iraqi Freedom and Operation Enduring Freedom. *J Trauma*. 2006;61:1366–1372.

CONCLUSION

Military history is defined as much by advances in technology as courage on the battlefield. Military *medical* history is no different. From the founding of our republic until today, US military health professionals have championed clinical and technological advances that have saved lives, prevented countless cases of disability, and preserved our nation's fighting strength. Table 2.1 provides a consolidated list of advances to casualty care without differentiation among those that grew from prewar civilian research, those that were the contributions of civilians in uniform, and those that resulted primarily from military innovation. In nearly every case, innovations forged in the crucible of war were quickly brought back to civilian healthcare, where they have benefitted millions of Americans. Because military technology, tactics, and terrain constantly evolve, military medicine must evolve as well to ensure that those our nation sends into harm's way will always receive the best care possible. (See "Learning from 'Blackhawk Down.'")

Notes

1. Chernow R. *Washington: A Life.* New York, NY: Penguin Group US; 2010.
2. Letter of J.M. Browne to the chief of the Bureau of Medicine and Surgery. In: *Report of the Secretary of the Navy, 1864.* Washington, DC: Department of the Navy, 1865: 633–635.
3. National Academy of Sciences. *Accidental Death and Disability: The Neglected Disease of Modern Society.* Washington, DC: National Academy Press; 1966.

Recommended Reading

Devine S. *Learning from the Wounded.* Chapel Hill, NC: University of North Carolina Press; 2014.

Lederer S. *Flesh and Blood: Organ Transplantation and Blood Transfusion in 20th Century America.* Oxford and New York: Oxford University Press; 2008.

Murray CK, Hitter SR, Jones SL. Army Medical Department at War: lessons learned. *Army Med Dep J.* 2016;Apr–Sep:1–3

Slater L. *War and Disease: Biomedical Research on Malaria in the Twentieth Century.* Brunswick, NJ: Rutgers University Press; 2009.

Smith DC. War and medicine. In: Slotten HR, ed. *The Oxford Encyclopedia of the History of American Science, Medicine and Technology.* Vol. 2. Oxford and New York: Oxford University Press, 2014: 567–586.

Smith DC. Extremity injury and war: a historical reflection. *Clin Orthop Relat Res.* 2015;473:2771–2776.

Woodward TE. *Armed Forces Epidemiological Board: The First Fifty Years.* Washington, DC: Borden Institute; 1990.

CHAPTER three

Educating Military Health Leaders

CRAIG LLEWELLYN, MD, MPH; JERRI CURTIS, MD; and BRIAN V. REAMY, MD

MILITARY MEDICINE

MILITARY PHYSICIANS SERVE TWO PROFESSIONS: the profession of medicine and the profession of arms. As a result, their education must address the application of medical and public health science to military populations and situations. Military medicine is largely organized around the same medical and surgical disciplines that define civilian medicine, plus some military-specific subspecialties such as aerospace, undersea, and operational medicine. However, it differs from civilian medicine in several important respects. These unique dimensions receive little thought in the civilian world (beyond practitioners of trauma surgery and emergency medicine), but military medicine has ancient roots, a rich history, and a dynamically evolving body of knowledge.

MEETING THE HEALTHCARE NEEDS OF AN "ALL-VOLUNTEER FORCE"

From the American Civil War through the end of America's involvement in Vietnam, the ranks of the US military were filled with a mix of volunteers and draftees. But in 1972, the decision was made to suspend the draft. This presented the Department of Defense with the challenge of recruiting enough highly trained physicians to meet the needs of the "all-volunteer force." In response, Congress created two programs that offer physicians-to-be substantial financial assistance to attend medical school in exchange for varying lengths of military service[1] (Table 3.1):

> " *The Department takes great pride in the fact that the [Uniformed Services University of the Health Sciences] graduates have become the backbone of our Military Health System. The training they receive in combat and peacetime medicine is essential to providing superior force health protection and improving the quality of life for our service members, retirees and families.* "

The Honorable Donald Rumsfeld, Secretary of Defense
Letter to the Chairman of the Uniformed Services
University Board of Regents, March 22, 2001

- The armed forces' **Health Professions Scholarship Program** (HPSP), administered by the Army, Navy, and Air Force, offers civilian medical students a signing bonus, a full scholarship, payment of fees, and a monthly stipend in exchange for a four-year commitment to practice military medicine after graduation and completion of a residency training program. Although most HPSP students separate from the military shortly after fulfilling their service obligation, enough remain in the ranks to make this program the major source of military physicians.

- The **Uniformed Services University of the Health Sciences** (USU) serves as the leadership academy of the military health system. Students admitted to USU are commissioned by their sponsoring service, attend tuition-free, and are paid the salary of a junior officer by their sponsoring service (Army, Navy, Air Force, or Public Health Service). In return for receiving a high-quality medical education and supplemental training in military medicine and leadership, USU graduates commit to a minimum of seven years of military service after residency training. Most willingly serve 20 years or longer.

"AMERICA'S MEDICAL SCHOOL"

The Mayo brothers, Drs. William J. and Charles H., first proposed the establishment of a "uniformed services university." They envisioned an institution devoted to educating a dedicated corps of military medical officers. Years later, Representative F. Edward Hébert, a long-serving Louisiana congressman who chaired the powerful House Armed Services Committee from 1971 to 1975, made it his lifelong goal. Representative Hébert believed that new doctors entering military service through the HPSP would benefit from interacting with colleagues steeped in the traditions and values of military medicine,

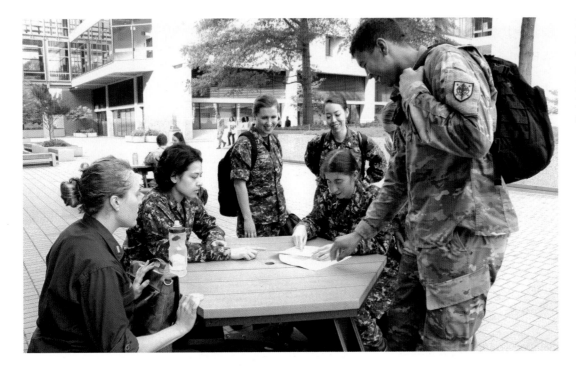

FIGURE 3.1. Medical students on the main campus of the Uniformed Services University of the Health Sciences, the leadership academy of America's Military Health System. Photo by Tom Balfour, Uniformed Services University of the Health Sciences.

much as Reserve Officers Training Corps (ROTC) students benefit from interacting with graduates of the Army, Navy, and Air Force academies. Hébert's efforts were so instrumental in bringing the university into being that when it opened its doors in Bethesda, Maryland, in 1976, Congress named the new medical school in his honor. Today, more than 5,200 graduates later, USU's F. Edward Hébert School of Medicine has clearly fulfilled Congress's intent by providing a steady supply of highly capable, adaptable, and innovative military medical officers[2] (Figure 3.1).

In addition to being the only medical school in America that charges no tuition or fees, USU's school of medicine differs from civilian medical schools in at least five important respects:

1. **Many students have military experience.** Approximately one-third of USU medical students have a prior military background as graduates of a service academy, ROTC, or prior active duty service in a

BUSHMASTER'S LEGACY

My "Bushmaster" experience as a Uniformed Services University of the Health Sciences (USU) medical student served me well during my first deployment to Iraq in 2003 as a regimental surgeon with the 2nd Armored Calvary Regiment. When we crossed the border and entered Iraq, we did not know what to expect. We had trained to provide the best possible care, including treating wounds from weapons of mass destruction. We also knew we would probably need to care for civilians on the battlefield. Bushmaster gave me my first experience with both.

When we reached Baghdad, our unit was assigned to Sadr City, an area that encompassed over 3 million of the city's poorest inhabitants. Early on, our biggest problem was the absence of critical infrastructure, including functioning hospitals. These had either been destroyed or completely looted of equipment and supplies. Thanks to my experience as a USU medical student, working daily with civilians and classmates from the Navy, Air Force, and Public Health Service, I was comfortable collaborating with the Iraqi Ministry of Health (MOH), nongovernmental organizations, the US Department of State, and my fellow military medical officers scattered across Baghdad. Over the next year, we renovated two public hospitals, sixty public health clinics, and the two nursing schools in our sector so the Iraqis could care for their own people.

Soon after arriving, the security situation began to unravel. On one of my trips to the Iraqi MOH, our convoy was struck by a well-coordinated attack involving machine guns and rockets. The vehicle in front of me was hit by a rocket-propelled grenade and was engulfed in flames. My Bushmaster training immediately took over. Under fire, my team and I successfully extracted and evacuated our wounded.[1]

In the days that followed, conditions continued to deteriorate. The United Nations compound was attacked by a massive vehicle-borne improvised explosive device that resulted in over 170 casualties and the death of the UN envoy. My unit was less than a half-mile away when we both heard and felt the concussion of the explosion. We reached the scene within minutes, joining medics and providers from other units in the vicinity, some of whom were fellow USU alumni. I had never seen so many casualties at one time. Were it not for my foundational training and the constant drilling of my team, I might have been mentally and emotionally overwhelmed by the carnage. Instead, working as a team, we cleared the scene within 90 minutes.

Bushmaster taught me to expect the unexpected, and to prepare and train for the worst because anything that can go wrong likely will go wrong—at the worst possible moment. It also taught me to improvise, to seek unique solutions to seemingly unsolvable problems, and to work in multi-service teams to achieve our shared goal: to provide "good medicine in bad places" under the most challenging circumstances.

It is my sacred privilege to care for our nation's sons and daughters who are serving in its defense. I have done so in locations and circumstances that few of my civilian counterparts could imagine, much less manage. The events I've recounted were the first of several wartime and operational deployments. Without my foundational education at USU and field exercises like Bushmaster, my subsequent success would have been far from assured. Fortunately, USU taught me essential military medical skills and instilled in me the virtues of service above self. It opened the door to my career as a military physician and a contributor to the remarkable teams with whom I have had the honor and privilege to serve.

Colonel Kelly A. Murray
Chief, Medical Corps Branch
Health Services Division
US Army Human Resources Command
USU Class of 1992

Note

1. For her actions in the ambush on her convoy, Colonel Murray received the Bronze Star with a "V" for valor, one of four Bronze Stars she earned for her work in Iraq.

TOPIC	TRAINING FOCUS	WHEN
Military Field Practicum 101	Teamwork, leadership, military core values, and identity formation as military medical officers. Basic field medical skills.	1st y
Military Field Practicum 102	Advanced military medical skills in a team capacity. Expanded knowledge of rapid combat trauma assessment and treatment, medical operational planning, multimodal combat pain control, and crisis communication.	2nd y
Military Field Practicum 201, "Gunpowder"	1.5-day field course at USU focused on Tactical Combat Casualty Care, small unit leadership, and medical platoon drills.	3rd y
Military Contingency Medicine and Military Field Practicum 202, "Bushmaster"	2 weeks of contingency medicine with a 4-day field course at Ft. Indiantown Gap, PA. Serves as "capstone" course that brings all the training together in mass casualty scenarios and drills.	4th y

TABLE 3.1. Supplemental Military Medicine and Leadership Curriculum at the Uniformed Services University of the Health Sciences

wide range of roles. As a result, in USU classrooms, college kids and former Peace Corps volunteers study with former fighter pilots, submariners, Army Rangers, and Navy SEALs. The maturity and perspective of "prior service" students helps their classmates adapt to military life.

2. **A national campus.** In addition to clinical clerkships at nearby military hospitals such as Walter Reed National Military Medical Center, USU students rotate to major military treatment facilities from Portsmouth, Virginia, to Honolulu, Hawaii. Many participate in overseas electives as well.

3. **Military-specific curriculum.** In addition to a standard medical education, USU medical students receive more than 700 hours of instruction in combat casualty care, posttraumatic stress, tropical medicine, the law of armed conflict, humanitarian and stability operations, detainee care, global health engagement, and military leadership[3] (Table 3.1 and Figure 3.2).

4. **Simulation education.** USU was an early adopter of medical simulation, an educational approach that uses robotic manikins, task-trainers, and human actors role-playing patients to teach students critical clinical and interpersonal skills in a safe and controlled setting. USU's Simulation Center

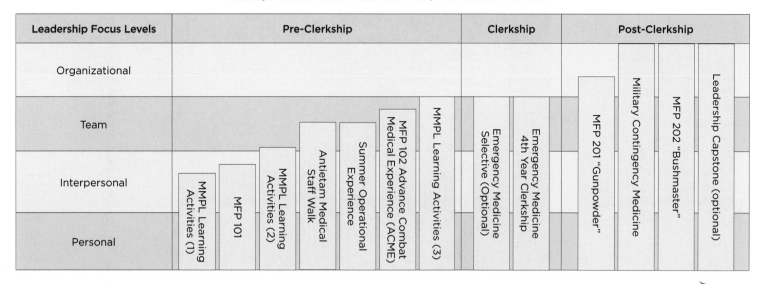

USU SCHOOL OF MEDICINE DEPARTMENT OF MILITARY AND EMERGENCY MEDICINE
Military Medical Practice and Leadership Curriculum Overview

Leadership Focus Levels	Pre-Clerkship							Clerkship			Post-Clerkship			
Organizational											MFP 201 "Gunpowder"			
Team					Antietam Medical Staff Walk	Summer Operational Experience	MFP 102 Advance Combat Medical Experience (ACME)	MMPL Learning Activities (3)	Emergency Medicine Selective (Optional)	Emergency Medicine 4th Year Clerkship		Military Contingency Medicine	MFP 202 "Bushmaster"	Leadership Capstone (optional)
Interpersonal		MMPL Learning Activities (1)	MFP 101	MMPL Learning Activities (2)										
Personal														

LEADERSHIP EDUCATION AND DEVELOPMENT →

also features a unique "wide-area virtual environment" that enables individual students and teams to practice combat casualty care in a walk-in virtual reality space that can put them in an urban ambush, the passenger bay of a MEDEVAC helicopter, a Critical Care Air Transport Team (CCATT), or a combat support hospital (Figure 3.3).

5. **Field exercises.** USU students not only learn to provide care in a clinic or hospital, they also learn how to practice in austere settings and combat zones. To impart these skills, at four different points in their four-year education, students participate in a series of progressively challenging field exercises, culminating with Operation Bushmaster, a multi-day, simulated deployment of hundreds of medical personnel in support of a major US military operation (Figures 3.4 and 3.5). Conducted

FIGURE 3.2. In addition to educating students in the biomedical sciences and clinical skills, USU educates its students to be leaders. Over four years, key competencies are progressively developed through the personal, interpersonal, team, and organizational dimensions of care.

MMPL: Military Medical Practice and Leadership
MFP: Medical Field Practicum

FIGURE 3.3. USU medical students at USU's Val J. Hemming Simulation Center practice combat casualty care in the "wide-area virtual environment." Photo by Tom Balfour, Uniformed Services University of the Health Sciences.

FIGURE 3.4. [*Opposite*] USU's "Operation Bushmaster," a large-scale, simulated deployment of a medical unit to a foreign battlefield, is held every October at the Pennsylvania National Guard's large training base at Fort Indiantown Gap, Pennsylvania. Photo by Eric Goolsby, Uniformed Services University of the Health Sciences.

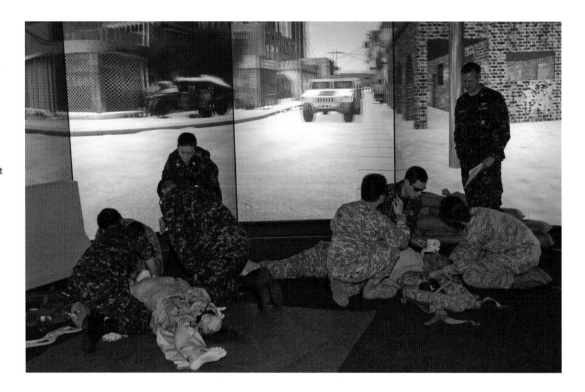

each fall at a large National Guard training base, Operation Bushmaster involves two full classes of USU medical students, 20 to 25 international medical students, graduate nursing students, experienced military faculty who fly in from around the country to teach and grade them, and more than 200 supporting enlisted staff, reservists, and National Guard members (Figures 3.6 and 3.7).

Unlike the service academies, USU students learn in a *tri-service* educational environment. This ensures that future leaders of the Army, Navy, and Air Force medical corps (and the US Public Health Service) study and train together under the watchful eye of uniformed and civilian faculty and staff. Daily interactions with strong role models; regular interdisciplinary sessions with graduate nursing, public health, and biomedical research students; and multiple clinical rotations at top Army, Navy, and Air Force teaching hospitals produce graduates who are comfortable working in interdisciplinary and joint service teams.

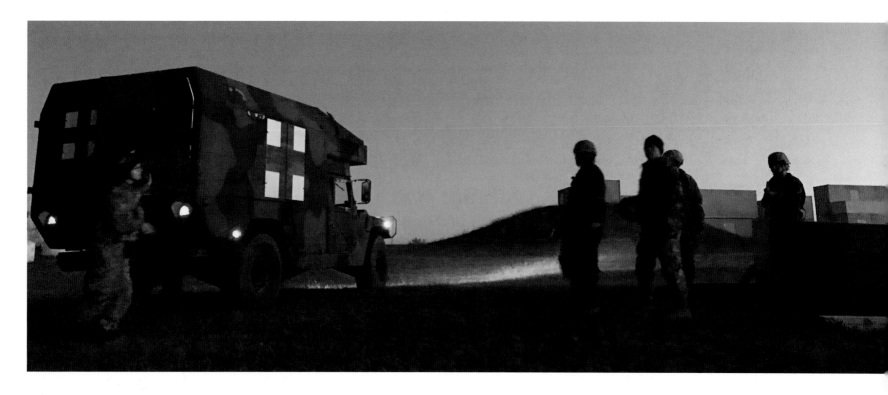

TRAIN FOR THE MISSION; EDUCATE FOR A LIFETIME

Five decades after USU opened its doors, the university's emphasis on military medicine and leadership
has proven its worth. USU graduates performed effectively in the First Gulf War and the Balkans
conflicts in the 1990s, and came into their own during Operation Enduring Freedom, Operation Iraqi
Freedom (OEF/OIF), and Operation New Dawn (see "Bushmaster's Legacy"). The university's tri-service
approach to education paid off as well. When deployed, it was not unusual for USU graduates in Iraq
and Afghanistan to coordinate care with classmates staffing CCATT flights, surgical services at Landstuhl
Regional Medical Center, and subsequent definitive care at Brooke Army Medical Center, Walter Reed, or
the National Naval Medical Center in Bethesda (see "One Team, One Fight" in Chapter 15). The bonds of
trust fostered in USU's classrooms one to two decades earlier helped foster tri-service cooperation in Iraq

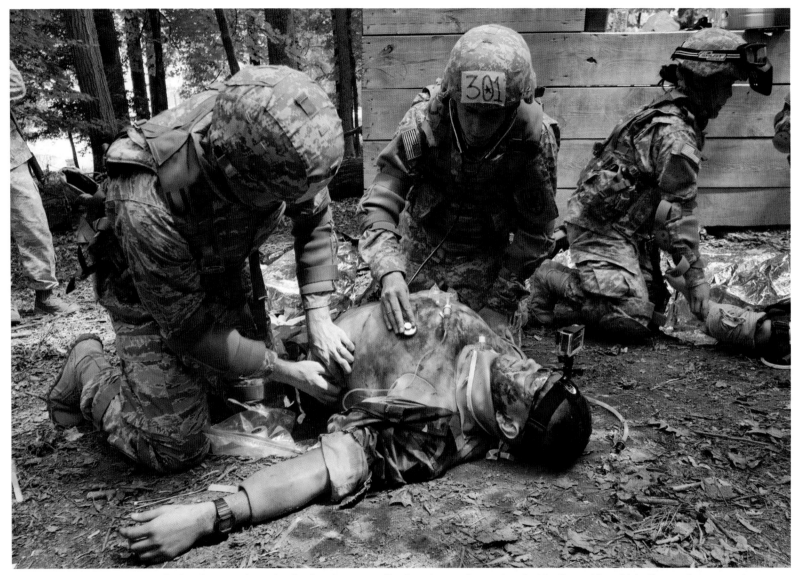

FIGURE 3.5. USU medical students treating a simulated patient—an enlisted service member equipped with a "cut suit"—which allows trainees to perform invasive, life-saving procedures without fear of harming the actor. The service member's head camera is capturing the action on video so the students and their instructor can subsequently review their performance from the patient's perspective. Photo by Tom Balfour, Uniformed Services University of the Health Sciences.

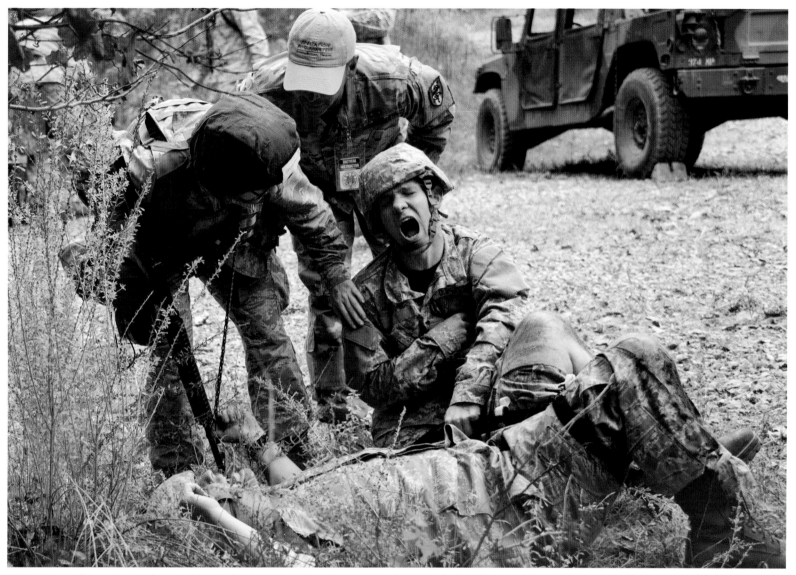

FIGURE 3.6. "Operation Bushmaster," Fort Indiantown Gap, Pennsylvania. A fourth-year medical student is treating two first-year medical students role-playing casualties of an improvised explosive device attack. An observer-instructor (wearing ball cap) looks on. Photo by Tom Balfour, Uniformed Services University of the Health Sciences.

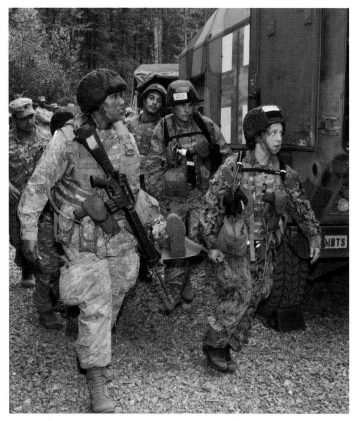

FIGURE 3.7. "Operation Bushmaster," Fort Indiantown Gap, Pennsylvania. Fourth-year medical students prepare to load a simulated casualty into a Humvee ambulance. Photo by Tom Balfour, Uniformed Services University of the Health Sciences.

and Afghanistan (Figure 3.8). This ensured seamless care from the point of injury on the battlefield to major Role 4 hospitals in Germany and the United States and subsequent rehabilitation.

USU's culture of national service has paid off as well. Graduates of the university's school of medicine serve in uniform four times longer, on average, than graduates who enter the military from civilian medical schools. As a result, although USU produces only 10 to 12 percent of doctors who enter military service each year, one-fourth of all active duty physicians, and more than a third of senior leaders, are USU alumni.[4,5] A 1995 report by the Government Accountability Office observed that "GAO's review of DoD retention data suggests that University graduates are likely to provide DoD with a cadre of experienced physician career officers. Scholarship program physicians, who comprise the majority of new physician accessions, are retained in the military for shorter periods, on average, than University graduates."[6]

GRADUATE MEDICAL EDUCATION IN THE MILITARY HEALTH SYSTEM

All newly minted military physicians must complete a residency program to learn the details of their chosen specialty. In addition to teaching the essential knowledge and clinical skills of their respective specialties, military residency programs teach essential military skills uniformed doctors need to effectively function as providers in the medical corps of the Army, Navy, and Air Force. For example, all interns complete a rigorous "Combat Casualty Care Course" (C4) as well as a course in "Military Medical Humanitarian Assistance." Military interns and residents must master the tenets of officership, including military bearing, professional conduct, and the fundamentals of leadership. Also, unlike civilian physicians, military physicians must maintain their physical fitness in order to demonstrate that they can deploy worldwide.

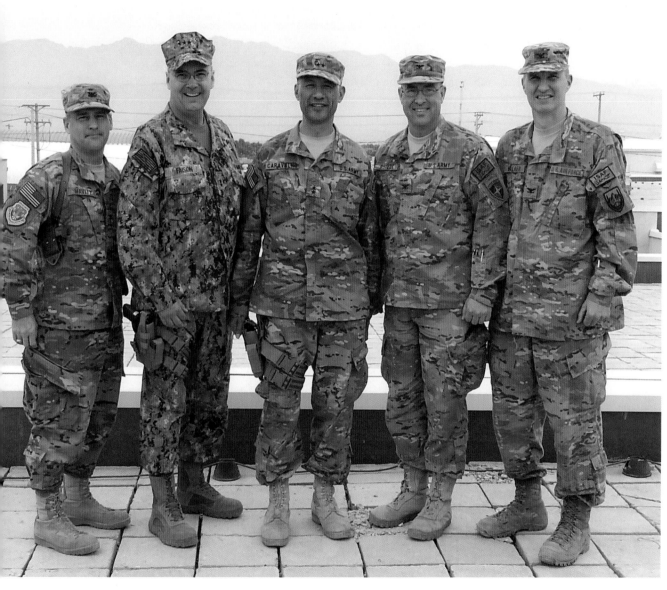

FIGURE 3.8. USU alumni, taken on the rooftop of Craig Joint Theater Hospital, Bagram Air Base, Afghanistan, May 8, 2014. Pictured, left to right:

- Colonel Mark Mavity (USU '88), then Central Command Surgeon; now Air Force Surgeon General Special Assistant for Invisible Wounds and Wounded Warrior Programs.
- Vice Admiral Forrest Faison (USU '84), then US Navy Deputy Surgeon General; now Navy Surgeon General.
- Major General Joe Caravalho (USU '83), then US Army Deputy Surgeon General; now Joint Staff Surgeon.
- Colonel David Ristedt (USU '95), then International Security Assistance Force Joint Command and US Forces–Afghanistan Surgeon; now US Army Pacific Command Deputy Surgeon.
- Colonel Gary Walker (USU '84), then Commander, Craig Joint Theater Hospital, and Commander, US Air Force 455th Expeditionary Medical Group; now retired from the military.

Photo courtesy of Vice Admiral Forrest Faison.

Graduate Nursing Education

The US military depends on far more than doctors for medical care. Military nurses play a vital role as well. In the late 1980s and early 1990s, growing requests for humanitarian assistance missions prompted the military to expand its ranks to include advanced practice nurses and nurse educators. In 1992, Rear Admiral Faye Abdellah, the recently retired chief nurse of the Public Health Service, led a task force that concluded, "Civilian colleges of nursing can prepare nurses for the military, *but they cannot prepare military nurses*" [emphasis added].[2] On the strength of this report, the services asked USU to establish a graduate school of nursing to educate advanced practice nurses. Rear Admiral Abdellah agreed to serve as founding dean, and the school opened its doors in 1996.

Over two decades, USU's Graduate School of Nursing steadily expanded from 15 family practice and nurse anesthesia students to more than 160 today. Along the way, the school added programs to train perioperative clinical nurse specialists and behavioral health specialists, and began a PhD program in nursing science. In 2014, it joined a national movement among graduate nursing programs by shifting its educational model to doctorate degrees. In 2014, the school was officially named the "Daniel K. Inouye Graduate School of Nursing" in honor of the late senator from Hawaii and Medal of Honor recipient, who was a lifelong champion of military nursing.

Graduate Dental Education

Full force readiness requires oral health. For years, the military has directly recruited dentists after they finished dental school. However, the need for many military dentists to work in isolated environments led to the expansion of graduate dental education programs across the services, encompassing such specialized skills as prosthodontics, periodontics, oral surgery, orthodontics, endodontics, facial pain, and comprehensive general dentistry. By 2010, USU was asked to enhance dental readiness training, academic rigor, and research by organizing 19 military graduate dental programs into a postgraduate dental college. Major General (Retired) Patrick Sculley, a former Army Dental Corps chief, agreed to serve as founding dean. The enhanced training and research these students undertake qualifies them for a master's degree in oral biology and certification in one of the dental specialties.

FOUR DECADES OF PROGRESS

Today, more than 40 years after the suspension of the draft, USU and the HPSP have ensured that America's all-volunteer force attracts dedicated and capable military health professionals. HPSP provides nearly 90 percent of the military's new doctors, and USU focuses on preparing a cadre of master clinicians and military health leaders. Together, these two programs, plus the small number of "direct accessions" who are commissioned out of civilian practice, help the military buffer downturns in one source or the other. The value of this strategy was apparent during OEF/OIF, as noted by a former Army surgeon general:

> Throughout the Afghanistan and Iraq conflicts of the past 13 years, Army Medicine was consistently and heavily relied upon to deploy physicians and other health care professionals into the combat zone, often on a recurring basis and for protracted periods (12–15 months). As Chief of the Army Medical Corps (2002–2005) and as Army Surgeon General and Commanding General of the Army Medical Command (2007–2011), I was intimately involved with the challenges of recruiting, career-developing and retaining highly qualified and committed Army physicians. While recruitment into Army HPSP scholarships waned during the height of fighting in the past decade, USU never failed to meet their obligation to recruit, educate & train and provide highly qualified Army physicians to the Army Medical Department. In addition, these were often graduates bound for much-needed primary care, emergency medicine and surgery careers—among the most needed specialties in these conflicts.
>
> —Lieutenant General (Retired) Eric B. Schoomaker
> 42nd Surgeon General, US Army (email to BVR, January 9, 2017)

HONORING REPRESENTATIVE HÉBERT'S VISION

Military medicine is more than the practice of medicine in a uniform, and USU is more than a "schoolhouse" to train military doctors, nurses, dentists, and public health practitioners. The university's faculty and staff conduct high-impact military-relevant research on a wide range of topics, from the neurobiology of traumatic brain injury to global health (Table 3.3). Learning in an environment

TABLE 3.3. Uniformed Services University of the Health Sciences interdisciplinary centers and institutes for research and education.

Center for Global Health Engagement
National Center for Disaster Medicine & Public Health
Center for Neuroscience and Regenerative Medicine
Tri-Service Center for Oral Health Studies
Center for Military Family Health
Center for Deployment Psychology
Center for Disaster and Humanitarian Assistance Medicine
Center for Health Disparities
Center for Prostate Disease Research
Center for the Study of Traumatic Stress
Center for Rehabilitation Sciences Research
Consortium for Health and Military Performance
Defense and Veterans Center for Integrative Pain Management
Infectious Disease Clinical Research Program
Murtha Cancer Center
Surgical Critical Care Institute

focused on scientific inquiry encourages USU's medical, nursing, dental, and graduate students to develop into innovators and problem-solvers. This philosophy paid off, as USU alumni teamed up with their HPSP counterparts to overcome multiple clinical and operational problems in the early years of OEF and OIF (Chapter 6). This was one of the foundational factors that drove the remarkable chain of healthcare innovations and improvements that ultimately transformed the US military's approach to combat casualty care.

Notes

1. Daubert VL, Relles DA, Roll CR Jr. *Medical Student Financing and the Armed Forces Health Professions Scholarship Program*. Santa Monica, CA: RAND Corporation; 1982.

2. Kinnamon KE, ed. *The Uniformed Services University of the Health Sciences: First Generation Reflections*. Bethesda, MD: Uniformed Services University of the Health Sciences; 2004.

3. Alter WA III, Lllewellyn CH, Haddy FJ. Teaching military medicine as a basic science: military applied physiology. *Mil Med.* 1985;150:334–335.

4. Reddy S, Torre DM, Boulet JR, van der Vleuten C. Celebrating 40 years of medical education at the Uniformed Services University of the Health Sciences. *Mil Med.* 2012;177:9.

5. Durning SJ, Artino AR Jr, Dong T, et al. Findings from the Long-term Career Outcome Study (LTCOS) and related work. *Mil Med.* 2015;180:4.

6. US Government Accountability Office. *Military Physicians: DoD's Medical School and Scholarship Program*. Washington, DC: GAO; September 1995. GAO/HEHS-95-244.

CHAPTER four

Combat Casualty Care Research

DAVID G. BAER, PHD; ANDREW P. CAP, MD, PHD; and TODD E. RASMUSSEN, MD

"REQUIREMENTS-DRIVEN" HEALTH RESEARCH

THE NATIONAL INSTITUTES OF HEALTH (NIH) and most other federal research agencies mainly sponsor "investigator-initiated" research. This process challenges research scientists to compete to present the most compelling idea, backed by a well-designed approach. The hope is that over time, this approach to the funding and conduct of medical research will build a critical mass of knowledge or trigger major discoveries that advance science and improve health. Researchers awarded funds through NIH mechanisms have considerable latitude over the projects they can pursue and the time frame over which they pursue them.

The military's approach to health research is different. Rather than funding science for science's sake, the Department of Defense (DoD) pursues "requirements-driven" research.[1,2] Instead of inviting researchers to pitch their ideas within a broad area of interest (such as lung cancer or heart failure), the DoD describes a specific problem or "requirement"—such as an urgent need for effective technologies to control bleeding or replace blood loss on the battlefield—and challenges researchers to develop a practical solution.

Direction starts with the National Security Strategy, a document the executive branch prepares for Congress, outlining how the government plans to address major national security priorities. The National Military Strategy further elaborates this vision, and it is ultimately refined in a series of service-specific documents.[2] These specific areas of need inform the DoD's research agenda.[3]

MEETING THE CHALLENGE OF COMBAT CASUALTY CARE

During the wars in Iraq and Afghanistan, the military health system's research focused mainly on improving combat casualty care. For example, at the outset of Operations Enduring Freedom (OEF) and Iraqi Freedom (OIF), there was no overarching, tri-service system to coordinate or monitor the delivery and outcomes of trauma care or provide real-time input to the DoD's Combat Casualty Care Research Program (CCCRP). The rising number of battlefield injuries spotlighted the need for better information.[4]

To better coordinate care and collect information on combat injuries, surgical treatment, survival, and outcomes,[4] the Army, Navy, and Air Force in 2004 created the Joint Trauma System (JTS), dedicated to improving trauma care (see Chapter 8). One of the first actions it took was to create a "Joint Theater Trauma Registry" (JTTR). Modeled after civilian trauma registries such as the American College of Surgeons' National Trauma Databank, the JTTR compiled treatment data, documented outcomes, and provided a resource to analyze and improve clinical performance. Using this trauma registry— now renamed the "Department of Defense Trauma Registry" or DoDTR—the JTS identified specific requirements that the DoD research community needed to address.[4,5]

THE MILITARY'S "LEARNING HEALTHCARE SYSTEM"

The DoD's requirements-driven approach, which systematically collects data to determine what works and what does not, and uses these insights to frame a research agenda to improve medical care, has been termed a "learning healthcare system." The National Academy of Sciences recently recognized this approach's success in a healthcare delivery system that spans the globe, calling it a model for continuous quality improvement.[6]

During OEF and OIF, the US military used battlefield data, collected through the JTTR, to inform the CCCRP, which is part of the Army's Medical Research and Materiel Command at Fort Detrick, Maryland. The CCCRP coordinates its work with a global network of Defense Centers of Excellence (DCoEs)—including the JTS—which perform clinical performance improvement and provide expert care (Table 4.1).

Working with the CCCRP, the DCoEs combine new insights and discoveries into useful products and clinical guidelines. The knowledge and materiel products developed through the DoD health research process quickly reach the education programs of the Uniformed Services University (USU) and other military health training platforms (Chapter 3).[6]

We can depict the relationship between these entities with a "books and bookends" illustration (Figure 4.1). The left bookend represents clinical entities that provide input to the DoD's research activities or institutions, which are represented by the individual books.[7] These research programs endeavor to produce knowledge and materiel solutions that are integrated by the DoD's clinical entities, represented by the other bookend. Besides using registry information to improve performance, the DCoEs, in conjunction with the relevant specialty consultants to the surgeons general, are the primary developers of clinical recommendations and guidelines.[7] The model rests on a foundation of medical education and leadership development provided by the USU and the enlisted training centers that produce Army medics, Navy corpsmen, and Air Force medical technicians—the backbone of battlefield care. This knowledge-based, requirements-driven learning healthcare system propelled most of the innovations that advanced combat casualty care during the recent wars.

THE MILITARY'S COMBAT CASUALTY CARE RESEARCH PROGRAM

The CCCRP, funded through the Army and the Defense Health Program, is one of DoD's largest medical research programs. It strives to optimize wounded warriors' chances of survival and recovery in current and future operational scenarios. To advance this mission, it sponsors an ambitious portfolio of research aimed at improving management of trauma from point of injury through medical evacuation to facility-based care.[7,8] In contrast to the big NIH research institutes, the CCCRP's budget is relatively modest, amounting to about $200 million per year. In fact, the DoD's entire annual investment in medical research (about $1 billion per year) is less than 1/30th the size of NIH's annual budget. Moreover, according to a 2013 interagency assessment,[9] the US military sponsors more than 80 percent of our nation's annual investment in research for trauma and injury care. In the field of trauma research, if the DoD doesn't fund it, it probably won't get done.

REQUIREMENTS AND GUIDANCE

DoD requirements guide the CCCRP's funding decisions. These are largely based on overarching documents like the National Defense Strategy and refined with input from DoD working groups and advisory committees. The capabilities documents that inform the process are written by the individual services or as part of the Joint Capabilities Integration

TABLE 4.1. Knowledge or materiel solutions resulting from military research and the continuously learning health system in trauma

TOPIC AREA OR PORTFOLIO	KNOWLEDGE OR MATERIEL PRODUCT
Hemorrhage Control	**Knowledge** • Defined the epidemiology and specific anatomic categories of hemorrhage • Described in detail the impact of hemorrhage on risk of mortality • Published guidance on the timing of extremity tourniquet application • Assessed the value of an endovascular approach to non-compressible torso hemorrhage **Materiel** • Tested, evaluated, and fielded extremity tourniquets and hemostatic bandages • Developed resuscitative endovascular balloon occlusion of the aorta (REBOA) technology • Developed XStat (Revolutionary Medical Technologies, Wilsonville, OR) topical hemostatic agent and applicator
Resuscitation	**Knowledge** • Determined benefit of blood product-based resuscitation • Defined specific and optimal ratios for blood component-based resuscitation • Demonstrated the mortality benefit from tranexamic acid in combat trauma resuscitation • Described the value of cold preservation of platelet products for resuscitation **Materiel** • Fielded a dried plasma product for reconstitution and use in resuscitation • Fielded prehospital blood products in a "golden hour" box • Developed modern interosseous access devices for trauma resuscitation • Fielded a cold-stored platelet product for trauma resuscitation
Forward Surgery	**Knowledge** • Defined the ischemic threshold of the limb and the utility of shunts in vascular trauma • Defined the value and importance of timing in performing an extremity fasciotomy • Defined the effectiveness of negative pressure therapy in treating soft tissue injuries • Demonstrated the value of extracorporeal support in the management of organ failure • Determined the value of "damage control" laparotomy and delayed abdominal closure **Materiel** • Developed a burn resuscitation decision support tool

| Neurotrauma (TBI) | **Knowledge**
• Defined the incidence and spectrum of severity of wartime TBI (epidemiologic study)
• Optimized resuscitative strategies for combat-related TBI
• Established a progressive return to activity pathway for mild TBI
• Determined the usefulness of existing pharmacologic therapies for TBI
• Formed multi-center consortia to provide insight into TBI definitions and endpoints

Materiel
• Developed noninvasive neuro-diagnostic devices for mild TBI
• Advanced preclinical and clinical development of pharmacologic agents to treat TBI |
| En-Route Care | **Knowledge**
• Defined mortality benefit linked to medical readiness and training level of flight crews
• Determined the mortality benefit of on-board resuscitation capability
• Optimized use of existing hemostatic devices during en-route care scenarios
• Optimized use of existing analgesics for en-route pain control

Materiel
• Developed a medical monitor (compensatory reserve index) to diagnose shock |

TBI: Traumatic Brain Injury

and Development System. Products of this process include validated capability-defining documents that provide the mandate for researchers and product developers to allocate resources to specific efforts. Periodically, additional guidance comes from the Office of the Assistant Secretary of Defense for Health Affairs, the civilian leadership of the military health system. Sometimes, additional funding for military trauma research comes from Congress through "congressional special interest" add-ons, or CSIs. These typically include language directing resources to specific projects or topic areas. Additional input into the CCCRP's programmatic decisions comes from clinical entities such as the DCoEs, specialty consultants to the Army, Navy, and Air Force surgeons general, and military doctors and nurses in the field.

CCCRP staff responds to this guidance with active program management that includes planning, programming, budgeting, and oversight of appropriated dollars. Because the CCCRP handles both Defense Health Program and Army research funds, it is responsive to both organizations and is supported by two chartered committees that provide input on how it manages its portfolio: the Joint Program Committee-6 and a US Army "integrating, integrated product team." Both groups include representatives from the clinical community, relevant DCoEs, civilian experts, and advanced developers.

FIGURE 4.1. The military's learning system in trauma depicted as books and bookends. The left bookend represents the clinical platforms that provide input to the research platforms (represented by the individual books). The research platforms programs are primarily Program-6 (P6; research, development, testing, and evaluation) funded and endeavor to produce knowledge and materiel solutions that are integrated by the clinical entities, represented by the bookend on the right. The clinical platforms are primarily Program-8 (P8; operations and maintenance) funded and operate registry-based, performance improvement (PI) and clinical investigation (CI) activities. The clinical programs are also the proprietors of clinical guidelines. The activities in this model rest on the academic, educational, and training foundation provided at the Uniformed Services University of the Health Sciences and enlisted medic training centers.

DCoE: Defense Center of Excellence
DoD: Department of Defense
O&M: operations and maintenance
RDT&E: research, development, testing, and evaluation

Figure modified from: Rasmussen TE, Reilly PA, Baer DG. Why military medical research? *Mil Med.* 2014;179(8):1-2.

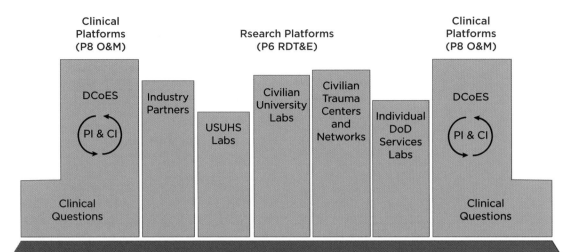

Advanced developers are particularly important because they spearhead the transition of promising discoveries from the science and technology (S&T) phase to the advanced development (AD) phase. This process includes studies to demonstrate product effectiveness, clearance of regulatory hurdles, and subsequent commercialization and delivery of products. Failure to coordinate the steps from S&T to AD can strand a promising product or technology in the "valley of death," where good ideas falter due to lack of planning and funding.[10]

Importantly, the CCCRP's active program management functions continue from the original research through subsequent partnership with military contracting agencies. This maximizes delivery of the desired knowledge and materiel solutions to the front-line providers who need them. The CCCRP also provides input into annual congressional appropriations planning relevant to military trauma. This ensures that the military's priorities for trauma research—including hemorrhage control, resuscitation, forward surgical care, traumatic brain injury, and other topics—are reflected in funding decisions so taxpayer dollars are well spent.

THE LIFE CYCLE OF RESEARCH

The CCCRP and other DoD research partners fund projects that span the spectrum of biomedical research, from basic to applied research, clinical trials, effectiveness studies, and the follow-on activities required to achieve regulatory approval and bring a product to market. S&T funding, managed by CCCRP staff, supports early pre-clinical and applied research aimed at advancing knowledge and materiel products. Promising efforts to develop impactful knowledge products continue under CCCRP management, while regulatory trials for materiel development (eg, drugs, devices, and technologies) are transitioned to AD. These AD teams work to sponsor the clinical trials and accomplish the regulatory approval work required to bring drugs, devices, and technologies to market and to the service member (Table 4.2). This coordinated, life-cycle approach optimizes the likelihood that research funds are allocated to create genuinely useful solutions in the shortest possible time.

As the centerpiece of the DoD's learning healthcare system for trauma care, the CCCRP delivers advances in trauma and injury care at a rapid pace and at a relatively modest cost. A number of these advances directly contributed to advances in combat casualty care achieved during OEF/OIF and Operation New Dawn.[11,12] A comprehensive list of the products produced by the CCCRP during the recent wars is beyond the scope of this chapter, but Table 4.1 lists several notable examples.

CONCLUSION

Trauma and injury research in the DoD is managed like a large materiel acquisitions organization. Thus, funding decisions are linked to specific clinical and programmatic requirements. The program is tightly managed to ensure that projects address specific needs or requirements in the shortest time possible. During the wars in Afghanistan and Iraq, much of the military's requirements-driven research portfolio was invested in improving combat casualty care (Figure 4.2). By aligning the investment of the CCCRP with the JTS and the DCoEs, the US military produced a learning healthcare system. Despite the pressure of treating thousands of severely injured casualties on the other side of the Earth while continuing to meet the healthcare needs of military beneficiaries and retirees here at home, America's military healthcare providers produced a remarkable series of advances in trauma care in a short amount of time.[9] How these advances were achieved, and the impact they had on the lives of individual service members, are described in the subsequent chapters of this book.

TABLE 4.2. Nomenclature for program elements of Department of Defense medical research, development, testing, and engineering dollars

MATURITY OF LIFE CYCLE RESEARCH		PROGRAM ELEMENT	DEPARTMENT OF DEFENSE VERBIAGE	IMPLICATION FOR MEDICAL RESEARCH
Science and Technology		6.1	Basic research that produces new knowledge in a scientific or technological area of interest to the military.	Research on fundamental principles—including cellular and molecular biology and medical genetics—aimed at understanding the cellular, molecular, and physiologic mechanism underpinning human health and injury
		6.2	Applied research supporting exploratory development and initial maturation of new information or technologies or further developing existing information or technologies	Applied or preclinical research—including animal models—preparing the ground for clinical research with patients
		6.3	Advanced knowledge or technology development supporting larger scale that can demonstrate the capability (knowledge or materiel) in more operationally realistic settings	Translational research focusing on iterative loops between basic and clinical research domains to accelerate (make more efficient and relevant) knowledge or materiel translation; includes applied and clinical methodology
Advanced Development		6.4	Demonstration and validation supporting the initial development and demonstration of a knowledge or materiel product designed to meet an agreed-upon set of performance standards associated with a validated operational need	Single or multi-center clinical research— including pragmatic, observational, and comparative effectiveness studies—that deliver knowledge products for translation or prepare materiel products for regulatory phase
		6.5	Engineering, manufacturing, and/or refinement of a specifically designated product (knowledge or materiel) that has demonstrated it can meet performance requirements, including developing necessary manufacturing processes needed to build that product	Pivotal efficacy study for Investigational New Drug (IND), Individual Device Exemption (IDE), or Product License Application (PLA) and/or associated manufacturing and regulatory costs to achieve approval for a device, drug, biologic, or technology

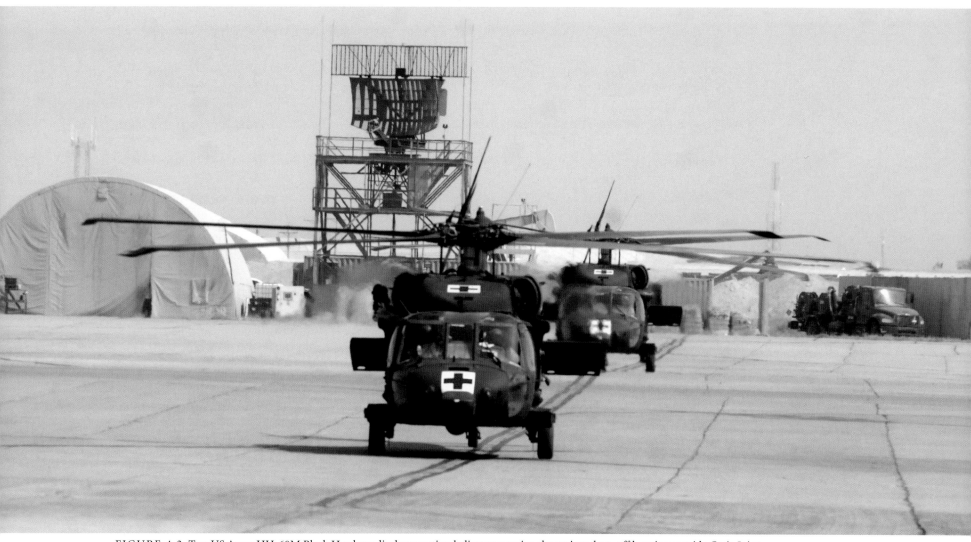

FIGURE 4.2. Two US Army HH-60M Black Hawk medical evacuation helicopters taxi to the patient drop-off location outside Craig Joint Theater Medical Hospital during a patient transfer mission at Bagram Airfield, Afghanistan, September 13, 2013. During Operations Enduring Freedom and Iraqi Freedom, much of the US military's requirements-driven medical research portfolio was invested in improving combat casualty care. US Army photo by Captain Peter Smedberg/Released. Reproduced from: https://www.dvidshub.net/image/1017283/10th-cab-medical-evacuation-crews-conduct-patient-transfers.

Notes

1. US Department of Defense. Defense Acquisitions Portal. https://dap.dau.mil/aphome/ppbe/Pages/Default.aspx. Accessed May 22, 2016.

2. US Department of the Army. *The US Army Operating Concept: Win in a Complex World, 2020–2040.* Fort Eustis, VA: Training and Doctrine Command; October 31, 2014. TRADOC Pamphlet 525-3-1. http://www.tradoc.army.mil/tpubs/pams/TP525-3-1.pdf. Accessed May 15, 2016.

3. Camp and base solutions: the silver lining of war. *Defence Procurement International Magazine.* 2014;Summer:190–192.

4. Blackbourne LH, Baer DG, Eastridge BJ, et al. Military medical revolution: military trauma system. *J Trauma Acute Care Surg.* 2012;73:S388–394.

5. Bailey JA, Morrison JJ, Rasmussen TE. Military trauma system in Afghanistan: lessons for civil systems? *Curr Opin Crit Care.* 2013;19:569–577.

6. The National Academies of Science, Engineering and Medicine. Activity: military trauma care's learning health system and its translation to the civilian sector. NAS website. http://www.nationalacademies.org/hmd/Activities/HealthServices/LearningTraumaSystems.aspx. Accessed May 22, 2016.

7. Rasmussen TE, Reilly PA, Baer DG. Why military medical research? *Mil Med.*2014;179:1–4.

8. Rasmussen TE, Baer DG, Doll BA, Caravalho J. In the "golden hour": combat casualty care research drives innovation to improve survivability and reimagine future combat care. *Army AL&T Magazine.* 2015;January–March:80–85.

9. Rasmussen TE, Kellermann AL. Wartime lessons—shaping a national trauma plan. *N Engl J Med.* 2016;375(17): 1612–1615.

10. Pusateri AE, Macdonald VW, Given MB, Walter SF, Prusaczyk KW. Bridging the technology valley of death: joint medical development. *Army AL&T Magazine.* 2015;November–December:40–45.

11. Kotwal RS, Howard JT, Orman JA, et al. The effect of a golden hour policy on the morbidity and mortality of combat casualties. *JAMA Surg.* 2016;151:15–24.

12. Rasmussen TE, Rauch TM, Hack DC. Military trauma research: answering the call. *J Trauma Acute Care Surg.* 2014;77:S55–56.

CHAPTER five

Futurist Thinking: Military Health Services System 2020

PATRICK SCULLEY, DDS, and WILLIAM R. ROWLEY, MD

I N 1995, AFTER TOURING THE NEWLY COMPLETED Brooke Army Medical Center at Fort Sam Houston in San Antonio, then Army Surgeon General Alcide LaNoue wondered if the gleaming facility was already obsolete due to rapid changes in healthcare that had occurred during the decade of its planning and construction. His facilities planners replied that to develop future facilities they would need a cogent description of the healthcare system these facilities would serve. So the Department of Defense (DoD) chartered a group to envision the long-term strategic requirements of what we now call the Military Health System, or MHS. Planners hoped it would not only influence future facility designs but also transform the military's approach to peacetime and wartime healthcare delivery.

The effort, named "Military Health Services System 2020," or *MHSS 2020*,[1-4] was meant to envision what the MHS would look like in 25 years. It involved 300 participants from the medical departments of the Army, Navy, and Air Force, along with representatives of other government agencies and civilian experts. It had three main objectives: (1) help the MHS explore future possibilities and propose strategies that would succeed in a range of potential future conditions; (2) train a generation of military health futurist leaders to navigate the threats and opportunities to come; and (3) make recommendations to redesign the MHS to meet tomorrow's challenges.

Today, 21 years later, the effort has proven its worth. Many of *MHSS 2020's* ideas and recommendations remain highly relevant. The report prompted military health leaders to look beyond daily concerns and envision potential opportunities and threats looming ahead. Perhaps *MHSS 2020's* greatest legacy was to encourage the powerful and sometimes parochial cultures of the Army, Navy, and Air Force medical corps to look beyond their differences, embrace advances in technology, and transform how they approach healthcare delivery. By doing so, *MHSS 2020* set the stage for the rapid-cycle improvements that transformed combat casualty care during the wars in Iraq and Afghanistan.

When the process got started in 1996, the group's thinking was strongly influenced by recent military events: the Beirut Marine barracks bombing, US military interventions in Panama and Grenada, the Persian Gulf War, Somalia, Hurricane Andrew relief in Florida, and military actions in Haiti and Bosnia. These events and the insights they generated were frequent topics of "Chautauquas" (online discussions) with expert and visionary military medical leaders such as PK Carlton, James Peake, and Michael Cowan, who later became surgeons general of the Air Force, Army, and Navy, respectively.

YEAR ONE (1996): ENVISIONING THE FUTURE TO DIRECT TODAY'S RESOURCES

During the first year of *MHSS 2020*, expert facilitators oriented participants to the process of futurist thinking. Then participants were divided into 20 workgroups and told to collaborate via the online Chautauquas. Each group analyzed a variety of medical, military, and global forces and developed potential forecasts for up to 25 years into the future. During the second half of year one, participants were assigned to one of ten interdisciplinary workgroups and told to weave the threads of their prior discussions into four scenarios of how the future might unfold.

The first scenario, "The Third Wave," was a positive extrapolation of the present. It contained potentially dangerous developments, but generally painted an optimistic view of the future. The second scenario, "The Dark Side," forecast a more dangerous and alarming future than we usually like to contemplate. The third scenario, "Global Mind Change," challenged traditional assumptions about what a successful future might look like. Under this scenario, cooperative efforts to resolve and suppress conflicts and promote cooperative sustainable development are substantially successful, prompting a fundamental rethinking of the role of military force and by extension, military medicine. The final scenario, "The Transformation," was initially left sketchy so participants could fill it in with ideas about what the "outer edge" of the possible might look like in 2020, given transformative technology and highly positive social circumstances.

After developing these scenarios, the workgroups identified nine key forces likely to influence the future role of military health: (1) social values, (2) technological change, (3) economic development, (4) environmental impacts, (5) political change, (6) demographic shifts, (7) medical progress, (8) organizational development, and (9) level of military readiness. A two-day Futures Symposium involving the senior leaders and 250 guest participants reviewed the four scenarios, developed a shared definition of the identity of military medicine (see below), crafted a vision of a preferred future, and set audacious goals for nine years hence (at that point, 2005).[1]

STATEMENT OF IDENTITY

"We are the healers who walk with warriors in unison. We are on a journey to do what must be done. We are a community of healers who know health is a wholeness. Our caring runs as deep as the pain of war. We take those who are broken and make them whole. We serve through a system of values, our roots reaching down to a stream flowing from generation to generation. Duty, honor, loyalty, and courage to sacrifice are the bonds that hold us together. We are an awesome force of warriors and healers protecting the values of home."[1]

YEARS TWO THROUGH FOUR (1997–1999)

In the three years that followed, *MHSS 2020* contributors sequentially focused on three high-impact topics. During the second year, 40 participants conducted a six-month in-depth study of advances in the emerging fields of biotechnology, genomics, and nanotechnology.[2] In the third year, a larger group devoted substantial time to envisioning the future of MHS involvement in small-scale conflicts and non-combat humanitarian missions.[3] In the fourth and final year of the project, participants used their training to envision the MHS of the future.[4] Today, we can see how this visioning exercise influenced subsequent innovations in battlefield casualty management as well as military operations other than war (MOOTWs), and the provision of healthcare services to service members in garrison. (The term MOOTW has since been replaced by other terminology such as low intensity conflict, stability actions, and global engagement. The *MHSS 2020* report envisioned a central role for health services across the spectrum of these actions irrespective of terminology.)

MILITARY OPERATIONS OTHER THAN WAR

A major theme that emerged was something participants called the "paradox of peace." Following the collapse of the Soviet Union in 1991, America faced no major enemies on the world stage. However, the Soviet Union's fall did not bring about the "end of history" as some had predicted. Instead, the United States found itself enmeshed in multiple small conflicts with different adversaries and objectives. Participants in *MHSS 2020* noted that many early 21st century military operations would be quantitatively and qualitatively different than large-scale war, at least as the term was applied to conventional military conflicts (Table 5.1). The list of differences proved prescient in describing the global security environment that evolved over the next 20 years.

MOOTWs are on the low end of conflict intensity, and include activities such as disaster relief, humanitarian assistance, peacekeeping, and evacuation of noncombatants. These missions have a strong health component and often require organized military medical forces to sustain the effort. In MOOTWs, military health personnel often serve as the "tip of the spear" because they are welcomed when other forces are not. For this reason, MOOTWs can also be a critical element in helping stabilize a nation, thereby avoiding the need for subsequent counter-terrorism or counter-insurgency operations. Given signs in 1997–1998 that MOOTWs would be more common in the future, *MHSS 2020* participants considered what the MHS needed to support operations of this type. Rather than base the group's planning on a single "best guess," several potential missions were envisioned through the lens of the four scenarios described above. Today, the widening Middle East conflict following the Arab Spring best fits forecasts based on the Dark Side scenario, confirming the value of modeling alternate futures, rather than a single (and potentially inaccurate) best guess.

Based on the expectation that the number of MOOTWs would grow, *MHSS 2020* participants concluded that robust medical department resources, capabilities, and organizational flexibility would be needed to support US armed forces in a variety of non-combat as well as combat operations. To envision requirements, the group applied the military's "DTLOMS" framework (the acronym stands for "Doctrine, Training, Leader Development, Organization, Materiel, and Soldier"). This enabled the group to create a comprehensive set of requirements to ensure needed capacity.

In addition to logistics and manpower, the group developed a list of leadership competencies required to provide health services support for MOOTW engagements in the 21st century. The US military still uses this list in its leadership development courses.

COLD WAR	EARLY 21ST CENTURY
Bipolar world (simple)	Multipolar world (complex)
Winning wars	Preventing chaos
Soviet Union is US peer competitor	No peer competitor capable of mounting broad strategic challenges
War between sovereign states	Intrastate wars; terrorism; conflicts with extremists, paramilitaries, drug cartels, organized crime
Symmetric conflicts (eg, tanks vs tanks)	Adversaries use asymmetrical means (eg, airliners, roadside bombs, targeted assassinations)
Military is target of conflicts	Civilians often the targets of violence
Preparations geared to global war with the Soviet Union; more recently to two near simultaneous major theater wars	Global war unlikely; scope and scale of threat diminishing in many areas of potential regional conflict but proliferation of unconventional threats
Deterring communist aggression	Shaping world events to foster peaceful, sustainable development leading to greater national and global security
Protecting national border and territories from foreign nations	Protecting against threats to common security: arms proliferation (especially nuclear); spreading conflict and disorder; environmental catastrophe; crimes against humanity; natural disasters
Military operations other than war detract from the central mission of deterrence	Military operations other than war are important for shaping world events and responding to the full range of threats
Willing in certain circumstances to accept inequality and support dictators to prevent the spread of communism	Need to promote fairness and encourage democracy to address grievances that can lead to terrorism, intrastate wars, and chaos
Medical resources for combat support	In addition to combat support, medical resources are a fundamental asset for achieving national objectives; widening range of health roles

TABLE 5.1. Characteristics of Cold War Versus 21st Century Conflict

- **Moral constancy.** Ability, amid chaos and rapid change, to provide predictability by striving to do the "right thing" and establishing a climate of caring, integrity, and trust.

- **Visioning.** Ability to clarify aspirations, establish a vision, and inspire and empower others to attain that vision; set long-term goals and act proactively to achieve them.

- **Flexibility.** Ability to rapidly adapt to, and thrive in, changing conditions, and to alter strategies and restructure organizations with minimum disruption.

- **Systems thinking.** Ability to grasp the "big picture," see interrelationships between forces, consider alternative possibilities, and anticipate long-term consequences of actions.

- **Cultural and historical appreciation.** Ability to appreciate other cultures and differences in ethnicity and religion, and to feel comfortable working in other cultures.

- **Technological sophistication.** Understanding and appreciation of leading-edge technological capabilities with an ability to discriminate useful technology from bad.

- **Acknowledging uncertainty.** Ability to accept uncertainties and create an atmosphere of trust so other people can share uncertainties and focus learning on important areas of uncertainty.

- **Embracing error.** Ability to take innovative risks, identify and correct mistakes without hesitation, and learn from them within a culture so others can do likewise.

- **Boundary spanning.** Ability to effectively relate to people in other organizations and volatile situations, to tolerate ambiguities, and to value and reward others who possess these abilities.

DID *MHSS 2020* GET THINGS RIGHT?
ASSESSING ACHIEVEMENTS AND RECOMMENDATIONS

Objective 1: Propose strategies that will be successful across a range of
potential future conditions.

- The process helped planners recognize that alternative futures can be managed with preparation and flexibility. Leaders can shape a desired future with a shared vision and appropriate strategies. This allowed a military culture very resistant to change to embrace advances in technology and the societal changes that are transforming the culture and processes of modern health delivery.

- Frequent conversations among participants helped leaders appreciate the key role each service plays, while highlighting the need for cross-service cooperation to improve efficiency and boost the impact of their efforts.

- Looking back, the scenarios envisioned in 1997 are still relevant. All four forecast events that have come to pass.

- The *MHSS 2020* project embraced the characteristics of a "learning organization" as articulated in 1990 by Peter Senge: systems thinking; personal mastery; mental models; shared vision and team learning.[5]

- Today, nearly 20 years later, the MHS reflects many of the principles promulgated in *MHSS 2020*. In particular, it recognizes "the need for continued development towards an integrated *learning health system* as a critical enabler and a key characteristic of an integrated health system" [emphasis added].[6]

Objective 2: Train military health futurist leaders.

- Many of the mid-career participants in *MHSS 2020* later assumed senior leadership roles in their respective service. Six achieved flag/general officer rank, including three surgeons general. These visionary officers used the view they gained of our rapidly changing world to make decisions that shaped the course of military medicine.

- One *MHSS 2020* participant who later served on the staff of the House Committee on Armed Services, Colonel (Retired) Jeanette James, noted that "participating in the process redirected my way of thinking about military health care and the need for the MHS to be a thinking and an anticipatory organization."

- The Joint Staff surgeon at the time, and later the 34th Navy surgeon general, Vice Admiral (Retired) Michael Cowan recalls, "*MHSS 2020* was highly influential. It helped me grow as a leader, and it laid the groundwork for future joint warfighting medical capabilities."

Objective 3: Make recommendations for redesigning the MHSS.

- "Create a Virtual Community of Practice for creating an MHS-wide rapid-response capacity." *MHSS 2020* introduced a mechanism for collaboration in the virtual space and across service lines via information technology tools. However, the services opted to keep individual control of doctrine development and training for their respective roles in MOOTWs. Nonetheless, the improved collaboration and integration fostered by *MHSS 2020* contributed to the subsequent development of a joint concept for health services.[7]

- "Develop a comprehensive Military Health Strategy through a major restructuring of the MHS to leverage flexibility across a spectrum of health services and military operations." Although the services have retained separate control of their programs, they have learned to collaborate down range to provide a broad spectrum of health services in support of MOOTW demands. *MHSS 2020* emphasized the importance of health promotion and health protection especially for achieving resilience during combat. Lieutenant General (Retired) Eric Schoomaker, an *MHSS 2020* participant who later became Army surgeon general, used these ideas to develop the Army Well Being Initiative.

- "Elevate the status of MOOTW and make it a distinct item in Defense Planning Guidance." The detailed analyses conducted in the course of this project informed MHS leadership and improved collaboration between the services' operational medicine specialists. Participants presented the final MOOTW report to the commander in chief, US Special Operations Command, who embraced it. Although MOOTW did not become a separate component of defense planning guidance, global health engagement to address a variety of health threats is now a vital capability. A recent example is the DoD's deployment of 3,000 troops to Liberia to build field hospitals, set up laboratories, provide security, and train medical personnel.

- "Develop and integrate across the MHS a leader development program." Although the services did not embrace the creation of a joint leader development program, MHSS 2020 showed the value of bringing mid-career officers together for planning and teambuilding. However, the Uniformed Services University of the Health Sciences, as the leadership academy for military health, partially takes on this role by providing leadership development to all of its medical, nursing, dental, and public health students, and by supporting graduate medical education in the National Capitol Region. The Uniformed Services University has also incorporated the 21st century leadership competencies identified by *MHSS 2020* into its MedXellence program, which is taught to mid- and senior-grade MHS leaders at various sites around the world.

- "Build global and local relationships and cultural appreciation to work with other parties during MOOTW operations." Today, the services fully embrace the importance of global health. So do many of our international partners. Recently, at the request of DoD leadership, the Uniformed Services University formalized its commitment to this objective by establishing the University Center for Global Health Engagement.

MHS 2020 thoughts about MOOTWs strongly influenced military operational medicine's transformation, setting the stage for the rapid pace of transformation that followed during Operation Iraqi Freedom (OIF) and Operation Enduring Freedom (OEF). The US Navy went into the Persian Gulf War with large, cumbersome fleet hospitals. By the time OEF began, the Navy had transitioned to small, nimble, forward resuscitative surgical systems that fit on a truck and trailer and can keep up with fast-moving Marines. (Chapter 14). The US Air Force transformed aeromedical evacuation to the point that it flies critically injured warfighters halfway around the world to major military hospitals in Germany and the United States as soon as 48 to 72 hours after injury. (Chapter 25) The Army upgraded the training of combat medics to the standard of civilian emergency medical technicians (Chapter 11). As a result of these and many other innovations, operational medicine in OEF and OIF was far more joint, agile, and capable than in the Persian Gulf War. These changes did not occur by chance. They were the fruit of the interservice cooperation and leader development *MHSS 2020* fostered nearly two decades ago.

Notes

1. *MHSS 2020: Envisioning Tomorrow to Focus Today's Resources.* Fort Sam Houston, TX: US Army Medical Department Center and School; 1996.
2. *MHSS 2020: Focused Study on Biotechnology & Nanotechnology.* Fort Sam Houston, TX: US Army Medical Department Center and School; July 29, 1997.
3. *MHSS 2020: OOTW Report.* Fort Sam Houston, TX: US Army Medical Department Center and School; July 31, 1998.
4. *MHSS 2025: Toward a New Enterprise.* Fort Sam Houston, TX: US Army Medical Department Center and School; December 28, 1999.
5. Senge PM. *The Fifth Discipline: The Art & Practice of The Learning Organization.* New York, NY: Currency; 2000.
6. *Military Health System Health Benefit Delivery Concept of Operations.* Draft v2.10. Washington, DC: Office of the Assistant Secretary of Defense for Health Affairs; Defense Health Agency. December 11, 2015.
7. *Joint Concept for Health Services.* Washington, DC: Joint Chiefs of Staff; August 31, 2015.

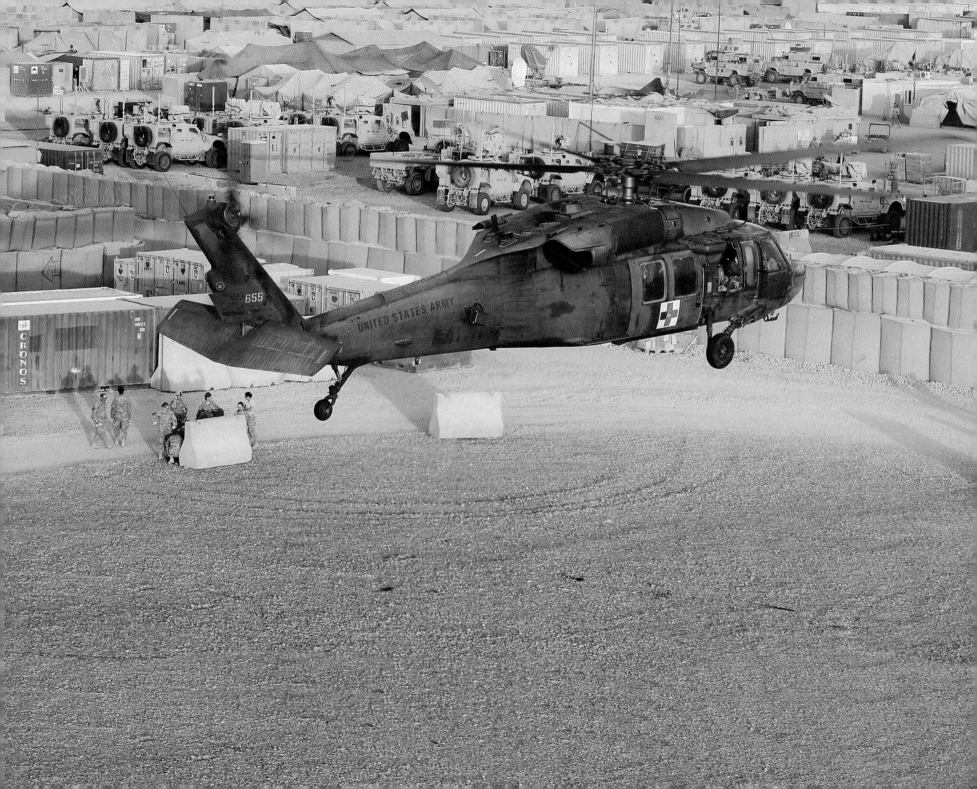

SECTION TWO

Innovations

[*Section Two image*] A US Army MEDEVAC
helicopter from Charlie Company, Sixth Battalion, 101st Airborne Combat Aviation Brigade, Task Force Shadow, prepares to land to
pick up a wounded US Soldier at a forward
operating base near Kandahar, Afghanistan,
June 22, 2010. Photo by Justin Sullivan/Getty
Images. Reproduced with permission from
Getty Images.

CHAPTER six

The Health Challenges of Operation Enduring Freedom and Operation Iraqi Freedom

STEPHEN L. JONES, MD, and CLINTON K. MURRAY, MD

H EALTHCARE ON THE BATTLEFIELD IS A COMPLEX, risk-filled endeavor. Medical teams serve far forward to provide immediate treatment to wounded troops. They deliver care in austere and extreme conditions, frequently under fire. As a result, care delivered in combat is emotionally charged and full of uncertainty. Planning for military healthcare is influenced by the mission, the enemy, and environmental and political factors. Each war presents unique challenges for medical planners and providers, as shown by the recent operations in Afghanistan and Iraq.

OPERATION ENDURING FREEDOM

The war in Afghanistan began unlike any other. Small teams of special operations forces worked with Afghan militias to overthrow the Taliban regime and rout al-Qaeda from their safe havens. In just over six weeks, the Northern Alliance, 100 Special Forces soldiers, and US airpower defeated the Taliban in northern Afghanistan. In the south, 200 Army Rangers parachuted into a small desert airfield 50 miles southwest of Kandahar. They took Kandahar and Kabul, conventional forces entered the country, and the remaining organized Taliban and al-Qaeda opposition was destroyed in Operation Anaconda in March 2002. The conflict then entered a new phase aimed at restoring stability and creating a new

" Today, a severely

wounded service

member in Afghanistan

is more likely to survive

his or her injuries than

an equally injured

trauma victim in

many parts of the

United States. "

government. Coalition forces began training the Afghan National Army and Police, and establishing provincial reconstruction teams to assist interagency nation-building efforts.

In the summer of 2006, increased fighting led Coalition forces to implement a comprehensive counter-insurgency strategy. As the Afghan National Army's capability grew, it assumed greater responsibility for the country's security. A formal ceremony in Kabul on December 28, 2014, marked the official end to Operation Enduring Freedom (OEF).[1] Total US military casualties included 1,843 killed and 20,071 wounded.[2]

THE HEALTH CHALLENGES OF OPERATION ENDURING FREEDOM

Operations in Afghanistan challenged medical staff in unique ways. Small units fighting across an area the size of Texas were often isolated at the end of extended lines of communication. The war in Iraq drew much of the US military's attention and resources, limiting the number of forward surgical teams and MEDEVAC helicopters available to US forces in Afghanistan. As a result, in the early years of the conflict, medical evacuation to field hospitals sometimes took hours.

As the conflict progressed, the Taliban began employing increasingly powerful improvised explosive devices (IEDs). Effective body armor and the quick application of tourniquets saved many lives, but Soldiers and Marines patrolling on foot often sustained devastating injuries. Many were seriously wounded, with multiple amputations, complex abdominal and genitourinary trauma, and traumatic brain injuries.[3]

Afghanistan is a country of environmental extremes. Operation Anaconda was fought in mountains that rose to 10,469 feet, higher than any other battle in US history.[4] The heavy loads troops carried up and down ridgelines took a physical toll that accumulated during multiple deployments. In the southern provinces, troops fought in deserts where temperatures frequently exceeded 120°F. They also fought in river valleys with lush vegetation, where blast wounds were contaminated with environmental molds that caused invasive fungal infections.

With 14 ethnic groups, Afghanistan's culture is as diverse as its physical environment.[5] An Afghan's loyalty typically is to family, clan, and tribe rather than to the central government. Afghans are a modest people who value privacy and are reluctant to share personal information. Many Afghan women are virtually confined to their homes, and greatly restricted from interacting with men who aren't close relatives. To overcome this barrier, military humanitarian assistance teams included female healthcare providers.

At the onset of OEF, the health status of Afghans was among the worst in the world. Life expectancy for men was 44 years; for women, only one year longer. One in twelve Afghan women died during childbirth and one of every four Afghan infants died before age five. Sadly, many of these deaths were from preventable causes, including measles, diarrhea, tuberculosis, and respiratory infections.[6] The US Agency for International Development led efforts to restore civilian healthcare by providing basic healthcare services. In areas of the country deemed too dangerous for international organizations to work, military healthcare teams supported the effort.

OPERATION IRAQI FREEDOM

Operation Iraqi Freedom (OIF) started with air strikes on March 19, 2003, aimed at eliminating Iraq's leadership. The ground campaign began the next day with the limited forces on hand. Three weeks of tough fighting followed as Coalition units advanced toward Baghdad. On April 9 a small contingent of Marines and a crowd of jubilant Iraqis pulled down Saddam's statue in Baghdad's Firdos Square.[7]

After the Coalition Provisional Authority disbanded the Iraqi Army, reconstruction began amid lawlessness and looting. In 2004, Sunni insurgents, the Shia Mahdi Army, and al-Qaeda in Iraq increased the frequency and intensity of their attacks. Intense urban combat followed in cities across the country, and by 2006 sectarian violence rose to the level of a civil war.[7] To increase forces on the ground, the US Army implemented 15-month rotations for Soldiers in the summer of 2006, and troop levels eventually reached 170,000.

To counter the IED threat, the United States modified many of its existing armored vehicles (Chapter 9) and deployed thousands of mine-resistant ambush-protected (MRAP) vehicles. Coalition forces moved into neighborhoods to provide security, Sunni tribes joined as part of the "Anbar Awakening," and US special operations forces mounted an effective counter-terrorism campaign.

As violence fell, the Coalition transitioned responsibility for security to Iraqi forces. The final US troops withdrew from Iraq on December 18, 2011, officially ending OIF.[8] US military casualties in Iraq totaled 3,481 killed and 31,951 wounded.

THE HEALTH CHALLENGES OF OPERATION IRAQI FREEDOM

The health challenges of OIF began before the first units deployed. Medical teams prepared to treat chemical casualties because of the threat of weapons of mass destruction. At Fort Campbell alone, medical staff administered 160,000 immunizations for anthrax, smallpox, and other threats to 30,000 members of the 101st Airborne Division and Tennessee National Guard. As deployments began, some units were cut to keep troop levels down. This decision, and the invasion's rapid start, meant that not all medical units were in place when the war began.[7]

Environmental conditions in Iraq were also challenging. Summers were brutally hot, with temperatures rising to 145° F. Occasional sandstorms reduced visibility and prevented medical evacuations.[5] Cultural considerations were similar to those in Afghanistan, particularly with regards to the treatment of women.

Although years of sanctions had degraded Iraq's infrastructure, it was far more developed than Afghanistan's. The challenge in both countries was to rebuild healthcare capacity without creating lasting dependency on the United States. Again, the focus was on restoring basic healthcare services rather than installing advanced equipment too difficult to maintain. Iraq's hospitals had a limited capacity to treat critical cases and severely injured civilians. Coalition hospitals often cared for Iraqi Security Forces. Unfortunately, many of these patients were colonized with multi-drug-resistant bacteria (see Chapter 27). US medical personnel recognized the problem and implemented strict infection control measures.

MEETING THE HEALTHCARE DEMANDS OF TWO WARS

Medical and operational commanders collaborated to provide effective force health protection and casualty treatment. Noncommissioned officers conducted rigorous training and instilled the discipline required for warriors to consistently wear their body armor (Chapter 9) and eye protection (Chapter 21), and to treat wounded comrades (Chapters 10 and 11). Leaders also enforced measures that reduced disease and non-battle injury rates to historic lows (Chapter 7).

Cooperation among the military services contributed to historically high casualty survival rates. A Marine critically wounded in Afghanistan or Iraq might be treated by a Navy corpsman and evacuated on an Army MEDEVAC helicopter to a field hospital staffed by personnel from multiple services. The most severely injured were promptly flown out of the war zone on Air Force C-17s staffed by Critical Care Air Transport Teams (Chapter 25) to the Army's Landstuhl Regional Medical Center, and from there to major military treatment facilities in the United States.

Analysis of casualty information by the Joint Trauma System provided real time improvements in care (Chapter 8). The Joint Trauma Analysis and Prevention of Injury in Combat program reviewed operational and medical data to improve protection for service members. Studies by armed forces medical examiners of service members killed led to improvements in both protection and casualty treatment (Chapter 9). Mental health advisory teams deployed to Iraq and Afghanistan to bolster behavioral health support (Chapter 30).

Rapid translation of insights generated by the military's "learning healthcare system" led to improved frontline care as well as better care at military medical centers back home. Combat units developed new tactics, wore more effective personal protective equipment, and fielded better vehicle designs, such as the Stryker double-V hull (Chapter 9). Medical staffs acquired better equipment and steadily refined their approach to the resuscitation, treatment, and rehabilitation of wounded warriors (Chapters 26–31).

Improvements in care were captured in joint standards and training programs. Corpsmen, medics, and infantry received training in Tactical Combat Casualty Care (Chapter 11). Medical staff from all three services attended the Combat Casualty Care Course, Joint Trauma Management Course, Emergency

War Surgery Course, Trauma Nursing Care Course, and Joint Enroute Care Course. Medical units reorganized and adapted new procedures to work more efficiently and effectively. Combat support hospitals were split and positioned to reduce medical evacuation times (Chapter 13). Forward surgical teams were also split and strategically positioned to provide lifesaving surgical care in remote locations (Chapter 14).

MEETING THE HEALTHCARE CHALLENGES OF HOME

Casualty care is a continuum that extends from the battlefield through evacuation to definitive care and rehabilitation. In 2007 *The Washington Post* published two lengthy articles that criticized the care wounded warriors received at Walter Reed Army Medical Center. These stories led to a close examination of care by independent teams established by President Bush and the Department of Defense. In their reports, the teams noted that the military was delivering world-class care from the battlefields of Iraq and Afghanistan to the operating rooms, intensive care units, and inpatient wards of Walter Reed. Unfortunately, once patients improved enough to be released from the hospital, a complex bureaucracy made coordination of care, including transition to the Department of Veterans Affairs (VA) healthcare system extremely difficult.

Confronted with these findings, the services took swift action. They immediately enhanced administrative support for wounded warriors and families, facilitating the scheduling of follow-up appointments and easing the transition to VA care. They worked to provide care that was more interdisciplinary, collaborative, and patient-centered (Chapter 31). They improved handoffs from inpatient to outpatient teams and sought greater family participation in treatment decisions (Chapter 33). To ensure that these improvements would be institutionalized, the Military Health System established "Centers of Excellence" for comprehensive, interdisciplinary care at military treatment facilities across the country. It created specialized centers for amputee care, traumatic brain and psychological injuries, vision, hearing, and chronic pain (Chapter 29). These centers not only provide state-of-the-art treatment, they also conduct clinical research to advance care.

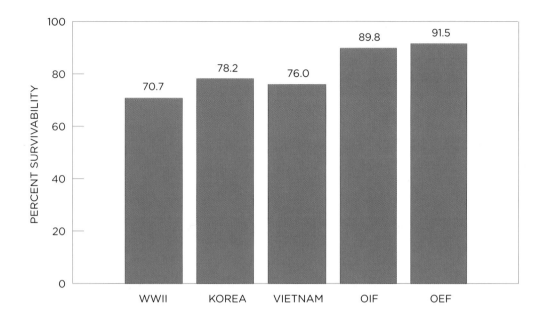

FIGURE 6.1. Improving casualty survivability. Operation Enduring Freedom (OEF): October 7, 2001– March 26, 2014; Operation Iraqi Freedom (OIF): March 19, 2003– August 31, 2010. Figure courtesy of Dr. Michael J. Carino, Office of The Surgeon General.

CONCLUSION

Military healthcare has changed dramatically since Vietnam. Leaders developed new approaches to treatment including Tactical Combat Casualty Care, balanced resuscitation, damage control surgery, and improved pain control. Paramedics and critical care nurses were added to tactical MEDEVAC aircraft, and Critical Care Air Transport Teams transported severely injured warriors to medical centers back home. By the end of the conflict, casualty survival rates approached 92 percent. That's vastly better than the rate of 76 percent achieved in Vietnam (Figure 6.1). Without these improvements, an additional 6,000 service members would have died rather than return home to their families.

Today, a severely wounded service member in Afghanistan is more likely to survive his or her injuries than an equally injured trauma victim in many parts of the United States. Many of the techniques developed during OEF and OIF were so effective that civilian trauma centers and emergency medical systems are adopting them here at home (Chapter 45).

The health challenges encountered in Iraq and Afghanistan were very different from those of prior conflicts. Future wars will present new problems (Chapter 34). To ensure that America's warriors receive the best possible care in future battles, we must learn the lessons of the current conflicts, and sustain the problem-solving capacities required to meet the challenges of the next.

Notes

1. *Dismounted Complex Blast Injury. Report of the Army Dismounted Blast Injury Task Force.* Fort Sam Houston, TX: Dismounted Complex Blast Injury Task Force; June 18, 2011. http://armymedicine.mil/Documents/DCBI-Task-Force-Report-Redacted-Final.pdf. Accessed January 23, 2016.

2. Wright DP, Bird JR, Clay SE, et al. *A Different Kind of War: The United States in Operation Enduring Freedom (OEF), October 2001–September 2005.* Fort Leavenworth, KS: Combat Studies Institute Press; 2010.

3. Council on Foreign Relations. US War in Afghanistan, 1999–present. 2014. http://www.cfr.org/afghanistan/us-war-afghanistan/p20018. Accessed January 23, 2016.

4. US Department of Defense. Defense Casualty Analysis System. US military casualties—Operation Enduring Freedom (OEF) casualty summary by casualty category. January 21, 2016. https://www.dmdc.osd.mil/dcas/pages/report_oef_type.xhtml. Accessed January 22, 2016.

5. Central Intelligence Agency. The world factbook. https://www.cia.gov/library/publications/the-world-factbook, Accessed January 23, 2016.

6. World Bank, Asian Development Bank, United Nations Development Programme. *Afghanistan: Preliminary Needs Assessment for Recovery and Reconstruction.* Washington, DC: World Bank; January 2002. http://reliefweb.int/report/afghanistan/afghanistan-preliminary-needs-assessment-recovery-and-reconstruction. Accessed January 23, 2016.

7. Stewart RW, ed. *American Military History, Volume II: The United States Army in a Global Era.* Washington, DC: Center of Military History; 2010.

8. Council on Foreign Relations. Timeline: the Iraq War, 2003–2011. 2014. http://www.cfr.org/iraq/timeline-iraq-war/p18876. Accessed January 23, 2016.

Recommended Reading

Jones SL. Wounded, ill, and injured challenges. *Army Med Dep J.* 2016;Apr–Sep:71–76.

CHAPTER seven

Force Health Protection: Preventing Deployment-Related Diseases and Non-Battle Injuries

MARK S. RIDDLE, MD, DRPH; JOHN W. SANDERS, MD, MPH; and
BONNIE SMOAK, MD, PHD

THE MARCH TO BAGHDAD, 2003

IN THE LATE DAYS OF MARCH, the US Army 3rd Infantry Division and the US Marine Corps 1st Marine Expeditionary Force (a combined force of about 150,000) were given the objective to move forward from the northern Kuwait border and march northwest toward Baghdad (225 miles). Military planners worked feverishly to prepare for this mission. Medical intelligence reports suggested that harsh environmental exposures and infectious diseases (plus feared chemical and biological weapons attacks) could threaten the troops. Planners studied lessons from the wars in Vietnam, the Persian Gulf, and elsewhere, and devised strategies to guard against these formidable threats. The expeditious and massive mobilization demonstrated the US military's amazing capability to quickly move large numbers of personnel, equipment, and supplies. Commanders applied best practices in public health and disease prevention to safeguard the fighting forces. Despite all the planning and preparation, things did not go well. Each month, about 30 percent of US troops fell ill with diarrhea. One in five were too ill to perform their duties. To reduce the risk of outbreaks, MREs (meals, ready-to-eat) and other military rations were supplied, and the troops were instructed to eat only from approved sources. However, sometimes military provisions were short, or the troops found it easier (or tastier)

FIGURE 7.1. To avoid the chance of setting off improvised explosive devices on the path, Staff Sergeant John Nickerson of Pontiac, Michigan, wades through an irrigation ditch while leading his patrol through the farmland around Forward Operating Base Hassanabad, Afghanistan. Photo by Chuck Liddy/Raleigh News & Observer. Reproduced with permission from Getty Images.

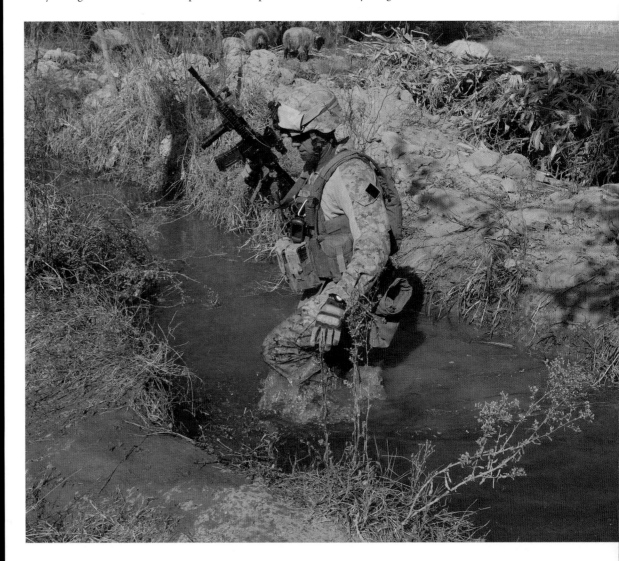

" Good doctors are no use without good discipline. More than half the battle against disease is fought, not by the doctors, but by the regimental officers. "

Lieutenant General William Slim
Commander-in-Chief
British 14th Army in Burma,
World War II

to access food from the local economy. Sanitary water supplies were provided through reverse osmosis units, field mobile storage tanks ("water buffalos"), and bottled water. However, given the choice of warm, chlorine-treated water or a refreshing drink from local municipal sources or the Euphrates River, too many troops picked the latter. Finally, combat operations often required troops to dive into ditches and seek shelter in abandoned farm buildings where they couldn't avoid fecal contamination (Figure 7.1). The situation was so notorious they dubbed one city along the march "Al Diarrhea." Baghdad was captured, but the number of troops who were unable to fight due to disease or non-battle injuries (DNBIs) was deeply concerning. Something had to be done.

THE PROBLEM

The threats faced by deployed Soldiers, Sailors, Airmen, and Marines are not limited to enemy bullets, artillery, missiles, and improvised explosive devices. They include deadly or disabling infectious diseases and non-combat injuries. If these health threats are not held in check, they can sicken or kill service members before, during, or after deployment.[2] In fact, in every conflict from the Mexican-American War through World War I, the US Army lost more soldiers to disease and non-battle injuries than to combat operations (Figure 7.2). Even in recent conflicts, disease and non-battle injuries account for a substantial share of deployment-related deaths.

Nonfatal cases are important as well. The best-trained pilots or tank crews cannot perform their jobs when they are experiencing bouts of vomiting and diarrhea due to gastrointestinal (GI) illness. If the illness or injury is serious enough, they may be lost from the fight. Their absence may compromise the mission and cost lives.

One need only look at the number of air medical evacuations by cause during the US military's recent campaigns in Iraq to understand the importance of protecting a force's health. Even during wartime, cases of disease and non-battle injuries accounted for most medical evacuations from theater (Figure 7.2). Recognizing this, the Military Health System redoubled its efforts to strengthen unit resilience and protect warfighter health.

FIGURE 7.2. Ratio of deaths due to combat versus disease or nonbattle injury in historical and modern times. Blue line: disease and non-battle injury deaths (truncated for the Mexican and Civil Wars to allow for better graphical discrimination of trends); red line: combat deaths.

OIF: Operation Iraqi Freedom
OEF: Operation Enduring Freedom

Data sources:
1. Cirillo VJ. Two faces of death: fatalities from disease and combat in America's principal wars, 1775 to present. *Perspect Biol Med.* 2008;51:121–133.
2. Murray CK, Jones SL. Army Medical Department at war: healthcare in a complex world. *US Army Med Dep J.* 2016;Apr-Sep:199–206.

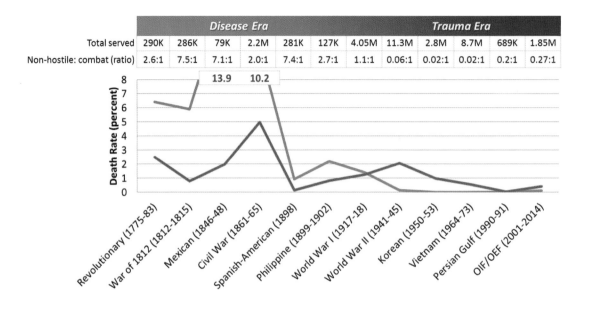

	Disease Era						Trauma Era				
Total served	290K	286K	79K	2.2M	281K	127K	4.05M	11.3M	2.8M	8.7M	689K	1.85M
Non-hostile: combat (ratio)	2.6:1	7.5:1	7.1:1	2.0:1	7.4:1	2.7:1	1.1:1	0.06:1	0.02:1	0.02:1	0.2:1	0.27:1

THE INNOVATION

Over the past century, the military has focused on protecting the health and fitness of the force so personnel are ready to deploy, whenever and wherever needed, to defend our nation. Once units are deployed, commanding officers and their supporting medical officers strive to preserve fighting strength by minimizing preventable diseases and non-battle injuries. Because America's modern, high-tech military relies on relatively small numbers of highly trained personnel to fill many mission-critical roles, it is more important than ever to maintain their health. Force health protection is more important than ever before.

THE CONCEPT OF "FORCE HEALTH PROTECTION"

"Force health protection" applies to measures that promote, improve, or conserve the mental and physical well-being of service members.[3] It is not new. In fact, 150 years ago, Dr Jonathan Letterman, medical director of the Army of the Potomac, provided a compelling rationale for the importance of force health protection:

> A corps of Medical officers was not established solely for the purpose of attending the wounded and sick; the proper treatment of these sufferers is certainly a matter of very great importance, and is an imperative duty, but the labors of Medical officers cover a more extended field. The *leading idea*, which should be constantly kept in view, is to strengthen the hands of the Commanding General by keeping his army in the *most vigorous health*, thus rendering it, in the highest degree, efficient for enduring fatigue and privation, and for fighting [emphasis added].[4]

As with other military activities, force health protection is governed by doctrine, policies, and guidance. This guidance directs programs and processes to promote and sustain a healthy and fit force, prevent injury and illness, protect the force from health hazards, and deliver the best possible medical and rehabilitative care to sick and injured troops anywhere in the world.[5] Typical efforts to meet these objectives include programs to promote nutrition, physical fitness, and dental health; discourage tobacco use; control weight; prevent injuries; vaccinate against infectious diseases; and provide chemoprophylaxis against malaria. Force health protection also includes planning before deployment; ongoing surveillance to identify emerging health threats on the battlefield; and delivery of preventive medicine and healthcare in support of combat operations. To ensure that commanders and their medical officers take these tasks seriously, a unit's DNBI rate is constantly monitored and used as a benchmark to assess their performance.

DISEASE AND NON-BATTLE INJURY SURVEILLANCE: THE "VITAL SIGNS" OF A DEPLOYED FORCE

In the language of public health, the term "surveillance" describes the regular collection, analysis, and interpretation of health-related data. It is done to monitor the health of the force and quickly spot outbreaks of disease and injuries so effective countermeasures can be taken. In many cases, public health surveillance also includes monitoring to prevent unhealthy environmental and occupational exposure to respiratory, water-borne, and foodborne threats that might produce long-term health problems. During large-scale deployments, Department of Defense policy dictates that DNBI surveillance must be conducted on a daily basis. It is, in effect, the "vital signs" of the deployed force.

In addition to detecting emerging health threats, DNBI surveillance provides commanders with a measure of the overall effectiveness of disease and injury prevention efforts. Examples include military logistics (supplying clean food and water) and preventive medicine activities such as routine camp hygiene and vaccinations.

IMPACT

As a result of concerted efforts to protect the health of service members deployed to Iraq and Afghanistan, units involved in Operations Enduring Freedom (OEF), Iraqi Freedom (OIF), and New Dawn had historically low rates of DNBIs compared to those involved in earlier conflicts (Figure 7.3). Nevertheless, at various points and in various units, diseases and non-battle injuries hindered operational effectiveness. Leading causes of DNBI in Iraq and Afghanistan included training and transport accidents, respiratory and dermatological conditions, and outbreaks of GI disease. Despite the progress that has been made, we must remain vigilant. Reports from a recent humanitarian and disaster response training mission, Continuing Promise 2011, remind us that the health of our forces can never be taken for granted (see Figure 7.3).

TECHNICAL CHALLENGES OF DISEASE SURVEILLANCE

1. Inconsistent Reporting

An important limitation to DNBI surveillance is variability in the methods used to collect data over time. Also, because DNBI surveillance is based on documented healthcare encounters, many cases are missed due to poor reporting. In some conditions, such as disabling knee or back injuries from training, service members usually seek care. However, in others (for example, bouts of GI illness), sick service members often attempt to treat themselves for hours or days before reporting the condition to a healthcare professional. Other causes of incomplete reporting include limited access to care during remote operations, relatively mild cases of illness, and a "Soldier strong" attitude that leads many to self-manage "nuisance" illnesses, or seek informal treatment from medics and corpsmen rather than getting formal medical care. Regardless of the reason, incomplete reporting can obscure or delay detection of important health threats. Also, because the military monitors and reports diseases differently from one conflict to the next, it is difficult to compare current data to earlier conflicts. It can even be difficult to compare DNBI rates in one theater of operations to another (Figure 7.4).

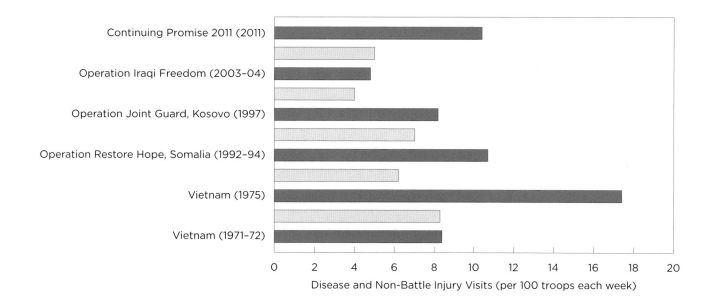

Continuing Promise 2011 (2011)

Operation Iraqi Freedom (2003–04)

Operation Joint Guard, Kosovo (1997)

Operation Restore Hope, Somalia (1992–94)

Vietnam (1975)

Vietnam (1971–72)

Disease and Non-Battle Injury Visits (per 100 troops each week)

2. Inadequate Follow-Up

"The reason for collecting, analyzing and disseminating information on a disease is to control that disease. Collection and analysis should not be allowed to consume resources if action does not follow."[6]

—William Foege

In military terminology, a "casualty" is any active duty service member lost to operations for health reasons, whether due to enemy action or not. But as noted in the opening vignette, it can be hard to motivate troops engaged in combat operations to follow mundane procedures such as drinking properly treated (but less tasty) water, consuming MREs instead of locally sourced food, and using hand sanitizer regularly to prevent human-to-human transmission of GI diseases. As a result, cases of preventable illness often spike during combat operations (see Figure 7.4).

FIGURE 7.3. Overall disease and non-battle injury rates by major historical and modern deployments.

Data sources:

1. Eaton M. *Non-battle Injury and Non-Battle Psychiatric Illness in Deployed Air Force Members* [dissertation]. Chapel Hill, NC: University of North Carolina; 2010. Chern A, McCoy A, Brannock T, et al.

2. Incidence and risk factors for disease and non-battle injury aboard the hospital ship USNS Comfort during a humanitarian assistance and disaster response mission, Continuing Promise 2011. *Trop Dis Travel Med Vaccines.* 2016;2(7):1–9.

FIGURE 7.4. Self-reported and clinic-associated disease and non-battle injury rates for selected health conditions by phase of combat, Iraq, 2003. Light bars represent clinic-associated cases; solid dark bars represent self-reported cases.

Data source:
Sanders JW, Putnam SD, Frankart C et al. Impact of illness and non-combat injury during Operations Iraqi Freedom and Enduring Freedom (Afghanistan). *Am J Trop Med Hyg.* 2005;73(4):713–719

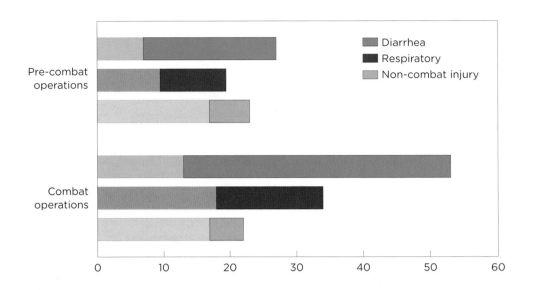

3. Smaller Units and More Specialized Personnel

In an era marked by multinational insurgencies and global terrorist networks, military operations are shifting from deployment of large conventional forces to small, highly mobile teams of Special Operations personnel. With relatively few team members involved in any particular operation, success depends on each individual's health. In addition, our modern Army is more technologically sophisticated than in the past. As a result, highly specialized training is required to fill key roles. Similar transformations have occurred in the US Navy and Air Force. Once, a Navy ship might have 20 or 30 crew members with the skills required to perform important tasks. Today, only two or three might be qualified to fill certain specialized roles. Instead of relying on large formations of bombers, our modern Air Force uses small numbers of highly sophisticated aircraft to deliver precision munitions on a target. Under such circumstances, the loss of key team members to illness or non-battle injury can compromise a mission and endanger the unit.

EMERGING INFECTIOUS DISEASES

Military preventive medicine officers face disease threats rarely confronted in the United States. In Iraq, these included leishmaniasis (transmitted by sand flies), Q fever, and invasive fungal wound infections (see Chapter 27). More recently, US military personnel in various parts of the world have confronted Ebola virus, chikungunya, dengue hemorrhagic fever, pandemic influenza, and drug-resistant malaria. All of these diseases, and many others, could one day threaten the health of the US population.

Historically, national outbreaks of infectious disease have often been linked to political instability (as either cause or effect). In severe instances, disease outbreaks can lead to civil disorder, the deployment of security forces, and ultimately, an urgent request for US military assistance. For this reason, American military health planners monitor a wide array of global disease threats.

Diseases that are endemic (ie, commonplace) in the local populations may go unrecognized until they spark an epidemic among deployed military personnel. Although outbreaks of this type were relatively well-controlled in the OIF and OEF theaters of operations, they still posed serious challenges to the health of our forces. For example, military health providers had to contend with the introduction of a multidrug-resistant *Acinetobacter* bacteria into our combat support hospitals (Chapter 27). This occurrence underscores the need to conduct ongoing laboratory-based disease surveillance of local human and animal populations to quickly pinpoint potential sources of disease.

UNRECOGNIZED LONG-TERM EFFECTS

Certain long-term health consequences of warfare, such as posttraumatic stress disorder and the loss of limbs, are widely understood. Other consequences are just being described. It now appears that certain conditions, such as infectious diarrhea and other GI conditions, may produce long-term consequences such as dysfunctional bowel syndrome and possibly inflammatory bowel disease. Over time, chronic disorders like these could significantly burden the Military Health System. To minimize long-term problems, it is critical to prevent as many of these infections as possible.

THE MILITARY VALUE OF PREVENTION

"Prevention of disease and injury has helped US forces avoid what historically has been the far greater cause of casualties than injuries inflicted by enemy combatants. Low DNBI rates are a true force multiplier. Fewer personnel affected by illness and injury yields a decreased requirement for replacements, and less demand for medical treatment and evacuation."[7]

—Ellen Embry, former Deputy Assistant Secretary of Defense

For more than a century, the US military has excelled at protecting the health of the personnel it sends into harm's way. As is true with other advances in military medicine, we must not take this progress for granted. Future conflicts will bring new challenges (Chapter 34). To protect the health of our armed forces, we must be ready to identify and counter health threats as swiftly as we counter adversaries on the battlefield. In this way, we will not only ensure the national security of the United States, we will ensure our nation's health security as well.

Notes

1. Slim WJS. *Defeat Into Victory*. New York: D. McKay; 1961.
2. Cirillo VJ. Two faces of death: fatalities from disease and combat in America's principal wars, 1775 to present. *Perspect Biol Med.* 2008;51:121–133.
3. US Joint Chiefs of Staff. *Department of Defense Dictionary of Military and Associated Terms*. Washington, DC: JCS; 1979. http://books.google.com/books?id=Bj_cAAAAMAAJ. Accessed October 11, 2016.
4. Letterman J. *Medical Recollections of the Army of the Potomac*. New York: D. Appleton; 1866.
5. Department of Defense. *Force Health Protection (FHP)*. Washington, DC: DoD; October 9, 2004. DoD Directive 6200.04.
6. Foege WH, Hogan RC, Newton LH. Surveillance projects for selected diseases. *Int J Epidemiol.* 1976;5:29–37.

7. Embry E. Statement by Ms. Ellen Embry, Deputy Assistant Secretary of Defense, Force Health Protection and Readiness, before the Subcommittee on Defense Appropriations Committee, US House of Representatives, May 1, 2007. http://www.dod.gov/dodgc/olc/docs/testEmbrey070501.pdf. Accessed March 26, 2016.

Recommended Reading

Baird C. Deployment exposures and long-term health risks: the shadow of war. *US Army Med Dep J.* 2016;Apr-Sep:167–172.

Garges EC, Taylor KM, Pacha LA. Select public health and communicable disease lessons learned during Operations Iraqi Freedom and Enduring Freedom. *US Army Med Dep J.* 2016;Apr-Sep:161–166.

Hauret KG, Pacha L, Taylor BJ, Jones BH. Surveillance of disease and nonbattle injuries during US Army operations. *US Army Med Dep J.l* 2016;Apr-Sep:15–23.

Wojcik BE, Humphrey RJ, Hosek BJ, Stein CR. Data-driven casualty estimation and disease nonbattle injury/injury rates in recent campaigns. *US Army Med Dep J.* 2016;Apr-Sep:8–14.

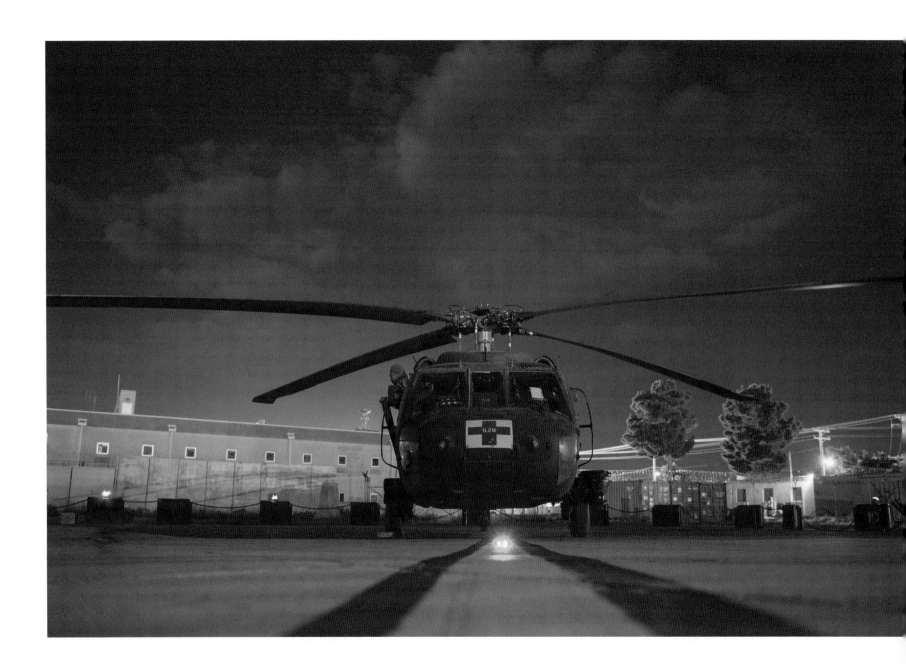

CHAPTER eight

The Joint Trauma System

JEFFREY BAILEY, MD; DONALD JENKINS, MD; and SUSAN WEST, BSN

THE PROBLEM

THE US MILITARY'S EXPERIENCE IN KOREA AND VIETNAM had amply demonstrated the benefits of rapid evacuation and early access to surgical care (see Chapter 2). On the strength of their success, military surgeons returning from Southeast Asia championed the development of organized trauma systems in civilian hospitals in many parts of the United States. Ironically, the US military did not follow suit. As a result, it began the wars in Iraq and Afghanistan with modern helicopters, mobile surgical units, and well-trained personnel, but no organized trauma system (Figure 8-1).[1]

TRAUMA CARE, BUT NO TRAUMA SYSTEM

In the latter part of 2003, the Army Surgeon General sent his designated Trauma Expert, Colonel John Holcomb, to Iraq to assess the performance of the Army's surgical teams. Colonel Holcomb found that during the initial invasion, medical units did a reasonable job of meeting injured troops' needs. Combat medics on the battlefield rendered point-of-injury (Role 1) care, and personnel who needed surgery were taken to nearby Role 2 field treatment facilities that offered limited surgical capability. However, when the Army began deploying larger, Role 3 hospitals with greater surgical capability to

FIGURE 8.1. [*Opposite*] UH-60, Bagram Airfield, Parwan, Afghanistan, May 21, 2016. Photo by Senior Airman Justyn Freeman, 455th Air Expeditionary Wing. Reproduced from: https://www.dvidshub.net/image/2606889/craig-joint-theater-conducts-mass-cal-exercise.

VIGNETTE >> Iraq, 2003: A truck packed with explosives detonated near a concentration of US troops. Many were injured, some of them severely. Because medical and surgical teams were established near the site, all of the injured were taken there, rather than to combat support hospitals with greater capability less than 30 minutes away. As a result, some of the injured Soldiers died of potentially survivable injuries.

Iraq, no effort was made to incorporate them into an organized trauma care system (Figure 8.2). As a result, critically injured troops sometimes failed to get "the right care at the right place at the right time." Colonel Holcomb's observations prompted the Army Surgeon General to send a team of nurses to Iraq to develop and implement a basic trauma system involving every service that was deployed in Iraq at the time: the result was the Joint Theater Trauma System or JTTS.[1,2]

THE INNOVATION: THE JOINT THEATER TRAUMA SYSTEM

As a result of these efforts, in November 2004, the military formally incorporated its five Role 3 facilities in Iraq into an overall system of care. Trauma nurses joined these facilities and immediately began systematically compiling data on injuries, treatment, and outcomes. Their efforts identified instances when injured troops were not always provided the most currently acceptable care or were not sent to the facility best suited to meet their needs. In response, guidelines were written to better direct care. The surgeon in charge of the effort visited all of the Role 3 facilities and captured their best practices of each. These were turned into authoritative Clinical Practice Guidelines and shared with the other Role 3 facilities. This swiftly brought every Role 3 hospital into alignment with the best practices of its peers. To ensure compliance, JTTS nurses monitored adherence with the guidelines on a daily, weekly, and monthly basis. Their efforts not only improved consistency: they documented better outcomes among injured troops.[2]

Based on this success, the US Army Institute of Surgical Research in San Antonio, Texas, stepped up its analysis and sharing of the clinical information being collected in Iraq. Consequently, the military health system's response to the next 90 bombings in Iraq was much more effective: casualties were properly distributed to Role 3 facilities. As a result, all injured service members received the right care at the right place at the right time.[2,3]

INSTITUTIONALIZING SUCCESS

Following this initial success, each new team of Trauma Nurses heading to Iraq was trained before deployment at the US Army Institute of Surgical Research. Ultimately, 21 consecutive JTTS teams were deployed.

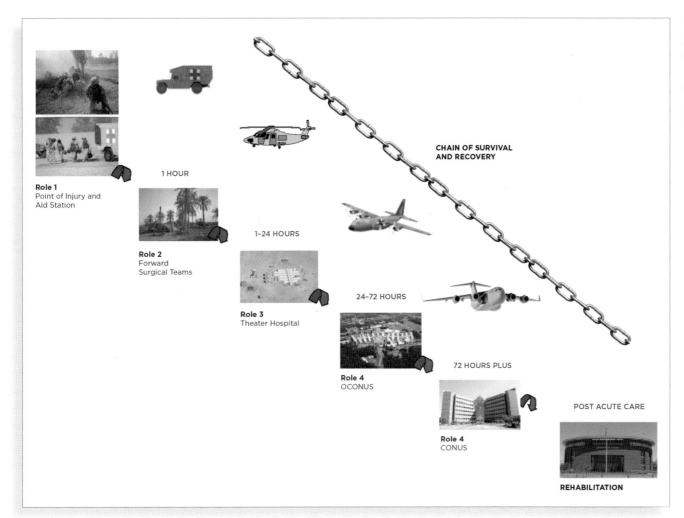

FIGURE 8.2.
Joint Trauma System
continuum of care.

OCONUS: outside
continental United States;
CONUS: continental
United States

**CHAIN OF SURVIVAL
AND RECOVERY**

1 HOUR

Role 1
Point of Injury and
Aid Station

1–24 HOURS

Role 2
Forward
Surgical Teams

24–72 HOURS

Role 3
Theater Hospital

72 HOURS PLUS

Role 4
OCONUS

POST ACUTE CARE

Role 4
CONUS

REHABILITATION

THE MILITARY'S "LEARNING HEALTHCARE SYSTEM"

For the past two years, I had the privilege of chairing a National Academy of Medicine (NAM) committee charged to review the trauma care system of the US military. In light of prior NAM reports describing the ideal properties of a so-called "learning healthcare system," my committee was asked to determine the extent to which military trauma care exhibits these properties, how it can be improved, and how our nation can speed lessons from the military to civilian trauma care sectors, and vice versa.

Frankly, I was surprised to be given this assignment. I am not a trauma surgeon nor have I ever served in the military. My main professional concern for the past 30 years has been the study and practice of modern methods of quality management and improvement as applied to healthcare systems throughout the world. I was co-founder and for 19 years served as President and CEO of the nonprofit Institute for Healthcare Improvement.

In my experience, the key to continual improvement in any organization lies in nurturing authentic curiosity; a relentless ambition to be better; and culture and processes that allow knowledge to come from experience, be reflected upon, and used in never-ending "plan–do–study–act" cycles. To a healthy, developing child, such learning-in-action comes naturally—watch the ball, swing the bat, observe what happens and why, change your stance, and swing again—over and over and over again. This sustained improvement learning is based on real-world experience.

While every child does this, most organizations do not. Tradition and habits straightjacket their ability to set bold goals; study their own work; formulate ideas for change; carry out frequent, informative tests of change; and accumulate knowledge over time. If they learn at all, they relegate the assignment to an "R&D" (research and development) shop or outside consultants, while most employees just continue to do the same job they have always done. This approach wastes the wisdom of the workforce. Fear, not ambition, dominates such workplaces: questions are seen as challenges to authority; gathering data is just a burden; testing change in the workplace is rare; and everyone asks the boss what to do rather than interrogating the facts to identify the best course of action.

The US military's trauma care system offers a clear and instructive counterexample.[1] Indeed, it is one of the finest examples of a learning organization that I have ever seen, inside or outside healthcare. It is far from perfect and far from being fully deployed (our report makes hard-hitting recommendations for its improvement). But, at its best, military trauma care over the past decade or more has come to illustrate vividly nearly every important characteristic of a learning system. Chapter 8 describes one jewel in its crown—the Joint Trauma System—that captures, reflects upon, and acts upon data in cycles of fast pace and wide workforce involvement. If learning designs like the Joint Trauma System were applied to healthcare generally, both inside and outside the military, performance would catapult to levels never before achieved. The military calls these pragmatic learning processes "focused empiricism." It is simpler to say "saving lives."

Donald M. Berwick, MD, MPP
President Emeritus and Senior Fellow
Institute for Healthcare Improvement
Cambridge, MA

Notes

1. Berwick D, Downey A, Cornet E, et al. *A National Trauma Care System: Integrating Military and Civilian Trauma Systems to Achieve Zero Preventable Deaths After Injury*. Washington, DC: National Academies Press; 2016. http://www.nationalacademies.org/hmd/Reports/2016/A-National-Trauma-Care-System-Integrating-Military-and-Civilian-Trauma-Systems.aspx. Accessed July 11, 2016.
2. For more information about the Institute for Healthcare Improvement please visit www.ihi.org.

As the tempo of combat operations grew, the teams increased to 16 people (from the original five). A typical JTTS team included physicians, nurses, and technicians from the US Air Force, US Army, and US Navy, plus nurses from Canada. In October 2007, the JTTS started sending team members to Afghanistan as well. When the operational tempo began to wind down, the teams scaled back their work. The last JTTS team left Iraq in the fall of 2009, and the final JTTS team in Afghanistan departed in November 2014. Over the course of their efforts, 43 Clinical Practice Guidelines were developed and disseminated within the Joint Trauma System (JTS).[3]

USING DATA TO DRIVE IMPROVEMENT

Data collection is the foundation of the military trauma system. The vehicle for collecting this data is the Department of Defense Trauma Registry (DoDTR), previously known as the Joint Theater Trauma Registry (JTTR). Data collection for the registry began in 2003 and continues at multiple sites. Beginning in October 2007, an electronic "store-and-forward" system allowed JTTS staff in Iraq and Afghanistan to compile and submit clinical data to the US Army Institute for Surgical Research in San Antonio in near real-time. The military's trauma registry now has more than 130,000 records.

VIDEO CONFERENCES LINK CAREGIVERS ACROSS THREE CONTINENTS

In 2005, military trauma staff began a weekly video conference with participants across the continuum of care from the point of injury in Iraq and Afghanistan, to MEDEVAC (medical evacuation) and initial surgery in the war zone, to Critical Care Air Transport to Landstuhl, Germany, and from there to the United States. The goal of these case conferences was to inform, improve, and educate. In 2012, the military began to reward participants with Continuing Medical Education (CME) and Continuing Nursing Education (CNE) credits. On February 18, 2016, the 500th conference was held.[3]

CREATION OF A JOINT TRAUMA SYSTEM

As the military trauma system matured, its leadership recognized that the team in San Antonio and the teams in the combat zones were in fact two distinct, yet interdependent, entities. The San Antonio team operated the DoDTR, analyzed registry data, and published evidence-based clinical practice guidelines.

It also trained and organized the theater teams prior to deployment, and provided them with ongoing operational support and guidance once they reached the combat area. The forward deployed teams worked with in-country trauma care providers to improve trauma system performance and outcomes by collecting data in military hospitals, promoting the use of Clinical Practice Guidelines, and monitoring compliance with best practices. Over the years, the San Antonio team became the central repository for lessons learned. This gave stability and support to the forward-deployed quality improvement teams as they cycled in and out of the combat zones.[3,4]

As the tempo of military activity in Iraq and Afghanistan wound down, concern grew that the JTTS would be moth-balled because its funding was tied to the conflicts. In hopes of finding sustainment funding, the San Antonio team rebranded itself as the "JTS" to distinguish its activities from the purely combat zone-based "JTTS." To further enhance the value of the JTS, the team expanded its scope from Role 3 through Role 4 hospitals to include prehospital trauma care (see Chapter 35), rotary wing MEDEVAC (see Chapter 13), and initial treatment by Forward Surgical Teams (FSTs) in Role 2 facilities (see Chapter 14). This gave the military health system, for the first time, visibility of the full continuum of combat casualty care, from point of injury to rehabilitation in the United States[4–6] (Figure 8.3).

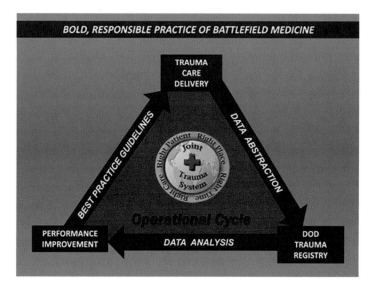

FIGURE 8.3.
Joint Trauma System operational cycle.

DoD: Department of Defense
Illustration: Courtesy of the US Army Institute of Surgical Research

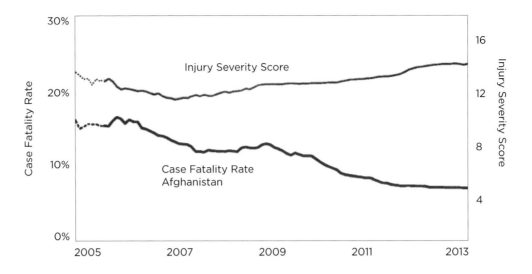

FIGURE 8.4.
Impact of military trauma care and research. Illustration: Courtesy of the US Army Institute of Surgical Research.

IMPACT

Civilian business and healthcare leaders have long embraced the adage that "You can't manage what you can't measure." Creation of the JTTS in Afghanistan and Iraq (and its subsequent evolution into the JTS) played a fundamental role in driving the rapid advances in technology, practice, and medical doctrine that transformed combat trauma care during Operation Enduring Freedom/Operation Iraqi Freedom/Operation New Dawn, and resulted in unprecedented rates of survival despite an overall increase in injury severity (Figure 8.4).

Data collected and shared by the JTS were used to identify numerous opportunities to improve care and evaluate the results in real time. Global voice and video conferencing allowed trauma surgeons, critical care nurses, critical care air transport teams, and other clinical experts to directly engage their counterparts providing care in the combat zone. As a result, the system adapted, evolved and in a few short years achieved the lowest death rate among combat casualties in human history. On December 3, 2015, the JTS was recognized as the "Best Medical Innovation" in combat casualty care to come out of the war by AMSUS (the Association of Military Surgeons of the United States).

Equally important, many of the JTS-guided innovations developed in the "crucible of war"—such as rapid application of tourniquets to stem bleeding from badly mangled extremities (see Chapter 10), administration of blood products in balanced proportions (see Chapter 16), and damage control surgery (see Chapter 15)—are now being embraced by civilian providers at a scale not seen since the end of the Vietnam War. More lessons will be shared over the next decade.[6]

NEXT STEPS

The most important opportunity to improve civilian care may come from understanding not only adopting "what" was learned, but also "how." (See The Military's "Learning Healthcare System.") To this end, on June 17, 2016, the National Academies of Sciences, Engineering, and Medicine (Washington, DC) released a landmark report titled *A National Trauma Care System: Integrating Military and Civilian Trauma Systems to Achieve Zero Preventable Deaths After Injury*.[6] The press release[7] that accompanied the report gave the following summary:

> *Given the military's success in reducing trauma deaths after injury, the civilian sector stands to reap tremendous benefits if best practices can be reliably adapted from the military, the committee said. A joint effort is needed to ensure the delivery of optimal trauma care to save the lives of Americans injured within the U.S. and on the battlefield. The committee envisioned a national trauma care system grounded in sound learning health system principles applied across all phases of trauma care delivery—from prehospital care at the point of injury to hospitalization, rehabilitation, and beyond. This will require synergized military and civilian efforts, committed leadership from both sectors, and a strategy that aims to reduce variations in care and outcomes while supporting continuous learning and innovation.*

If this vision takes hold, it will not only improve civilian trauma care: it will strengthen military trauma care. In times of relative peace, it is essential for the military health system to maintain the skills of its high-performing teams. Thus, they will be ready to deploy, whenever needed, to care for those who go in harm's way.

Notes

1. Eastridge BJ, Jenkins D, Flaherty S, Schiller S. Holcomb JB. Trauma system development in a theater of war: experiences from Operation Iraqi Freedom and Operation Enduring Freedom. *J Trauma.* 2006;61:1366–1372.

2. Perkins JG, Brosch LR, Beekley AC, Warfield KL, Wade CF, Holcomb JB. Research and analytics in combat trauma care: converting data and experience to practical guidelines. *Surg Clin N Am.* 2012;92:1041–1054.

3. Bailey J, Spott MA, Costanzo G, Dunne JR, Dorlac W, Eastridge B. *Joint Trauma System: Development, Conceptual Framework, and Optimal Elements.* San Antonio, TX: US Department of Defense, US Army Institute for Surgical Research; 2012: 51. http://www.usaisr.amedd.army.mil/pdfs/Joint_Trauma_System_final_clean2.pdf Accessed April 8, 2016.

4. *Emergency War Surgery. Fourth United States Revision.* Fort Sam Houston, TX: Borden Institute; 2013.

5. *Emergency War Surgery. Fourth United States Revision.* Chapter 35: Battlefield Trauma Systems. Fort Sam Houston, TX: Borden Institute; 2013: 497–502.

6. Berwick D, Downey A, Cornet E, et al. *A National Trauma Care System: Integrating Military and Civilian Trauma Systems to Achieve Zero Preventable Deaths After Injury.* Washington, DC: National Academies Press; 2016. http://www.nationalacademies.org/hmd/Reports/2016/A-National-Trauma-Care-System-Integrating-Military-and-Civilian-Trauma-Systems.aspx. Accessed July 11, 2016.

7. Public Release Webinar for the Report by the Committee on Military Trauma Care's Learning Health System and Its Translation to the Civilian Sector. https://www.nationalacademies.org/hmd/Activities/HealthServices/LearningTraumaSystems/2016-JUN-17.aspx. Accessed August 2, 2016.

CHAPTER nine

Devising Countermeasures: The Joint Trauma Analysis and Prevention of Injury in Combat Program

COLIN M. GREENE, MD, MPH

THE PROBLEM

OPERATION IRAQI FREEDOM BEGAN WITH MUCH OPTIMISM[1] but soon deteriorated into an insurgency. Month by month, attacks with conventional weapons and IEDs grew in number, power, and sophistication. The soft-sided Humvees in general use at the time were no match for these weapons, and those with hastily improvised armor did little better. The military needed countermeasures.

THE INNOVATION

In the January 2006 National Defense Authorization Act, Congress directed the secretary of defense to coordinate medical research on the "prevention, mitigation, and treatment of blast injuries."[2] Congress also specified the creation of a joint database to collect, analyze, and share information on the effectiveness of personal and vehicular equipment to protect against blast injury.[3] To understand the full context of the threats posed by blasts, the Army engaged medical, materiel, and information technology experts, as well as intelligence and operational personnel, to analyze classified information.[4]

THE JOINT TRAUMA ANALYSIS AND PREVENTION OF INJURY IN COMBAT PROGRAM

VIGNETTE >> Iraq, 2006: Somewhere in the hot, dry Iraqi countryside, an improvised explosive device (IED) explodes under the lead vehicle of a US convoy. Of the six crew members in the vehicle, one dies instantly, one dies shortly thereafter, and four require urgent evacuation by helicopter (Figure 9.1). Several service members in nearby vehicles suffer concussions or complain of headaches and other symptoms. The attack reminds all involved, from the convoy commander to senior military leaders in the province, that battlefield medical care can do only so much.

FIGURE 9.1. [*Opposite*] US Army Soldiers transport a trauma victim to a US Army medical helicopter in Tarmiyah, Iraq, September 30, 2007. The Soldiers are from Charlie Company, 4th Battalion, 9th Infantry Regiment, 4th Stryker Brigade Combat Team, 2nd Infantry Division, out of Fort Lewis, Washington. Photo by Navy Mass Communication Specialist 2nd Class Summer M. Anderson. Reproduced from: https://www.army.mil/e2/c/images/2012/01/20/232645/size0.jpg.

The seeds for interdisciplinary cooperation were sown before the congressional directive. As attacks in Iraq grew, US intelligence and operational personnel began working to understand and thwart insurgent tactics. Combat-zone medical providers examined their evacuation and surgical techniques. Materiel developers sought to enhance the protective capacity of personal equipment and vehicles. The Armed Forces Medical Examiner started sharing case information with the National Ground Intelligence Center. In one instance, this intelligence–medical examiner partnership clarified a lethal element of injury that helped the military devise safer seating arrangements in armored vehicles.

Soon, other groups joined in. Materiel organizations in the Army and Marine Corps began to collect and catalogue damaged helmets and body armor, known as "personal protective equipment" (PPE). Medical personnel in the war zones and in the United States gathered data on the severity and locations of wounds. This provided a better picture of enemy attack methods, damage to vehicles and PPE, and associated injuries to troops. The Army Research Laboratory conducted live-fire testing based on findings from combat. With this information, interdisciplinary teams could learn more details about how injuries occur, and use these insights to recommend changes in tactics, vehicle design, and protective equipment.

While these interactions were useful, most occurred on an ad hoc basis. In October 2006, the Army brought leaders of intelligence, materiel, medical, and operational organizations together at Fort Detrick, Maryland, to establish the "Joint Trauma Analysis and Prevention of Injury in Combat" (JTAPIC) program.

Mission and Structure

A new sense of urgency took hold. Longstanding attitudes about "my data" and "need to know" gave way to "our data" and "need to share."[4] The newly created JTAPIC program acquired three main missions:

1. **Materiel recovery and analysis** combined analysis of battle-damaged body armor and other PPE, ballistic fragments recovered from wounded and killed service members, and the corresponding medical and autopsy reports to pinpoint vulnerabilities and identify patterns of injury. The

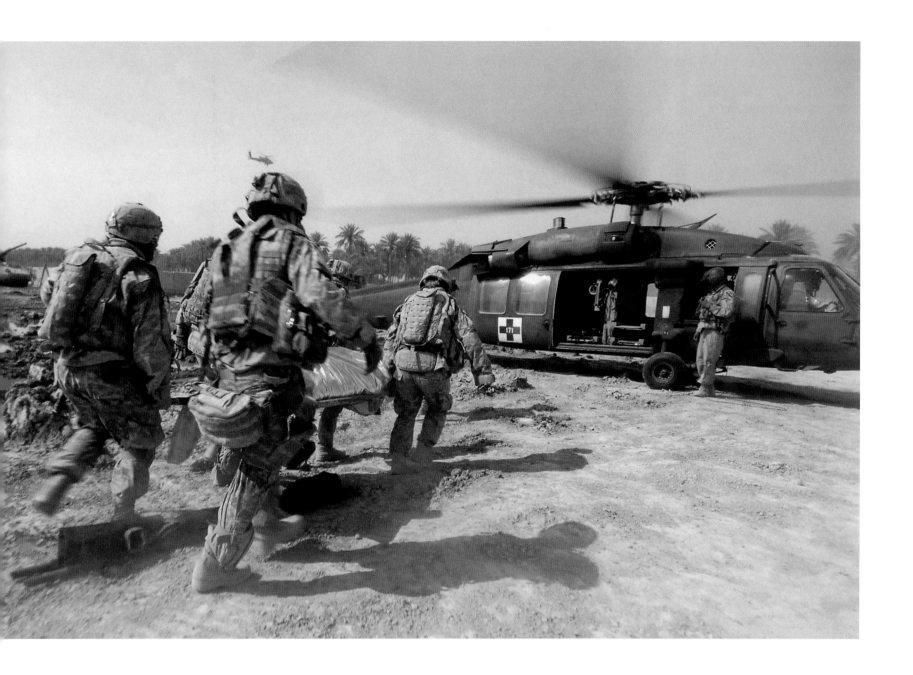

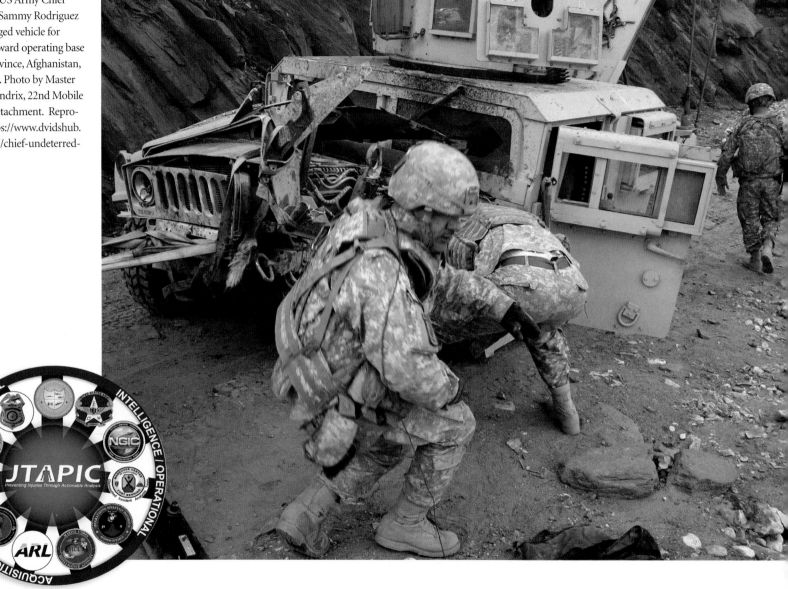

FIGURE 9.2. US Army Chief Warrant Officer Sammy Rodriguez prepares a damaged vehicle for recovery to a forward operating base in the Kunar province, Afghanistan, January 23, 2008. Photo by Master Sergeant Eric Hendrix, 22nd Mobile Public Affairs Detachment. Reproduced from: https://www.dvidshub.net/image/74767/chief-undeterred-after-ied-attack.

insights, subsequently validated by kinetic analysis and testing, helped designers create more effective armored vehicles and protective gear.

2. **Combat theater incident analysis** produced a "storyboard" of selected injury-causing events from different viewpoints: intelligence (enemy situation and weaponry); operational (friendly forces and mission); materiel (armor, PPE, and equipment fragments); and medical (wounds and causes of death) (Figure 9.2). Military personnel used the results of these analyses to adjust tactics, techniques, and procedures, and to make more informed decisions about needed upgrades to vehicles and protective equipment.

3. **Injury prevention analyses** were done in response to specific requests for information from personnel dealing with operations and acquisitions. Like analyses of combat-related matters, these generated critical insights for planned upgrades in vehicles, PPE, and tactics. Unlike combat incident analyses, however, injury prevention analyses apply more structured study designs and greater scientific rigor; they are also typically tailored to a specific requestor's needs.[4] These analyses take longer than other JTAPIC functions, but findings are typically available in one-tenth the time required to perform a formal research study (based on a typical ten-week or less turnaround time for a JTAPIC request for information analysis, versus the usual two-year span permitted for research, development, technology, and engineering project dollars).

Although JTAPIC is based at Fort Detrick, it interacts with a widely dispersed network of partners (Figure 9.3). The arrangement is codified in JTAPIC's charter[5] and has remained largely unchanged since the program was established.

Solving Information Technology Challenges

As a data-driven organization, JTAPIC requires substantial information technology support. The first challenge involved getting timely medical information from combat areas. Traditional methods could take up to six months, an unacceptable timeframe. To overcome this obstacle, a JTAPIC partner, the Naval Health Research Center, developed a method to query multiple databases to obtain medical data with minimal delays.

FIGURE 9.3. [*Opposite, bottom*] Graphic representation of the Joint Trauma Analysis and Prevention of Injury in Combat (JTAPIC) organization. The eleven partner organizations, clockwise from the top, are:
- Naval Health Research Center
- US Army Aeromedical Research Laboratory
- National Ground Intelligence Center
- Maneuver Center of Excellence Dismounted Incident Analysis Team
- Marine Corps Current Operations Analysis Support Team
- Marine Corps Intelligence Agency
- Army Research Laboratory
- Product Manager, Infantry Combat Equipment
- Program Executive Office–Soldier
- Joint Trauma Service
- Armed Forces Medical Examiner System

Center logo: JTAPIC Program Office

The second challenge was to store data about injuries in a standard format, so it could be analyzed by intelligence, medical, operational, and materiel experts. To accomplish this task, another JTAPIC partner, the National Ground Intelligence Center, developed a "datashare" system that allows collaborating partners to create standardized data fields for each event and ensure consistent terminology across disciplines.

The third challenge was to devise a secure way to efficiently gather, store, and examine large data sets and the resulting analyses. To solve this problem, a third JTAPIC partner, the Army Research Laboratory, stepped up. It created a system that allows secure, remote collaboration and analysis of specific data subsets, project tracking, and storage of final results in a product library.[6]

The Approach

To illustrate how the program works, consider the IED attack cited earlier in this chapter. As soon as possible after such events, JTAPIC technicians examine the vehicle, determine the precise location and extent of damage, note where each casualty was sitting and the injuries they received, and examine any PPE that can be recovered. Technicians also analyze operationally relevant circumstances of each attack (mission, weather, terrain, etc), as well as known intelligence about enemy actions and weapons used. With this information, JTAPIC seeks to answer several questions: Are certain crew positions in this particular vehicle more dangerous than others? If PPE was used, was it properly worn and did it function as intended? Did the attack produce a higher (or lower) than expected casualty rate, create a previously unseen pattern of injuries, or indicate use of a new weapon or tactic? When recurring patterns of injury or methods of attack are noted, it often indicates a potential vulnerability.

Once JTAPIC identifies a vulnerability, it develops a list of potential countermeasures. Examples include (*a*) vehicle upgrades or redesign; (*b*) changes in the construction or use of PPE; (*c*) modified procedures, such as safer ways to exit a damaged vehicle; and (*d*) possible modifications to tactical planning or operations. By producing prompt, evidence-based analyses and an array of options, JTAPIC helps leaders make better decisions (Figure 9.4).

Impact

Initially, JTAPIC focused on IED attacks directed at armored vehicles. Its findings prompted several upgrades to the Stryker combat vehicle, including modifications to the vehicle's hull and driver

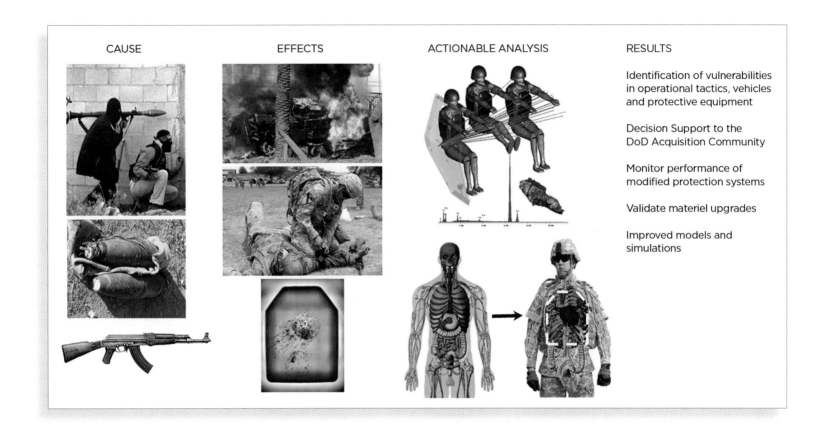

CAUSE	EFFECTS	ACTIONABLE ANALYSIS	RESULTS

RESULTS

Identification of vulnerabilities in operational tactics, vehicles and protective equipment

Decision Support to the DoD Acquisition Community

Monitor performance of modified protection systems

Validate materiel upgrades

Improved models and simulations

compartment (Figure 9.5). These improvements saved warfighters' lives and reduced the severity of combat injuries. In addition, an analysis of vehicle occupants' actions during and immediately after an IED attack prompted changes in design and procedures for exiting damaged vehicles (Table 9.1).

After these initial successes, JTAPIC was asked to expand its focus to examine injuries involving dismounted (foot patrol) personnel. These reviews prompted several upgrades to the design and use of PPE, including helmets, body armor, and urogenital protective gear, as well as development of hand-held counter-IED tools (Table 9.2).

FIGURE 9.4. The Joint Trauma Analysis and Prevention of Injury in Combat analysis process.
DoD: Department of Defense

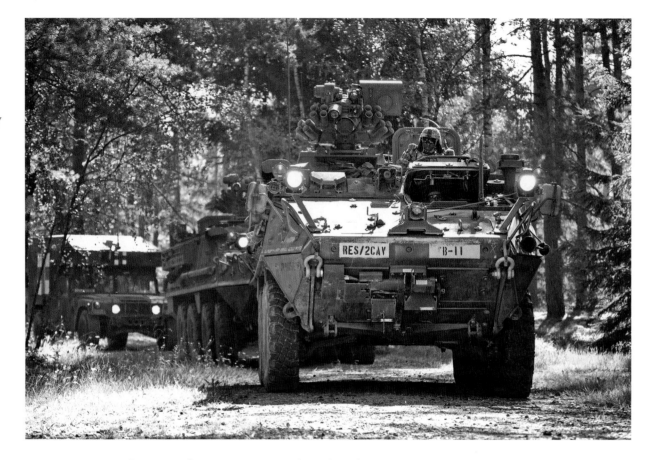

FIGURE 9.5.
Two Stryker armored vehicles, followed by a Humvee. 7th Army Training Command, Grafenwoehr, Germany, August 25, 2016. Photo by Gertrud Zach, Training Support Activity Europe. Reproduced from: https://www.dvidshub.net/image/2819511/2cr-res-trains-with-selectable-lightweight-attack-munition.

Since the program's inception in 2006, the military has repeatedly cited JTAPIC as an important initiative in helping prevent combat-related injuries and deaths in Iraq and Afghanistan. In addition, JTAPIC data helped guide Department of Defense planning and purchasing decisions. JTAPIC's ability to produce actionable information in weeks rather than years ensures that its products are timely, relevant, and useful.

JTAPIC's Future

With the recent decrease in combat operations, JTAPIC has shifted its focus from analyzing particular incidents to broader studies designed to prevent injuries and preserve force readiness. In 2015 the program initiated or contributed to several developments, including improving the design of forward operating bases; avoiding the expense of an unnecessary vehicle redesign; confirming a design concept for a combat-region manikin; guiding the design of future Army and Marine Corps vehicles; upgrading a bomb-protective suit worn by those who dispose of explosive ordnance; providing evidence-based redirection of spending on helmet sensors to detect mild traumatic brain injury; and forming a cooperative agreement with the Veterans Benefits Administration to identify and track service members injured in blasts.

CONCLUSION

JTAPIC's motto is "Preventing injury through actionable analysis." By bringing intelligence, medical, operational, and materiel experts together to study injuries in combat, JTAPIC identifies new and emerging hazards and generates actionable information to guide the development of countermeasures. At a time when our armed forces face a growing array of conventional and unconventional threats, JTAPIC provides a timely source of high-value information to prevent combat-related trauma.

TABLE 9.1. Vehicle design and survivability improvements based upon joint trauma analysis and prevention of injury in combat analysis

- Stryker "Double V" hull
- Stryker flat-bottom hull mine protection kit
- Stryker driver compartment improvement
- Mine-Resistant Ambush Protected (MRAP) vehicle underbody vulnerability mapping
- MRAP All-Terrain Vehicle (MATV) underbody improvement kit
- Cougar transfer case tie-down redesign
- Vehicle gunner egress (doctrinal change, multiple vehicles)
- MRAP egress trainer (redesigned restraints and egress handles)
- Breathing apparatus installed in MRAP vehicles

TABLE 9.2. Dismounted improvements based on joint trauma analysis and prevention of injury in combat analysis

- Identified training need to keep service members from stepping off of cleared path
- Fielding and use of "sickle sticks" as counter-improvised explosive device tools
- Urogenital injury analyses led to ballistic undergarment protection development
- Decision to use new plate carrier (lighter weight armor vs vulnerability)
- US Marine Corps modular armor system development
- Extensive analysis in support of helmet-test protocols

Notes

1. Author's personal service experience with the 28th Combat Support Hospital, Camp Speicher (Tikrit) and Baghdad, Iraq, 2003–2004.
2. National Defense Authorization Act for Fiscal Year 2006. Pub L No. 109-163, January 6, 2006. Section 256, Prevention, mitigation, and treatment of blast injuries.
3. US Department of Defense. *Medical Research for the Prevention, Mitigation, and Treatment of Blast Injuries.* Washington, DC: DoD; July 5, 2006. DoD Directive 6025.21.
4. US Department of Defense. *Efforts and Programs of the Department of Defense Relating to the Prevention, Mitigation, and Treatment of Blast Injuries.* Washington, DC: DoD; 2008. Annual report to Congress.
5. US Army Medical Research and Materiel Command. *Charter for the Joint Trauma Analysis and Prevention of Injury in Combat Program.* Ft Detrick, MD: USAMRMC; March 2013.
6. Greene CM. Program accomplishments for CY15. Presentation at: JTAPIC Program Annual Review; December 8–10, 2015; San Diego, CA.

CHAPTER ten

Battlefield Tourniquets

JOHN F. KRAGH, Jr, MD, and JOHN B. HOLCOMB, MD

THE CHECKERED HISTORY OF TOURNIQUETS

A T THE TIME US FORCES INVADED AFGHANISTAN IN 2001, warriors were taught that placing a tourniquet to control severe bleeding from extremity wounds was a measure of last resort.[1] Preferred methods of bleeding control included putting direct pressure on wounds, applying field dressings with pressure wraps, elevating the injured limb, and attempting to compress the bleeding artery at a pressure point.

The military's dim view of tourniquets probably dates back to World War I, a bloody conflict that produced huge numbers of extremity wounds. Because evacuation of wounded Soldiers could take hours or even days, a tourniquet might be left in place for prolonged periods, with predictably bad results. Although troops were taught that tourniquets should be used only to stop arterial bleeding and removed as soon as surgical control was obtained, mistakes continued to be made throughout World War II. Fortunately, during the wars in Korea and Vietnam, use improved, with positive results.[4,5]

THE PROBLEM: PREVENTABLE DEATHS FROM UNCONTROLLED BLEEDING ON THE BATTLEFIELD

Warned to minimize use of tourniquets, frontline medics, corpsmen, and other military health providers in Afghanistan and Iraq struggled to control bleeding from combat injuries using conventional

FOUR PATIENTS' STORIES

Afghanistan, January, 2002. During an intense firefight with the Taliban, two Special Operations team members were shot. The US intelligence officer's chest wound appeared graver than the bullet wound to the Special Forces Soldier's thigh, so the hard-pressed medic treated the chest wound first. Unfortunately, the Soldier's femoral artery had been severed. Without a tourniquet, he bled to death during the helicopter flight to a medical treatment area.[2] His bereaved Green Beret teammates said his death was preventable. Every Soldier, they said, should carry a tourniquet and know how to use it, especially on themselves.

Afghanistan, March, 2002. Shot while flying in combat, an Army helicopter pilot bled profusely from a severed artery near his wrist. He landed his helicopter amid a dramatic firefight, and an Army paramedic applied a tourniquet that stayed in place for the next 16 hours. The pilot survived, kept his arm and hand, and eventually returned to fly helicopters for his unit. (Snow was central to the pilot's survival because cooling prolongs the ability of tissue to withstand lack of blood flow and oxygen.[3])

Houston, 2012. When an industrial accident cut off a 25-year-old man's arm, coworkers applied pressure to control the bleeding. A medical helicopter soon arrived, and the nurse and paramedic crew saved the man's life by applying the civilian equivalent of a Combat Application Tourniquet, or CAT—while they transfused blood products. Considering his near-fatal injury, the man left the hospital in remarkably good condition.

Houston, 2013. After an adult suffered a deep cut to a forearm artery, a non-medical first responder controlled the bleeding with a civilian version of the CAT. The man survived.

measures. Worse, because of numerous casualties sustaining multiple wounds from gunshots, improvised explosive devices, and rocket-propelled grenades, there were not enough medics. An infantry platoon of 42 Soldiers typically has only one medic. If the platoon's four nine-person squads are widely dispersed at the start of a firefight, several people might sustain simultaneous life-threatening injuries at different points on the battlefield. In such situations, there is no way a single medic can treat everyone. As a result, uncontrolled bleeding from limb wounds was causing otherwise preventable deaths.

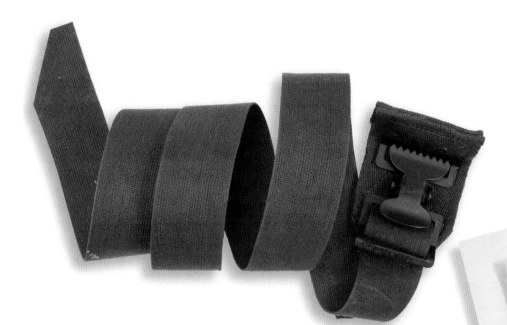

FIGURE 10.1. The standard tourniquets issued at the start of Operations Enduring Freedom and Iraqi Freedom were ineffective. Most employed an inadequate "strap and buckle" design dating back to World War II. Photographs courtesy of Francis S. Trachta, Army Medical Department Museum, Fort Sam Houston, Texas.

To make matters worse, the tourniquets issued at the start of Operations Enduring Freedom and Iraqi Freedom (OEF/OIF) were ineffective. Most employed an inadequate "strap and buckle" design dating back to World War II (Figure 10-1).[1] Others were nothing more than an elastic band with an "S" hook on both ends (see "Getting the Right Equipment Into Theater"). These tourniquets were difficult to apply, required two hands to use, and, more often than not, could not be sufficiently tightened to stop arterial bleeding. In fact, if a poorly applied tourniquet blocks venous flow without stopping arterial flow, it can cause more bleeding rather than less.

THE INNOVATION: DESIGN A BETTER TOURNIQUET AND MAKE IT A TOOL FOR FIRST AID

Grim reports from frontline providers in Afghanistan and Iraq forced military surgeons to rethink the tourniquet's proper role. Implementation of the Joint

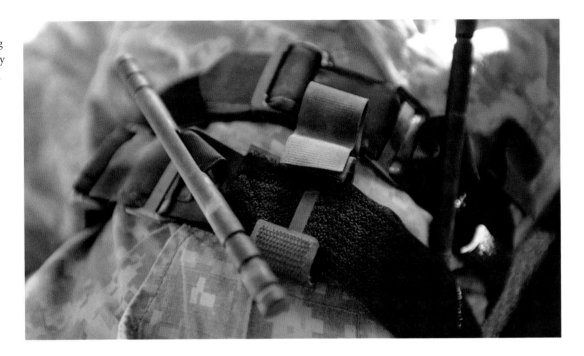

FIGURE 10.2. Tourniquets placed on a simulated wounded Soldier's leg during a mass casualty response exercise, January 23, 2010, Forward Operating Base Farah, Afghanistan. Reproduced from: https://www.dvidshub.net/image/245311/fob-farah-medical-personnel-put-test.

Theater Trauma System in Iraq and Afghanistan (Chapter 8) confirmed the need for better methods to control extremity hemorrhage. After a survey of preventable deaths in Special Operations personnel concluded that all combatants should carry tourniquets,[6] a policy was put into place in April 2005. Soon thereafter, better-designed tourniquets began to reach deploying personnel.

The decisive development was the invention of the Combat Application Tourniquet (CAT). Developed with support from the US Army Medical Research and Material Command (Chapter 4) and quickly refined to its current design, the CAT is lightweight, easy to use, and has a built-in windlass that enables it to be tightened enough to stop arterial bleeding (Figure 10.2). Importantly, this type of tourniquet can be applied with one hand, so a warfighter with a badly damaged arm can treat himself or herself on the battlefield, rather than waiting for help under fire.[1]

IMPACT

Widespread training boosted tourniquet use. Meanwhile, military surgeons gathered enough information about casualties to measure the risks and benefits of tourniquet use. These data were used to refine first aid practices. Evidence clearly showed that prompt application of tourniquets was saving lives with minimal risk. This dispelled old notions that using tourniquets leads to amputation of limbs that might have otherwise have been salvaged. .These findings spurred even greater awareness and training.[7,8] By 2009, researchers estimated that use of tourniquets on the battlefield had saved 1,000 to 2,000 US service members' lives (Figure 10-3).[9]

It did not take long for the military's findings about tourniquet use to begin changing civilian thinking about the best way to control bleeding from severely damaged limbs.[10] Troops returning to civilian life help spread awareness about the benefits of tourniquets as a fist aid tool.[11] Former military trauma surgeons John Holcomb, Dave King, and Don Jenkins brought these lessons to the Houston, Boston, and Minnesota areas, respectively. Their actions saved lives.

Whether the injuries stem from terrorism, as in the Boston Marathon bombings (see "A Message From Boston" in Chapter 28), or a severe automobile or motorcycle crash, evidence points to the value of encouraging tourniquet use by civilian emergency medical service (EMS) units and even trained bystanders. Still, recent surveys suggest that only one civilian EMS worker in five has applied a tourniquet to a patient. To increase civilian awareness of tourniquets and other techniques to control severe bleeding, the White House launched the "Stop the Bleed" campaign in October 2015 (Figure 10.4).

Today, more American service members are surviving severe limb wounds, thanks to tourniquets (Figure 10.5). Since tourniquet use became widespread, the odds of surviving battlefield wounds have climbed steadily. Compared to the start of OEF and OIF, the survival rate from isolated limb wounds has improved six-fold, even as wounds have become more severe. Clearly, tourniquets played an important role. Stopping or reducing bleeding before the patient reaches the hospital prevents or delays the onset of shock. This keeps a badly injured warfighter alive a bit longer, so the surgical team can save his or her life.

GETTING THE RIGHT EQUIPMENT INTO THEATER

The hard-won lessons of war are often forgotten, only to be relearned during the next conflict at great cost. The rediscovery of battlefield tourniquets is illustrative. This simple life-saving tool was used on the battle-field for more than 400 years. In 2001, the world's most advanced military went to war with a military-issue tourniquet invented during the Civil War. Although determined to be ineffective during World War II because it could not be reliably tightened to stop arterial bleeding sufficiently, it continued to be issued to US service members during the conflicts in Korea, Vietnam, Grenada, Panama, Desert Storm, Somalia, and until 2005, Iraq and Afghanistan. It was only replaced when a US Army medic developed a far more effective replace-ment. Even then, the Civil War-era strap and buckle device remained in the military inventory until 2008.

In July 1999, I was assigned to the Navy Special Warfare Development Group, a tier-1 special mission unit. Included in my supplied individual first aid kit (IFAK) was the strap-and-buckle tourniquet described above. During self-aid/buddy aid training, I would throw a device to someone in the audience with the instruction to apply an effective tourniquet within 30 seconds, lest they [the patient] lose consciousness by hemor-rhagic shock. The exercise was in effect a trick question, since there was no way to use the device to create an "effective tourniquet."

In January 2003, I was assigned to the 2nd Force Service Support Group as the senior medical officer of a shock trauma platoon in advance of our pending invasion of Iraq. The supplied IFAK did not contain the strap-and-buckle tourniquet, but did contain the TK-4 tourniquet, a 1-inch elastic band with an S-hook on either end. Although the device was totally ineffective at stopping arterial blood flow to a badly damaged leg or arm, it could create enough compressive force to block returning venous blood flow. As a result, if anyone tried to use the device on the battlefield, the resulting back-pressure produced in a damaged arm or leg would increase blood loss, rather than reduce it.

Seven years later, in August 2010, I was assigned to the II Marine Expeditionary Force (Forward) as the force surgeon in preparation for deployment to Helmand Province, Afghanistan, in support of Operation Enduring Freedom. Incredibly, the IFAK I received contained the same TK-4 tourniquet—the elastic band with S-hooks—only it was now reinforced with a composite canvas covering! During my in-call with the commanding general, I discussed the need to supplement the contents of the IFAK with materials recommended in the Tactical Combat Casualty Care (TCCC) guidelines, including two Combat Application Tourniquets (CATs). Through a series of authorizations, including message traffic in garrison and fragmentary orders in theater, we were able to acquire and supply the appropriate IFAK equipment to every Marine in Helmand Province. This requirement was later included in the operations order to ensure it endured after the completion of our tour in theater.

Since 2010, the Marine Corps has completed systematic reviews and refined the content of its IFAK to be in compliance with guidelines published by the Committee on TCCC and Defense Health Agency policy. All Navy medicine personnel assigned to the Marine units are trained in TCCC. All Marines are trained in the principles of TCCC, with special emphasis on combat lifesaver skills in hemorrhage control. A draft Marine Corps order on combat casualty care is being staffed to codify the requirement for training for medical and non-medical personnel.

Captain Jeffrey W. Timby, Deputy Commanding Officer,
Tripler Army Medical Center
Former Deputy Medical Officer of the
Marine Corps and Fleet Marine Force Specialty Leader

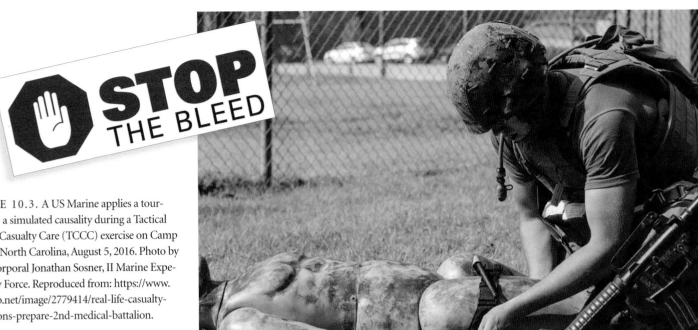

FIGURE 10.3. A US Marine applies a tourniquet to a simulated causality during a Tactical Combat Casualty Care (TCCC) exercise on Camp Lejeune, North Carolina, August 5, 2016. Photo by Lance Corporal Jonathan Sosner, II Marine Expeditionary Force. Reproduced from: https://www.dvidshub.net/image/2779414/real-life-casualty-simulations-prepare-2nd-medical-battalion.

FIGURE 10.4. "Stop the Bleed" is a nationwide campaign to empower individuals to act quickly and save lives. Reproduced from: https://www.dhs.gov/stopthebleed.

FIGURE 10.5. [*Opposite*] A wounded Afghan National Army soldier is carried on a stretcher to a US Army MEDEVAC helicopter from Charlie Co, Sixth Battalion, 101st Airborne Combat Aviation Brigade, Task Force Shadow, June 21, 2010, in Qandahar, Afghanistan. Photo by Justin Sullivan/Getty Images. Reproduced with permission from Getty Images.

The reappraisal of the role of tourniquets—a lifesaving lesson learned in the crucible of combat—is a military medicine revolution of the first rank. Tourniquets transformed combat casualty care in Afghanistan and Iraq. Today, they are helping to save lives back home.

Notes

1. Kragh JF Jr, Walters TJ, Ber DG, et al. Practical use of emergency tourniquets to stop bleeding in major limb trauma. *J Trauma.* 2008;64:S38-49; discussion S49-50.
2. Kragh JF Jr, Walters, TJ, Wastmoreland T, et al. Tragedy into drama: an American history of tourniquet use in the current war. *J Spec Oper Med.* 2013;13:5–25.

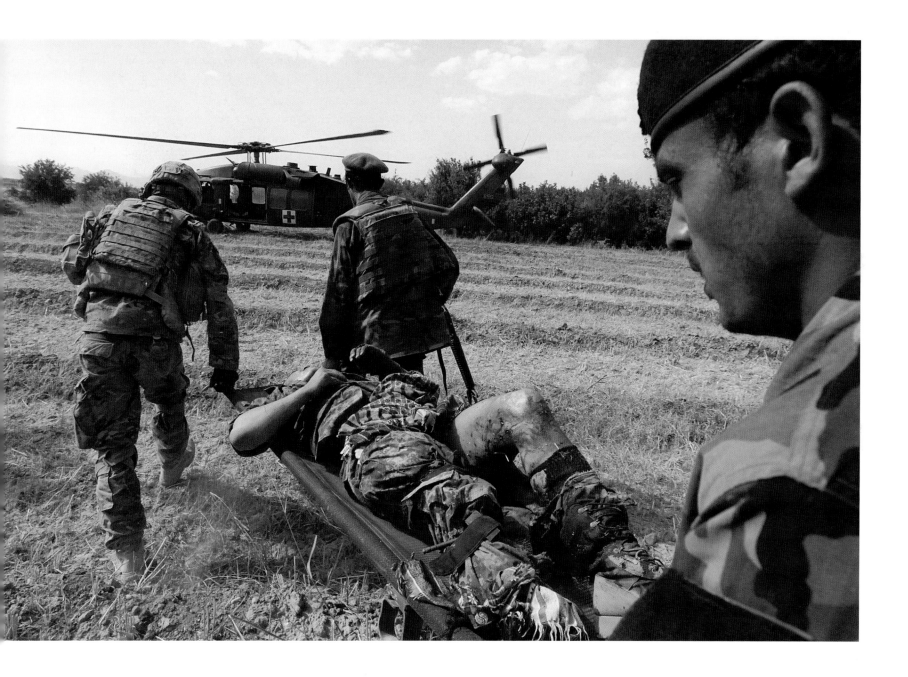

3. Kragh JF Jr, Baer DG, Walters TJ. Extended (16-hour) tourniquet application after combat wounds: a case report and review of the current literature. *J Orthop Trauma.* 2007;21(4):274–278.

4. Welling DR, McKay PL, Rasmussen TE. Rich NR. A brief history of the tourniquet. *J Vasc Surg.* 2012:55(1):286–290.

5. Kragh JF Jr, Swan KG, Smith DC, Mabry RL, Blackbourne LH. Historical review of emergency tourniquet use to stop bleeding. *Am J Surg.* 2012;203(2):242–252.

6. Holcomb JB, McMullin NR, Pearse L, et al. Causes of death in U.S. Specials Operations Forces in the global war on terrorism: 2001-2005. *Ann Surg.* 2007;245:986-991.

7. Beekley AC, Sebesta JA, Blackbourne LH, et al. Prehospital tourniquet use in Operation Iraqi Freedom: effet on hemmorhage control. *J Trauma,* 2008;64:S28–37.

8. Kragh JF Jr, Walters TJ, Baer DG, et al. Survivial with emergency tourniquet use to stop bleeding in major limb trauma. *Ann Surg.* 2009;249:1–7.

9. Andersen RC, Shawen SB, Kragh JF Jr, et al. Special topics. *J Am Acad Orthop Surg.* 2012;20:S94–98.

10. Jacobs LM, Joint Committee to Create a National Policy to Enhance Surviviability from Intentional Mass-casualty and Active Shooter Events. The Hartfort Consensus III: implementation of bleeding control. *Bull Am Coll Surg.* 2015;100:20–26.

11. Bulger EM, Snyder D, Schoelles K, et al. An evidence-based prehospital guideline for external hemorrhage control: American College of Surgeons Committee on Trauma. *Prehosp Emerg Care.* 2014;18:163-173.

Recommended Reading

Kragh JF Jr, Dubick MA. Battlefield Tourniquets: lessons learned in moving current care toward best care in an Army Medical Department at war. *US Army Med Dep J.* 2016;Apr-Sep:29–36.

CHAPTER eleven

Tactical Combat Casualty Care

FRANK K. BUTLER, MD, and ROBERT MABRY, MD

THE PROBLEM: UNCONTROLLED BLEEDING FROM EXTREMITY WOUNDS

WHEN US FORCES BEGAN OPERATIONS AGAINST AL-QAEDA and the Taliban in 2001, most of them did not have tourniquets. That's a major reason 8 out of every 100 US combat fatalities in the early years of the wars in Iraq and Afghanistan died as a result of uncontrolled bleeding from an arm or leg wound—bleeding that a tourniquet could have stopped (Chapter 10).

Most service members who die from combat wounds either do so immediately from a non-survivable injury, or shortly thereafter, before they reach a medical treatment facility with a surgical capability. This has profound implications for reducing fatalities. The best hospital-based care in the world can't bring a dead casualty back to life. Therefore, the greatest opportunities to save lives lie in improving the *prehospital* phase of combat casualty care.[1]

Unfortunately, in contrast to the many advances in modern medicine and surgery made before the onset of the war in Afghanistan, little had changed in how the US military delivers prehospital care on the battlefield in 140 years.[2]

> *"Your work is absolutely vital to helping us uphold our obligation, our sacred obligation, not only to our service members who fight, but also to the families and loved ones who support them ... you have quite literally saved thousands of lives ... I wish every single American understood just what you have done for our warriors. I wish they knew as much as I know; I wish they could see what I've seen about the heroic efforts you have made on behalf of our warriors."* [2]

Note from Vice President Joe Biden
On the tenth anniversary of the founding of the
Committee on Tactical Combat Casualty Care

THE INNOVATION: TACTICAL COMBAT CASUALTY CARE

Successful battlefield care must combine good medicine with effective small unit tactics. Unlike medical care provided in hospitals, clinics, and other fixed settings, which can be entirely focused on meeting the patient's needs, casualty care on a battlefield has three goals: (1) save the casualty, (2) prevent additional casualties, and (3) complete the mission. Consequently, effective delivery of battlefield care requires special skills and techniques that are largely unique to this life-or-death setting. The approach the US military developed to teach these skills is called "Tactical Combat Casualty Care," or TCCC.

Work on TCCC began in the early 1990s as a research effort by the Naval Special Warfare Command and the Uniformed Services University of the Health Sciences (see Chapter 4). Shortly thereafter, US Special Operations Command joined in. The partners sought to improve battlefield trauma care, with a special focus on front-line enlisted providers: Army medics, Navy corpsmen, and Air Force pararescuemen.

The up-front involvement of line leadership proved to be a key factor in TCCC's success because line commanders are responsible for all aspects of their units' actions on the battlefield—including the provision of medical care. For this reason, changing the military's approach to combat casualty care required more than getting the doctors on board: it required close coordination with line commanders, their medical advisors, and combatant commanders.

The TCCC research effort was different from other efforts to improve trauma care because its goal was broader than improving a single aspect of treatment or developing a new drug or device. Instead, it set out to develop a set of best-practice guidelines for the battlefield.

The effort began with a comprehensive review of all recommended elements of prehospital trauma care as taught in the military in 1993. The research considered these recommendations' usefulness in light of the realities of the tactical combat environment: extremes of temperature and harsh terrains; the possibility that the enemy is shooting at you as you attempt to render care; the possibility that evacuation will be significantly delayed; the probable skills, training, and experience of combat medical providers; equipment limitations; and the potential for mass casualties in situations when there is only one medic or even no trained provider to respond.

Proposed TCCC interventions initially focused sharply on treating the three major causes of preventable battlefield deaths: (1) uncontrolled external hemorrhage, (2) obstructed airway, and (3) tension pneumothorax (a form of collapsed lung that causes the rapid buildup of air pressure inside the chest, leading to impaired breathing and heart function). TCCC researchers evaluated the evidence to support existing prehospital trauma care guidelines, as well as any proposed changes.

After drafting the first set of TCCC guidelines, the researchers asked experienced combat medical providers to review their feasibility. The resulting first set of TCCC guidelines were published in 1996. In addition to offering guidance to prehospital providers, the paper called on the military to initiate a formal process to periodically update the TCCC guidelines to address new medical technologies and incorporate lessons learned on future battlefields.

TACTICAL COMBAT CASUALTY CARE IN THE WAR YEARS (2001–2015)

Initially, the military didn't widely accept TCCC. Four things happened in the early days of the conflicts in Afghanistan and Iraq to change that: (1) the benefit of TCCC principles became increasingly clear as units who used it reported better survival rates than those that did not; (2) careful analysis of the treatment provided to US combat casualties revealed opportunities to improve care; (3) military medical research

VIGNETTE >> Afghanistan, 2003: A Preventable Death. A Special Forces Soldier on a mission with his team was seriously wounded by a rocket-propelled grenade. Although his body armor protected his chest and abdomen, the explosion damaged his right arm and (particularly) his right leg, which bled profusely from a severed artery. The unit's medic was killed early in the attack, and other members of the Soldier's unit did not have the skills or equipment required to save his life. Desperate to stop his bleeding, they applied three improvised tourniquets without success. The Soldier bled to death from a survivable wound to his right knee. Had this Soldier's team members been trained and properly equipped to deal with severe bleeding, he would have lived, and after surgical repair and rehabilitation, returned to duty.

produced new devices and strategies designed to help combat medical providers save lives; and (4) the US Special Operations Command and the Naval Operational Medicine Institute jointly established the Committee on Tactical Combat Casualty Care (CoTCCC).

The creation of the CoTCCC brought improved methodology and additional experience to TCCC decision-making processes. Just as importantly, the explicit support of the Special Operations community gave it legitimacy in the eyes of combat medics and warfighters. Roughly a decade later, the CoTCCC became an integral element of the Joint Trauma System (Chapter 8). This further enhanced its access to data and strengthened its ability to oversee and improve prehospital combat trauma care.

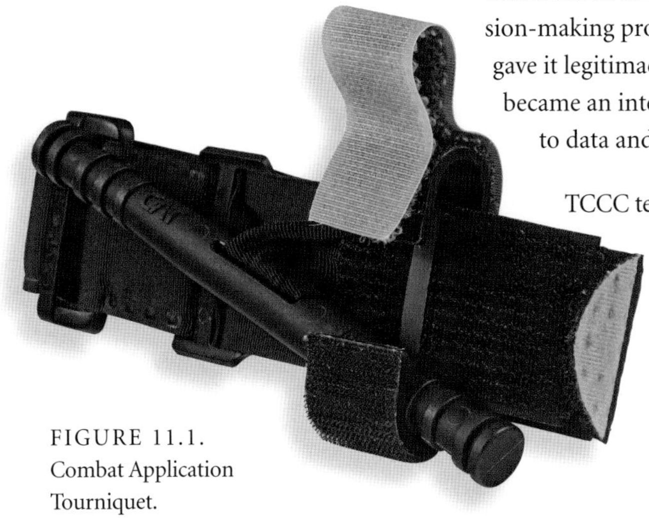

FIGURE 11.1.
Combat Application
Tourniquet.

TCCC techniques in widespread use today include the prompt application of tourniquets (Figure 11.1) and hemostatic dressings (see Figure 12.3) to control life-threatening external bleeding; "sit-up-and-lean-forward" positioning to protect the compromised airway of a warfighter with facial wounds; the insertion of a needle through the wall of the chest to relieve the buildup of air pressure from a tension pneumothorax when needed; and much-improved techniques to relieve pain from combat injuries. Table 11.1 summarizes key elements of battlefield trauma care pioneered by TCCC and now widely used throughout the US military and increasingly, in civilian care.

IMPACT

At the start of the wars in Iraq and Afghanistan, only a few elite units had TCCC training and equipment. Today, essentially the entire US military and most of our coalition partner nations train to this standard.

The most important measure of TCCC's cumulative impact is the striking reduction in the number of "potentially preventable" combat deaths. An example of a potentially preventable death is a Marine shot in the knee who bleeds to death on the battlefield from an arterial injury that could have been readily managed with a tourniquet. An example of a non-preventable combat death is a Soldier directly hit by a mortar round. Between these two extremes are deaths caused by injuries complex enough that determining whether better battlefield care might have prevented the loss of life must be carefully considered.

Two landmark papers from the recent conflicts demonstrate TCCC's positive impact: a large-scale study led by Colonel Brian Eastridge,[1] a trauma surgeon who directed the Joint Trauma System, and a paper by Colonel Russ Kotwal,[3] who for six war years served as the regimental surgeon for the 75th Ranger Regiment.

Eastridge's paper examined all 4,596 US combat fatalities sustained over 10 years in Iraq and Afghanistan.[1] During that time, 24 percent of US combat deaths were determined to be potentially preventable. Internal bleeding from torso (chest or abdomen) injuries was the primary cause of death in two-thirds of prehospital preventable deaths. It is noteworthy that, following the widespread use of tourniquets by combat forces, *deaths from uncontrolled extremity bleeding dropped by two-thirds*.

Kotwal's paper provided a dramatic example of what TCCC can accomplish when it is optimally applied. After implementing a Ranger First Responder program that ensured that every member of the regiment, not just medics, was trained and equipped to provide TCCC, the 75th Ranger Regiment achieved the lowest incidence of prehospital preventable deaths ever reported by a major combat unit: zero. Not a single Ranger in this unit died from external hemorrhage in 8.5 years of conflict.[3]

Other nations have also benefitted from TCCC. The Canadian military, which started training medical and non-medical personnel in TCCC in 1999, reported that its forces achieved their lowest combat casualty death rate in history. Canada attributed the success largely to adopting a "comprehensive, multileveled TCCC training package to both soldiers and medics."[4]

CONTINUED PROGRESS

At the start of Operations Enduring Freedom and Iraqi Freedom, the US military was not well prepared to treat casualties on the battlefield. Through the concerted actions of military medical innovators and leaders, the services swiftly closed this treatment gap by advancing practical knowledge and care. By the end of the war, US forces dramatically reduced the rate of preventable deaths and achieved the highest casualty survival rates in the history of warfare.

Now that major US combat operations in Iraq and Afghanistan have largely ended, the challenge for military medicine is to sustain these advances. Line commanders should ensure that every member of their unit is trained in TCCC and properly equipped to use it in combat. A medical rapid fielding initiative is needed to expedite delivery of newly recommended TCCC equipment, treatments, and training to deploying forces.[5]

Combat commander support was essential to TCCC's success. After all, line commanders own the battle space. Those who required their units to be trained in TCCC assured that anyone in their command who was wounded in combat would receive optimal prehospital care and would have a better chance of surviving.

Despite TCCC's documented benefits, it is not being taught as consistently as it should be. Line commanders typically act on the advice of their unit surgeons, and unfortunately, to date, few military physicians get formal training in TCCC. Today, medical students attending the Uniformed Services University of the Health Sciences are taught TCCC, as are military residents who attend the Combat Casualty Care Course, but many military physicians and surgeons have not been trained in TCCC. Many unit surgeons have limited experience overseeing delivery of prehospital trauma care. Training unit surgeons and other military physicians in TCCC is an important step in enabling them to better supervise corpsmen, medics, and pararescuemen and prepare them to perform TCCC on the battlefield.

TRANSLATION TO THE CIVILIAN SECTOR

In the past few years, through a strong partnership between the CoTCCC, the American College of Surgeons Committee on Trauma, and the National Association of Emergency Medical Technicians, prehospital interventions endorsed by the CoTCCC are gaining acceptance in civilian trauma care systems. These techniques include early use of tourniquets, hemostatic agents, intraosseous devices, hypotensive resuscitation, and modified spinal protection techniques.

A major example of military medicine's influence on the civilian community is the work of the Hartford Consensus, an effort led by the American College of Surgeons to reduce deaths from active shooter incidents and other events that cause civilian mass casualties.[6] Hartford Consensus messages call for

TABLE 11.1. Key Elements of Battlefield Trauma Care in Tactical Combat Casualty Care

- Structuring **battlefield trauma care** to be consistent with good small unit tactics.

- The aggressive use of **tourniquets** recommended by the Committee on TCCC (CoTCCC) to control life-threatening bleeding from arm or leg wounds.

- Use of CoTCCC-recommended **hemostatic dressings** to control life-threatening bleeding from locations that can't be treated with a tourniquet.

- Use of **junctional tourniquets** (customized pressure devices) to help control external hemorrhage from wounds to the groin area or axilla (armpit).

- **Sit-up-and-lean-forward positioning** of a casualty to protect the airway if the casualty is conscious and experiencing airway difficulty from facial wounds

- Ability to establish a **surgical airway** in casualties who have severe facial, oral, or throat wounds that are blocking their ability to breathe.

- Use of a 14-gauge, 3.25-inch **needle to decompress the chest** when a tension pneumothorax (collapsed lung under high air pressure) is suspected.

- **Intravenous (IV) lines are not started on all casualties.** Rather, they are used only when the casualty needs IV medication or blood or fluid resuscitation.

- If an IV is needed, but one cannot be easily started, use a specialized device called an **intraosseous needle** to bore a hole into a marrow-containing bone to deliver blood, IV fluids, or medication. Common sites include the breast bone (sternum) or the shin bone (tibia).

- Use of **tranexamic acid (TXA)**, a medication that increases survival in casualties at risk of death from hemorrhage. It is given as quickly as possible during battlefield trauma care to casualties at risk of hemorrhagic shock.

- Administration of **whole blood or "balanced resuscitation" with blood products** in a 1:1 ratio of packed red blood cells to plasma as soon as feasible, even in the prehospital environment.

- If blood products are not available, use **Hextend** (Biotime, Alameda, CA), a solution that stays in the bloodstream longer than electrolyte (salt water) solutions. Do not give too much fluid because this increases the risk of bleeding.

- **Safer, faster, and more effective pain relief** using the "triple-option" approach to battlefield analgesia, which emphasizes use of oral pain medication, ketamine, and oral fentanyl citrate lozenges rather than intramuscular morphine as was done at the start of the war years.

- **Prevent heat loss** through the use of both active and passive warming measures.

a number of civilian techniques that parallel those taught in TCCC. These include maintaining better situational awareness in active shooter incidents and swiftly applying tourniquets and topical hemostatic dressings to control massive external hemorrhage. The Hartford Consensus also emphasizes the value of engaging law enforcement officers and non-medical personnel in treating victims of mass-casualty events.

The Hartford Consensus's work was recently reinforced by the national launch of the "Stop the Bleed" campaign. Announced at a White House ceremony on October 6, 2015, this campaign encourages bystanders to help save lives following a shooting or terrorist bombing, mainly by controlling external bleeding. Through programs like these, TCCC may ultimately save far more American lives at home than it did on the battlefields of Iraq and Afghanistan.

ACKNOWLEDGMENTS

The authors gratefully acknowledge the sustained efforts of our colleagues at the Joint Trauma System and in the CoTCCC to provide the best care possible to our country's combat wounded.

Notes

1. Eastridge BJ, Mabry R, Seguin P, et al. Death on the battlefield (2001–2011): implications for the future of combat casualty care. *J Trauma Acute Care Surg.* 2012;73:S431–S437.
2. Butler FK, Blackbourne LH. Battlefield trauma care then and now: a decade of Tactical Combat Casualty Care. *J Trauma Acute Care Surg.* 2012;73:S395–S402.
3. Kotwal RS, Montgomery HR, Kotwal BM, et al. Eliminating preventable death on the battlefield. *Arch Surg.* 2011; 46:1350–1358.
4. Savage E, Forestier C, Withers N, Tien H, Pannel D. Tactical Combat Casualty Care in the Canadian Forces: lessons learned from the Afghan War. *Can J Surg.* 2011;59:S118–S123.
5. Butler FK, Smith DJ, Carmona RH. Implementing and preserving advances in combat casualty care from Iraq and Afghanistan throughout the US military. *J Trauma Acute Care Surg.* 2015;79:321–326.
6. Jacobs LM, Wade D, McSwain NE, et al. Hartford Consensus: a call to action for THREAT, a medical disaster preparedness concept. *J Am Coll Surg.* 2014;218:467–475.

Recommended Reading

Robinson JB, Smith MP, Gross KR, et al. Battlefield documentation of the Tactical Combat Casualty Care in Afghanistan. *US Army Med Dep J.* 2016;Apr-Sep:87–94.

CHAPTER twelve

Topical Hemostatic Agents

PATRICK GEORGOFF, MD; PETER RHEE, MD, MPH; and HASAN ALAM, MD

BACKGROUND

N MILITARY TRAUMA, HEMORRHAGE (BLEEDING) is the leading cause of preventable death. While the use of tourniquets has reduced blood loss in Soldiers with injured extremities, it can do little to stem bleeding from areas where a tourniquet cannot be applied, such as the chest, abdomen, groin, neck, and axilla (armpit). A recent study[1] of lethal combat wounds in Operation Iraqi Freedom (OIF) and Operation Enduring Freedom (OEF) showed that 87 percent of all battlefield deaths occurred before the injured person reached a medical treatment facility. Earlier treatment and, in particular, early bleeding control could have saved about one-quarter of these soldiers. In fact, 90 percent of these potentially preventable deaths were due to uncontrolled hemorrhage. Most of the fatal wounds were non-compressible or not amenable to tourniquet use.[1]

One approach to controlling bleeding of non-compressible injuries is to use topical hemostatic (clot-promoting) agents that can be applied directly to the wound. The term "hemostatic" has origins in Greek (hemo: blood, stasis: idle). Over the past 15 years, combat casualty researchers have developed and tested numerous such agents. Some of the best have been deployed on the battlefield.

VIGNETTE >> Iraq, 2005: While on routine patrol, a 27-year-old Marine suffered severe injuries (Figure 12.1) when his Humvee struck an improvised explosive device. A corpsman traveling in the same convoy provided immediate medical attention, and found that the Marine suffered extensive injuries to his back, buttock, and legs. The Marine's blood pressure was low and he was slipping in and out of consciousness. Tourniquets applied to his lower extremities slowed the bleeding from his legs. However, an injury to the right buttock continued to bleed profusely despite gauze packing and direct pressure.

In an attempt to control the bleeding, the corpsman applied the topical hemostatic agent QuikClot (Z-Medica, Wallingford, CT) to the wound. This, in combination with continuous pressure, stopped the bleeding. The Marine's blood pressure improved with fluid resuscitation, and he was soon evacuated by air medical transport. On arrival at the nearest military field hospital, he underwent surgery to definitively control the bleeding. The surgery was successful and the Marine went on to make a full recovery.

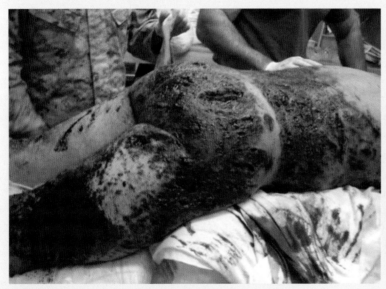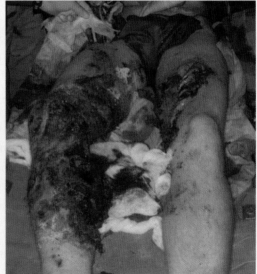

FIGURE 12.1. Case study: Marine wounded in Iraq, 2005.

HISTORY

Historically, battle dressings were used to compress wounds and absorb blood. The Carlisle bandage (Figure 12.2), which the US military used from the 1920s through World War II, consisted of an absorbent cotton pad and a linen wrap. The military slightly modified this standard-issue dressing after World War II, and renamed it the Army field bandage. While in use for almost 100 years, the military's standard dressings lacked any specific hemostatic features. Undoubtedly, many service members lost their lives due to the dressing's inability to immediately and effectively slow bleeding from non-compressible wounds.

TYPES OF TOPICAL HEMOSTATIC AGENTS

Recognizing the limitations of the original field bandage, the Department of Defense invested in an intensive research and development effort to produce battle-ready dressings with hemostatic properties. Today's topical hemostatic agents include novel compounds that can slow or even stop bleeding from non-compressible wounds.[2] While some compounds are applied to the wound as a powder, most are incorporated into the bandage gauze.

We typically divide topical hemostatic agents into three categories, based on their mechanism of action:

1. *Direct activation of the body's natural blood clotting factors.* One of the best-known topical hemostatic agents is QuikClot Combat Gauze (Figure 12.3). It is a rayon and polyester gauze impregnated with kaolin, an aluminum silicate mineral that triggers clot formation. At this time, Combat Gauze is recommended by the Committee on Tactical Combat Casualty Care (CoTCCC; Chapter 11) as their topical hemostatic agent of choice.

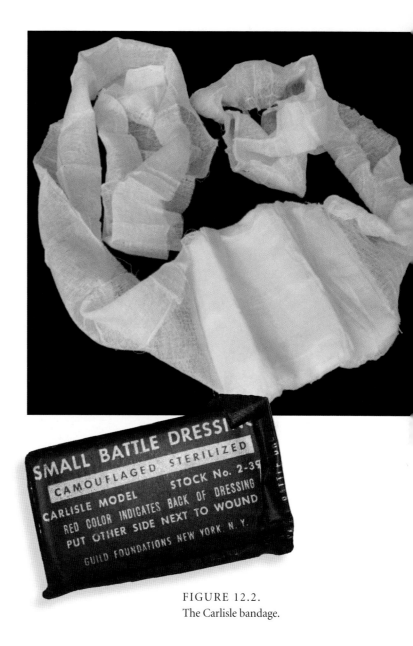

FIGURE 12.2.
The Carlisle bandage.

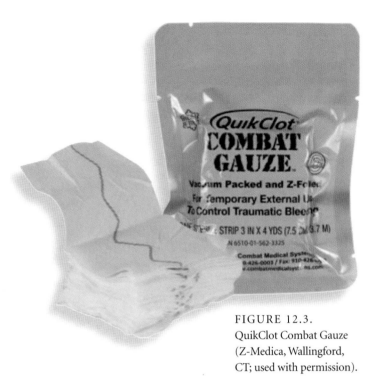

FIGURE 12.3.
QuikClot Combat Gauze
(Z-Medica, Wallingford,
CT; used with permission).

2. *Concentration of the body's natural blood clotting factors through rapid water absorption.* Two agents in this category are an early-generation version of QuikClot (Figure 12.4), which used a granular preparation of zeolite rock to absorb water, and TraumaDex (Davol Inc, Warwick, RI), which used a plant-derived starch to dehydrate the injury. By reducing the volume of water in and around the wound, the bandages concentrated clotting factors and platelets, indirectly enhancing clot formation. Both agents have been replaced by superior products and are no longer produced.

3. *Creation of an adherent seal over the injury.* These agents work independently of the body's clotting system by generating a physical barrier around severed vessels. To create this barrier, most currently available products use chitosan, a positively charged compound derived from the shells of shrimp and other marine arthropods. When chitosan comes into contact with blood, it swells, gels, and sticks together. It does not, however, activate the clotting cascade. Chitosan-based compounds include Celox (MedTrade Products Ltd, Crewe, UK) (Figure 12.5); HemCon (HemCon Medical Technologies, Portland, OR); and ChitoGauze (HemCon Medical Technologies). At this time, the CoTCCC recommends Celox and ChitoGauze as second-line hemostatic dressings.

These dressings share certain physical characteristics that make them effective in the battlefield. They are lightweight, durable, and cost-effective. They also have a long shelf life, are easy to use in austere conditions, and have been approved or cleared by the Food and Drug Administration. Today, the Army's individual first aid kit includes a tourniquet, rolled gauze, a compression dressing, and QuikClot Combat Gauze.

IMPACT

As researchers developed new topical hemostatic agents, they tested them in large animal models. Because these animals have anatomic and physiologic features similar to humans, these studies are vital to developing products useful to treat traumatic injury. Researchers tested 10 different hemostatic dressings versus the historical Army field bandage (ie, standard dressing), in which they examined rates of bleeding, blood pressure, and survival in a group of anesthetized pigs whose groin blood vessels were transected. When compared to a wide variety of topical hemostatic agents, the standard dressing resulted in worse outcomes, including decreased survival and a more rapid time to death. Figure 12.6 depicts the duration of survival in each group.[3] These findings are consistent with other, similarly designed studies.

Since the onset of OIF and OEF, many studies have examined effectiveness of different hemostatic dressings under battlefield conditions. While these studies have significant limitations because of the difficulties and danger of data collection in combat environments, first-responders and forward-operating trauma surgeons overwhelm-

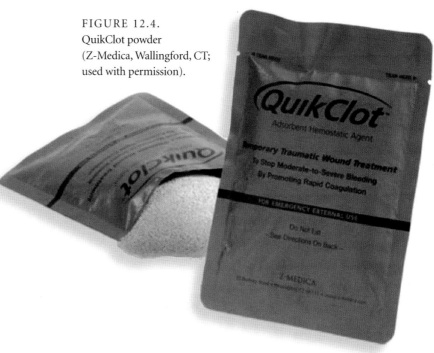

FIGURE 12.4.
QuikClot powder
(Z-Medica, Wallingford, CT; used with permission).

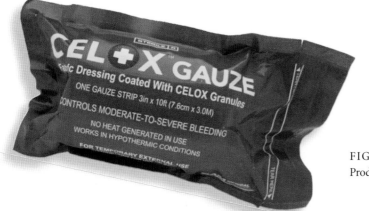

FIGURE 12.5. Celox gauze (MedTrade Products Ltd, Crewe, UK; used with permission).

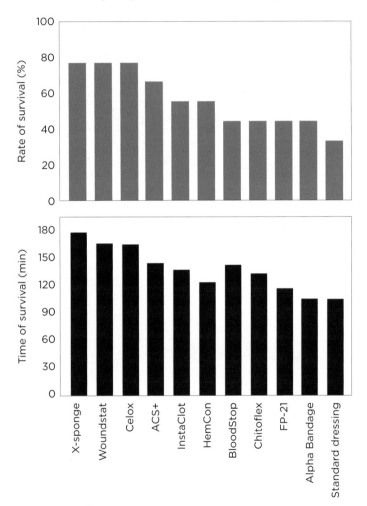

FIGURE 12.6. Rate and duration of survival in swine subjected to hemorrhage from groin vessels and treated with different topical hemostatic agents and bandages. Reproduced with permission from: Arnaud F, Parreno-Sadalan D, Tomori T, et al. Comparison of 10 hemostatic dressings in a groin transection model in swine. *J Trauma.* 2009;67:851.

ingly praise the effectiveness of topical hemostatic agents. In a review of 23 cases from OEF in which a hemostatic agent was applied in the absence of a tourniquet, 100 percent of first-responders felt the treatment was effective, and 57 percent of physicians who received these casualties identified the dressing as lifesaving.[4] In another study, two US Army emergency physicians collected and reviewed 64 unique cases in which medical providers used HemCon for combat injuries sustained in OIF and OEF. Most dressings were applied to injuries of the extremities caused by improvised explosive devices, gunshots, or indirect fire (eg, fragments from exploding mortar rounds or a rocket-propelled grenade). In at least two-thirds of these cases, medical personnel could not control bleeding with traditional dressings. Application of HemCon stopped the bleeding in all but two. The researchers noted that hemostatic dressings were most useful when a tourniquet could not be applied.[5]

Civilian medical personnel—including first-responders such as emergency medical services, police officers, and firefighters—also are being trained to use topical hemostatic agents. In one study, the Mayo Clinic's first responders were trained in the use of QuikClot Combat Gauze using a simple, computer-based learning module. In subsequent use in the field, QuikClot Combat Gauze was used in 62 injuries in which standard dressings failed to stop bleeding. The product halted hemorrhage in 59 cases (95 percent).[6] Today, many commercially available first-aid kits include topical hemostatic dressings. Products like QuikClot Combat Gauze are readily available online and in local pharmacies, and are advertised to participants in contact sports and outdoor activities.

CONCLUSION

Topical hemostatic agents—a class of products developed to improve casualty care on the battlefield—have proven to be so effective in the treatment of wounded service members that the technology was quickly adopted for civilian use. By rapidly reducing blood loss from non-compressible wounds, topical hemostatic agents help critically injured patients live long enough to reach definitive care. For many, like the Marine whose story opened this chapter, this treatment can make the difference between life and death.

Notes

1. Eastridge BJ, Mabry R, Seguin P, et al. Death on the battlefield (2001–2011): implications for the future of combat casualty care. *J Trauma Acute Care Surg.* 2012;73:S431–S437.

2. Kheirabad, B. Evaluation of topical hemostatic agents for combat wound treatment. *US Army Med Dep J.* 2011;Apr-Jun:25–37.

3. Arnaud F, Parreno-Sadalan D, Tomori T, et al. Comparison of 10 hemostatic dressings in a groin transection model in swine. *J Trauma.* 2009;67:848–855.

4. Lairet JR, Bebarta VS, Burns CJ, et al. Prehospital interventions performed in a combat zone: a prospective multicenter study of 1,003 combat wounded. *J Trauma Acute Care Surg.* 2012;73S38–42.

5. Wedmore I, McManus JG, Pusateri AE, et al. A special report on the chitosan-based hemostatic dressing: experience in current combat operations. *J Trauma.* 2006;60(3):655–658.

6. Zietlow J, Zietlow S, Morris D, et al. Prehospital use of hemostatic bandages and tourniquets: translation from military experience to implementation in civilian trauma care. *J Spec Oper Med.* 2015;15:48–53.

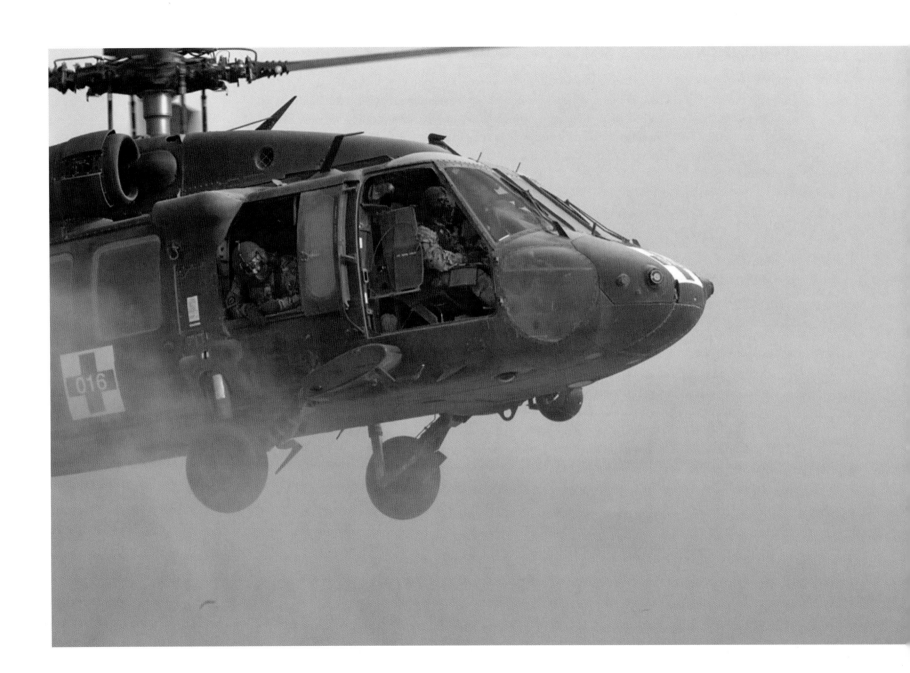

CHAPTER thirteen

MEDEVAC Lessons From the Iraq and Afghan Wars

ROBERT L. MABRY, MD

THE CHALLENGE

SINCE THE DAYS OF MAJOR JONATHAN LETTERMAN and the Army of the Potomac (Chapter 2), military doctors have recognized that rapid evacuation from the battlefield decreases suffering and saves lives. Helicopter evacuation (MEDEVAC) of seriously ill and injured patients during military operations came to the fore during the Korean War, and expanded significantly during the Vietnam War. The Bell UH-1 helicopter (or "Huey") was large enough to carry several patients plus a combat medic to provide basic trauma care en route to the hospital. The heroism of "Dustoff" crews, who regularly flew into firefights to rescue injured Soldiers, Marines, and Airmen, was widely recognized. Rapid MEDEVAC to surgical care was a principal reason that battlefield mortality was lower in Vietnam than in previous 20th century wars.

To retain the edge it had gained in Vietnam, the US military began, for a time, to use its MEDEVAC helicopters to transport injured civilians through the "Military Assistance to Safety and Traffic" (MAST) program. These local efforts helped spark rapid growth of civilian emergency medical services, or EMS, across the country. When local MEDEVAC helicopter units began deploying overseas, civilian air EMS services assumed the role previously played by MAST, and the military phased out its involvement. In time, these civilian aeromedical EMS services became the gold standard for transporting critically ill

FIGURE 13.1. [*Opposite*] UH-60 Black Hawk MEDEVAC helicopter with the 169th Aviation Regiment, New Mexico National Guard, performs a dust landing during a training flight on Camp Dwyer, Afghanistan, April 4, 2012. Photo by Captain Richard Barker, 25th Combat Aviation Brigade Public Affairs. Reproduced from: https://www.dvidshub.net/image/570533/life-camp-dwyer.

VIGNETTE >> Helmand Province, Afghanistan. In May, 2015, a Marine on foot patrol stepped on an improvised explosive device. The blast blew off his forearm and both legs below the knees, and threw him about 30 feet. He also sustained a concussion and internal injuries. Because he was bleeding profusely from the stumps of his amputated legs and arm, the unit's corpsman and fellow Marines immediately placed tourniquets on all three limbs. While the corpsman continued treatment, his platoon called for a MEDEVAC helicopter and secured a nearby landing zone. About 10 minutes later, an Army MEDEVAC helicopter staffed with a critical care paramedic and flight nurse arrived. After loading the badly injured Marine, they established intravenous (IV) access and began resuscitating him with a combination of packed red blood cells and plasma. The patient was sedated, intubated to protect his airway, and ventilated to ensure his brain got enough oxygen. Throughout the 20-minute flight to a forward surgical team (FST), the team continued to provide critical care. Shortly after the Marine received damage-control surgery (Chapter 15) at the FST, the MEDEVAC crew transported him a second time to the closest combat support hospital. During flight, the patient was supported by a mechanical ventilator and several intravenous medications, and he received two more units of blood. He survived his injuries and ultimately returned home.

and injured patients over long distances or difficult terrain. To assure a sustained level of excellence, most programs staffed their helicopters with two flight paramedics or comparably trained flight nurses.

Initially, the Army did not adopt this approach. Instead, it focused on enhancing the speed and performance of the airframe itself (Figure 13.1). As a result, our military went to war in Iraq and Afghanistan with better helicopters, but essentially the same staffing model it had used in Vietnam: a single combat medic trained to the level of a civilian basic emergency medical technician (EMT-B).

The operational environments encountered in Iraq and Afghanistan quickly exposed the inadequacy of this approach. Service members injured in remote, rugged areas (most of Afghanistan and large swaths of Iraq) often required advanced life support measures to survive even a brief flight to an FST. Also, because FSTs are not designed or staffed to hold postoperative patients for very long, air crews had to shuttle critically injured *postoperative* cases after their initial damage-control surgery. By necessity, many of these patients were sedated, intubated, and required multiple IV medications and blood products. On top of that, MEDEVAC crews were asked to transport unprecedented numbers of ill and injured civilians, including obstetric, pediatric, and geriatric cases (Figure 13.2). The medics staffing helicopters at the time lacked the training to properly care for these cases, particularly given the prolonged transport times some of these flights entailed.

THE INNOVATION

Initially, deployed units attempted ad hoc fixes and workarounds. FSTs would pull a nurse or physician from their team and put them

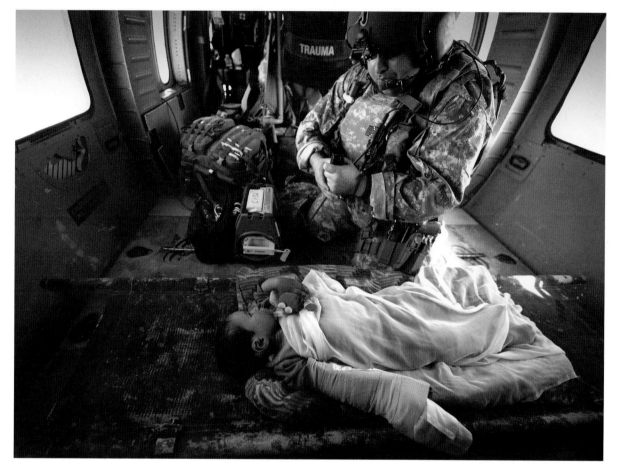

FIGURE 13.2. US army
flight medic Sergeant Bobby
Dorris (top) from Company
C, 1st Battalion, 52nd Aviation
Regiment MEDEVAC team,
treats an Afghan child with
burn injuries in flight on
their Black Hawk helicopter
in southern Afghanistan on
March 23, 2011. Photo by
Peter Parks/AFP/Getty Images.
Reproduced with permission
from Getty Images.

on the helicopter to care for their post-op patient. While this satisfied the immediate need, it took a valuable key team member away from the thinly-staffed FST. This put FSTs in a difficult spot: they could leave their team shorthanded during combat operations, or entrust their patient to a basic-level flight medic who had no training in critical care.

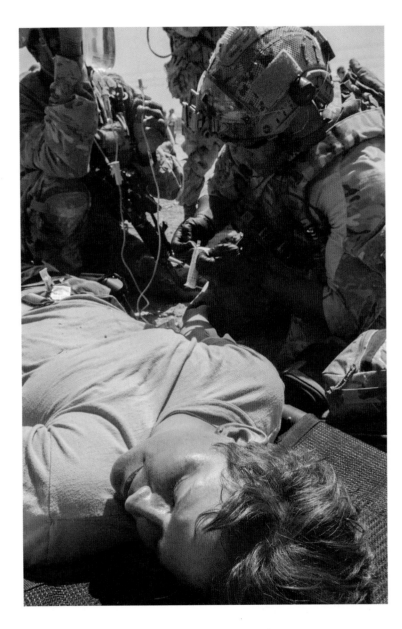

Operational elements quickly demanded better options. Some units, like the Army's 82nd Airborne Division and the 101st Air Assault Division, sent their flight medics to accelerated paramedic training courses between deployments. Only about 15 percent of these medics achieved paramedic certification, but the others were deemed "paramedic trained." This training expanded the range of flight medics' prehospital skills, but it did not address their equally pressing need for post-op and critical care expertise.

In 2009, Secretary of Defense Robert Gates triggered another major change by mandating that all combat casualties have access to surgical care within one hour (Chapter 14). To meet this standard, many FSTs had to split into even smaller units, making it impossible to spare a member to accompany a post-op patient. In response, the theater trauma director in Afghanistan formally requested that a detachment of critical care nurses be assigned to MEDEVAC units to fill the gap. These nurses, first deployed the following year, substantially augmented MEDEVAC units' in-flight critical care capabilities (Chapter 23).

Although Army MEDEVAC units performed the bulk of aeromedical evacuations in Iraq and Afghanistan, two other types of teams warrant comment.

1. **US Air Force Pararescue units**, or "PJs," were assigned the primary mission of rescuing downed pilots and crews from aircraft crashes. PJs combine the tactical and technical skills of a rescue specialist with the medical skills of an advanced emergency care provider (Figure 13.3).

FIGURE 13.3. An 83rd Expeditionary Rescue Squadron pararescue specialist gives an intravenous solution during a joint mass casualty and extraction exercise at Bagram Airfield, Afghanistan, June 16, 2016. Photo by Technical Sergeant Tyrona Lawson, 455th Air Expeditionary Wing. Reproduced from: https://www.dvidshub.net/image/2667959/others-may-live.

They operate in small teams and use special operations aircraft with enhanced, all-weather capabilities. In 2007, PJ units operating out of Bagram Air Field, Afghanistan, began flying MEDEVAC missions when weather prevented the launch of conventional MEDEVAC aircraft. That same year, the Air Force tasked "Guardian Angel" teams—a robust rescue package that includes two aircraft, five PJs, and a combat rescue officer— with a forward MEDEVAC role in Afghanistan.

In 2009, based on the PJs' success and Secretary Gates's "golden hour" directive, the Air Force directed that PJs expand their MEDEVAC activities. The Air Force added a tactical C-130 fixed-wing aircraft staffed with a flight surgeon and PJs to perform far-forward critical care evacuations. These missions typically occurred at night and often involved picking up patients from forward operating bases with a suitable runway for a C-130. Many of those transported had undergone emergency surgery and required ongoing resuscitation.[1]

2. **The United Kingdom's "Medical Emergency Response Team," or MERT,** originated during Operation Iraqi Freedom but evolved significantly when the UK deployed into Helmand Province, Afghanistan, in 2006. The MERT uses a CH-47 "Chinook" helicopter (Figure 13.4), a very large, tandem rotor helicopter capable of carrying a physician, nurse, multiple paramedics, and a security force. The MERT essentially brings a trauma team forward, allowing for rapid resuscitation of several severely injured patients from the point of injury to a combat support hospital. Immediate interventions include advanced airway management and the ability to rapidly transfuse multiple units of blood. Given Helmand Province's large size ($58,000 \text{ km}^2$) and the high incidence of complex blast injuries, physician-led MERTs provided highly advanced care to some of the war's most seriously injured fighters.[1]

IMPACT

Because hospital care has become so effective, most "potentially survivable" combat deaths occur at the scene of injury or en route to the hospital. This makes improving prehospital care the most promising avenue to improve rates of survival (Chapter 35).

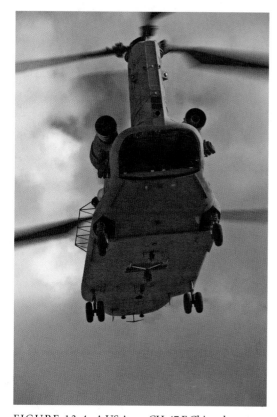

FIGURE 13.4. A US Army CH-47 F Chinook helicopter departs Forward Operating Base Wolverine, Zabul Province, Afghanistan, December 15, 2009. Photo by Technical Sergeant Efren Lopez. Reproduced from: https://www.dvidshub.net/image/233123/operation-enduring-freedom.

PREVENTING IN-FLIGHT HYPOTHERMIA ON MEDEVAC HELICOPTERS

In 2004, I was the officer in charge of a newly developed surgical shock trauma platoon in Taqqadum, Iraq (between Ramadi and Fallujah). The platoon was a combination of one shock trauma platoon and two forward resuscitative surgical systems, consisting of about 45 people. Our first mass casualty incident involved five Marines who had driven over an improvised explosive device in a Humvee that was not up-armored. The team did a great job of appropriately resuscitating the Marines and doing damage control procedures to stabilize them. We swiftly evacuated them to the combat surgical hospital (CSH) in Baghdad.

The next morning, in order to get feedback for our "how can we improve" conference, one of our general surgeons called the Baghdad CSH and got an earful. The surgeon in Baghdad wanted to know why our

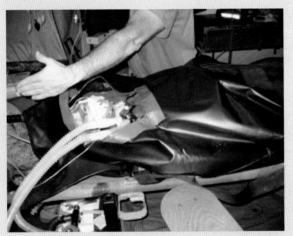

patients had arrived cold, coagulopathic, and unstable. We were dumbstruck, as it was 110 degrees in the shade and the helo [helicopter] ride from Taqqadum to Baghdad was 20 to 25 minutes at most. We quickly surmised that the helos were open to the environment (back ramp, machine gun ports) and that even flying at low altitude in high ambient temperature, the convection currents en route were cooling the patients off.

The "hot pocket." Photo by Rear Admiral Bruce Gillingham, Taqqadum, Iraq, 2004.

We stood there inside our Base-X [HDT Global, Solon, OH] tents brainstorming for 10 to 15 minutes trying to come up with ways to keep the patients warmer en route. We had standard wool blankets as well as space blankets and some heating blankets supplied by battery packs, but these were all inadequate. Finally, from the back of the tent a voice said, "body bags." There was a stunned silence and one of our ED [emergency department] docs derisively said, "We're not giving up on these patients!" The voice (I could not see him in the back of the tent) said, "No, I mean use the body bags as like a sleeping bag. Put the patient and their blankets inside." One of our other ED docs quickly produced a prototype. He cut a small hole for egress of ventilator tubing, and we put red duct tape in the shape of a cross on the chest area to identify the package as a living patient and not remains.

Long story short, the idea worked fabulously, and as chief of professional services, I shared it with the other four surgical units in Al Anbar under my supervision. It quickly spread to the Army units, and eventually made it to Afghanistan. Commercial versions are now available. The originator? An E-4 Navy corpsman who wasn't afraid to think out loud. There is no doubt in my mind that this idea improved outcomes and contributed directly to the outstanding DOW [died of wounds] rate we experienced. We originally called it "the Taqqadum Transport System" but it rapidly became known as the "Hot Pocket."

Rear Admiral Bruce L. Gillingham
Medical Corps, US Navy
Commander, Navy Medicine West

During Operations Enduring Freedom and Iraqi Freedom, several studies confirmed the value of enhancing the staffing of MEDEVAC helicopters.[2,3] In 2009, a group of Army doctors in Afghanistan took advantage of a natural experiment when an Army National Guard MEDEVAC (air ambulance) unit was deployed to their area. This unit was unique in that three-fourths of its flight medics were practicing, critical care-trained civilian paramedics in their regular jobs back home. This essentially put a modern, civilian air ambulance service in a combat zone. In addition to the unit's qualifications and experience (an average of seven years of paramedic experience), each aircraft flew with two providers instead of one, employed standardized protocols, and meticulously documented their care. In addition, the unit's supervisor was an experienced EMS physician who conducted regular quality assurance and quality improvement activities.

To assess the impact of this unit, the Army doctors compared the performance of the National Guard unit to that of legacy EMT-B–staffed MEDEVAC crews before and after the National Guard unit's rotation. The National Guard unit's mortality rate among severely wounded service members was 8 percent, compared to 15 percent in standard MEDEVAC units. After taking differences in case severity into account, the Army doctors determined that MEDEVAC flights staffed by Army National Guard paramedics reduced the odds of dying by 66 percent. On the strength of these findings, the Army changed its doctrine, and began training its flight medics to the level of a critical-care paramedic.[4]

With flight medic capability improved, and critical care flight nurses augmenting many teams, the US military added blood transfusion capability to selected Afghanistan MEDEVAC units in 2012. These double-staffed, blood-capable MEDEVAC missions, codenamed "Vampire," further boosted the critical care capability of these flights.

In addition to these findings, two studies demonstrated a survival benefit with the UK's MERT concept. One compared US and UK trauma registry data from Afghanistan and found that the MERT reduced time to surgery and mortality for certain moderate-to-severely injured casualties.[5] Another compared MERT responses to those made by conventional MEDEVAC units and paramedic PJs, finding that physician-led evacuations achieved higher survival rates.[2] However, these studies are limited because they could not control for important differences in the tactical situations. Also, since MEDEVAC capabilities were in a state of transition during this period, it is unclear how physician-staffed MERT units would stack up

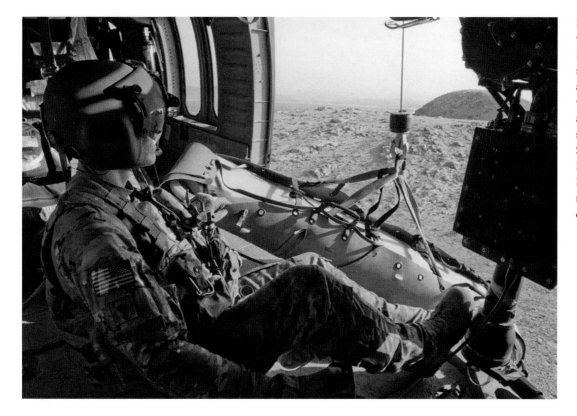

FIGURE 13.5. MEDEVAC crew chief with hoist near Forward Operating Base Fenty, Nangarhar province, Afghanistan, September 16, 2013. Using a hoist allows MEDEVAC crews to raise injured warfighters from remote or treacherous areas where landing the aircraft is impossible. US Army National Guard photo by Sergeant Margaret Taylor, 129th Mobile Public Affairs Detachment/RELEASED. Reproduced from: https://www.dvidshub.net/image/1023428/dustoff-medevac-crew-polishes-rescue-skills.

against MEDEVAC units with paramedics, critical care nurses, and blood capability. Nevertheless, the collective sense from these studies is that better-trained providers produce better outcomes.[1]

A recently published study by Russ Kotwal and colleagues confirmed the value of Secretary Gates's "golden hour" mandate. They found that following Gates's order, casualty evacuation time in Afghanistan fell from an average of 90 minutes to 43 minutes. The killed-in-action rate declined by 6 percent, and the risk of death among all injured decreased from 13 percent to 7 percent. Based on these findings, Kotwal's team estimates that Secretary Gates's mandate probably saved the lives of 359 service members (Figure 13.5).[5]

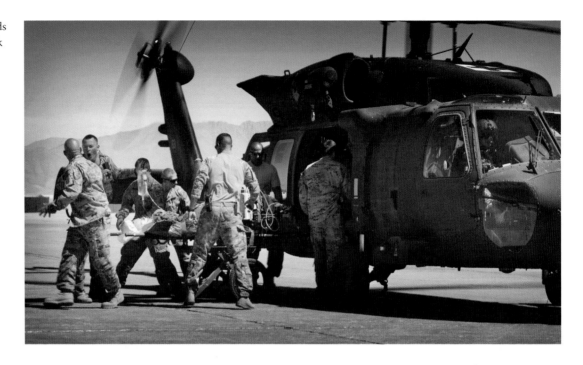

FIGURE 13.6. A Dustoff crew unloads a patient wounded in an insurgent attack on Forward Operating Base Salerno, Afghanistan, June 1, 2012. The MEDEVAC crews were airborne just minutes after receiving word of the incident. Bagram Air Field, Afghanistan. Photo by Sergeant 1st Class Eric Pahon, 82nd Combat Aviation Brigade. Reproduced from: https://www.dvidshub.net/image/613198/dustoff-rescue.

CONCLUSION

The US Army, which pioneered helicopter evacuation in Korea and Vietnam, can be justifiably proud of its role in creating civilian aeromedical EMS. Civilian services built on the Army concept by staffing their aircraft with highly skilled flight nurses and paramedics. After observing the benefits of the EMS approach in Afghanistan, the Army upgraded the staffing of its MEDEVAC aircraft with flight nurses and medics trained to the civilian standard (Figure 13.6). This innovation, and other advances in flight patient management championed by enterprising healthcare providers (see "Preventing In-Flight Hypothermia on MEDEVAC Helicopters") improved the care of battlefield casualties and created a highly flexible and effective medical evacuation system.

Notes

1. Olson CM Jr, Bailey J, Mabry R, et al. Forward aeromedical evacuation: a brief history, lessons learned from the Global War on Terror, and the way forward for US policy. *J Trauma Acute Care Surg.* 2013;75:S130–136.

2. Apodaca A, Olson CM Jr, Bailey J, et al. Performance improvement evaluation of forward aeromedical evacuation platforms in Operation Enduring Freedom. *J Trauma Acute Care Surg.* 2013;75:S157–S63.

3. Kotwal RS, Howard JT, Orman JA, et al. The Effect of a golden hour policy on the morbidity and mortality of combat casualties. *JAMA Surg.* 2015;30:1-10.

4. Mabry RL, Apodaca A, Penrod J, et al. Impact of critical care trained flight paramedics on casualty survival during helicopter evacuation in the current war in Afghanistan. *J Trauma Acute Care Surg.* 2012;73:S32–37.

5. Morrison JJ, Oh J, DuBose JJ, et al. En-route care capability from point of injury impacts mortality after severe wartime injury. *Ann Surg.* 2013;257:330–334.

Recommended Reading

Taylor AL, Corley JB. Theater blood support in the prehospital setting. *US Army Med Dep J.* 2016;Apr-Sep:43–47.

Davids NB. Shaping the flight paramedic program. *US Army Med Dep J.* 2016;Apr-Sep;48–51.

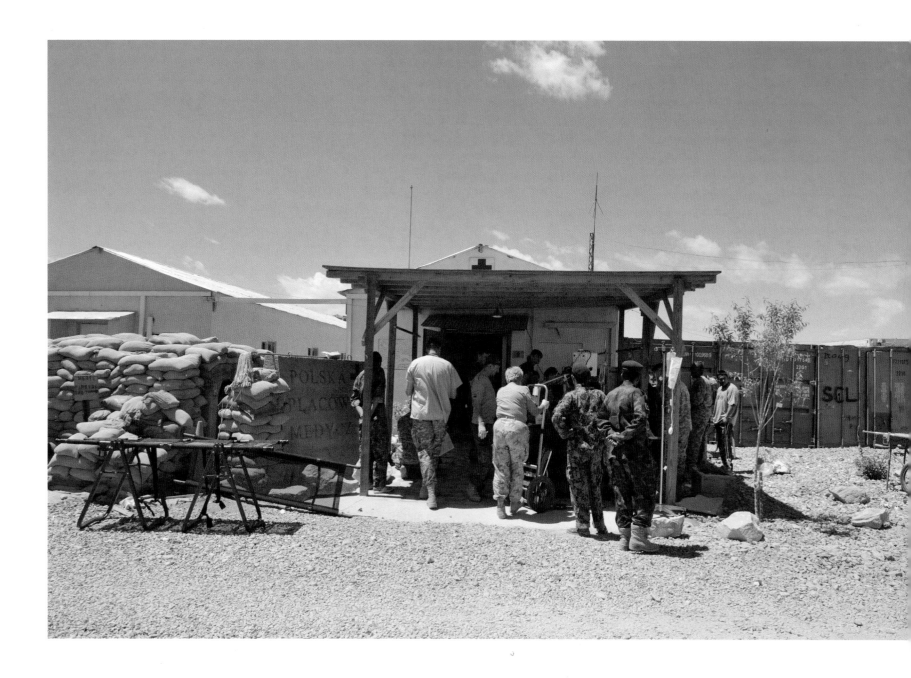

CHAPTER fourteen

The Forward Surgical Team

STEPHEN P. HETZ, MD

THE CHALLENGE

COMBAT MEDICINE IS DESIGNED TO GET WOUNDED SOLDIERS the care they need as quickly and as safely as possible. Treatment starts at the point of injury, with immediate first aid by combat medics or corpsmen. It continues all the way to sophisticated medical, surgical, reconstructive, and rehabilitative care at large medical centers in the United States. In America's military health system, there are four levels or "Roles" of care defined by the capabilities of the facility. Care starts with the front line medic (Role 1), and ends at a major military medical center (Role 4, see Figure 8.2).[1] Skilled medical evacuation from one level to the next is crucial to the system's effectiveness.

Historically, the first level of care where surgery was available was the Role 3 medical treatment facility (CSH or mobile Army surgical hospital).[1] The Role 3 facility was often located many minutes, if not hours, away from the fighting. Unfortunately, it was not uncommon for patients to die from a surgically correctable injury before they reached the nearest Role 3 facility.

MOVING SURGICAL CARE CLOSER TO THE BATTLEFIELD

The forward surgical team (FST) is designed to perform resuscitative surgery essential to stabilizing severely injured patients so they may be safely evacuated to the next level of medical care. During the

FIGURE 14.1. [*Opposite*] An outside view of the forward surgical team at Forward Operating Base Ghazni, Afghanistan, April 22, 2010. Reproduced from: https://www.dvidshub.net/ image/272854/ghazni-mass-casualty-operations.

American Civil War and World War I, military medical providers pushed lifesaving surgical teams close to the fighting (Chapter 2). With the advent of MEDEVAC helicopters in Korea and Vietnam, forward surgery fell out of favor, and the military began opting instead to transport casualties to the nearest Role 3 hospital.

In the 1980s, the idea of providing forward surgical care (now considered a Role 2 capability) with mobile, self-contained teams able to perform damage control surgery in austere settings began to take hold. Each service developed its own version. The Air Force, Navy, and Army versions were the MFST (Mobile Field Surgical Team), FRSS (Forward Resuscitative Surgical System), and FST, respectively.

The Special Operations community took a different approach. It created eight-Soldier teams anchored by two general surgeons that were able to perform damage control surgery in austere conditions *and* safely evacuate injured patients to a higher level of care. This allowed Special Operations forces to work far from the nearest Role 3 and well outside the range of transport required to reach conventional trauma care within the "golden hour" (Chapter 1).

FSTs sacrifice extensive surgical capability for mobility and proximity to the battlefield. They enable damage control surgical capability (Chapter 15) to closely follow and support brigade-sized units (about 5,000 troops) on the battlefield, but they cannot manage large numbers of critically injured casualties for extended periods of time (Figure 14.1).

FORWARD SURGICAL TEAMS IN IRAQ AND AFGHANISTAN

The first large-scale deployment of FSTs occurred during Operations Iraqi Freedom and Enduring Freedom. During the 2003 ground invasion of Iraq, this forward surgical system performed well. FSTs maneuvered with their assigned brigades and achieved good outcomes for wounded troops (Figure 14.2).

However, problems developed when the war's maneuver phase ended and the conflict evolved into an insurgency. This coincided with the development and positioning of robust Role 3 facilities. Initially, smaller units retained control of their FSTs and treated them as small hospitals. As a result, FSTs began performing operations that could be better handled at well-equipped CSHs only minutes (not hours)

VIGNETTE >> The forward surgical team (FST) was alerted only moments before a 24-year-old US Soldier who had been shot several times with an AK-47 assault rifle reached their base. The initial report stated the patient was conscious and able to maintain his airway, but had multiple gunshot wounds to his chest and legs. The FST immediately began preparing the blood products he'd need. When the Soldier arrived, the team noted he had an entrance wound in his right lateral chest and a markedly distended abdomen. Tourniquets placed on both legs had stopped the bleeding from gunshot wounds to his thighs. The patient was awake but confused. He had a rapid heart rate (150 beats a minute) and extremely low blood pressure—both indications of shock. Suspecting trapped air and blood in his chest, the team inserted a large bore tube. A sudden rush of air and blood confirmed their suspicion. Resuscitative treatment included a rapid transfusion of packed red blood cells and plasma in equal proportions, warmed to 40°C by a rapid blood infuser device.

Initial decision point: Can the patient be transported to the next level of care without immediate surgery? Answer: No.

Resuscitation continued as the wounded Soldier was moved to the adjacent operating room. After he was rapidly anesthetized, the surgical team members opened his abdomen, which was filled with blood. After controlling the bleeding with multiple surgical packs, the operating room team identified a large gunshot wound to the liver as the major source of bleeding.

Next decision point: What is required to stabilize the patient and allow safe transport to the next level of care?

As warmed blood products were infused, the surgical team isolated and controlled the sources of bleeding using a combination of clamps, sutures, and packing. Team members also identified and surgically addressed multiple injuries to the stomach, small bowel, and colon. Once that was done, they washed out the Soldier's abdominal cavity to reduce contamination, and performed a temporary surgical closure. Then they surgically explored the leg wounds and removed the tourniquets, which the patient tolerated well. Because the large bones of both legs were fractured, the team applied splints to avoid further injury. Then they dressed all open wounds. Over the course of his surgery, the Soldier received 12 units of fresh whole blood, 12 units of packed red blood cells, 13 units of plasma, and 5 units of clotting factors (Chapter 16).

As the patient was taken to the FST's small recovery area, his vital signs were stable, and he had no evidence of ongoing bleeding. Within an hour of this damage control surgery (Chapter 15), a second MEDEVAC helicopter was transporting the patient to the next level of care, a combat support hospital (CSH).

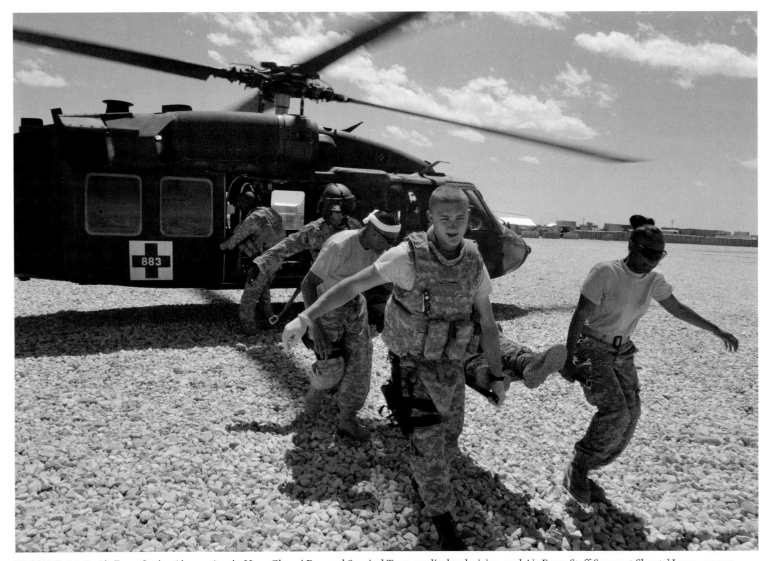

FIGURE 14.2. Air Force Senior Airman Austin Hess, Ghazni Forward Surgical Team medical technician, and Air Force Staff Sergeant Shante' Lopez carry a liter with an American Soldier from a MEDEVAC helicopter to Forward Operating Base Ghazni. April 22, 2010. Reproduced from: https://www.dvidshub.net/image/272860/ghazni-mass-casualty-operations.

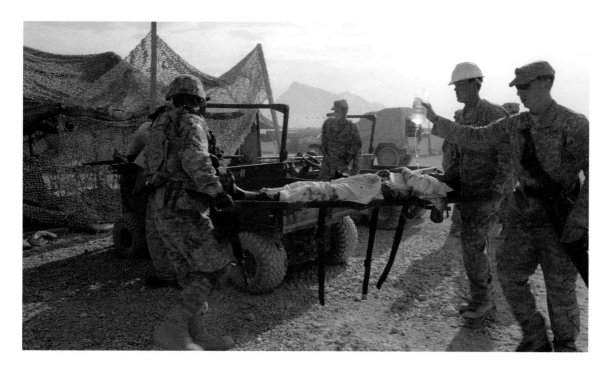

FIGURE 14.3. US Army Sergeant Justin White and Specialist Robert Cahill, both certified combat life savers from the 4-73rd Cavalry, 82nd Airborne, transport a suicide bomb victim to the triage tent outside the Forney Clinic located on Forward Operating Base Farah, Afghanistan, November 20, 2009. Reproduced from: https://www.dvidshub.net/image/225763/suicide-bomber-strikes-farah-city.

away. This resulted in an Army-wide directive to bypass FSTs in favor of the better-equipped CSHs. As a result, most wounded personnel in Iraq were transported to a CSH.

In Afghanistan, ground fighting was intense but sporadic, and occurred throughout a large, mountainous country (Chapter 6). Initially, only two FSTs accompanied US ground operations in Afghanistan, and no CSH was available during the campaign's first two months. With essentially no backup, these FSTs had to function as small hospitals (Figure 14.3). Eventually the military placed CSHs in strategic locations to help.[2,3]

To get surgical care closer to the widely dispersed fighting in Afghanistan, the military split the operations of CSHs and FSTs. This left each FST with only one anesthetist, and only one of the two "splits" had an orthopedic surgeon (Figure 14.4). Some feared these split teams would be unable to provide effective surgery. Fortunately, an analysis found that severely injured patients who received initial treat-

FIGURE 14.4. [*Opposite*] US Army
Major Neil McMullin, assigned to a
forward surgical team, holds bags of
saline while Majors Brian Helsel and
Matthew Hueman clean the broken
arm of an Afghanistan National Army
Soldier at Field Operating Base Shank,
Afghanistan, November 7, 2009. Reproduced from: https://www.dvidshub.
net/image/222953/operation-enduring-
freedom.

ment in an FST did as well as those treated in a CSH.[4] Likewise, FSTs performing split-based operations achieved excellent results, as long as they were staffed with experienced personnel and surgeons strictly adhered to damage control principles.[5]

TODAY'S FORWARD SURGICAL CAPABILITY

The current US Army Techniques Publication 4-02.5, *Casualty Care*, states, "The forward surgical team is a 20-Soldier team which provides far forward surgical intervention to render nontransportable patients sufficiently stable to allow for medical evacuation to a Role 3 combat support hospital."[6(p3-22)] ("Transportability refers to the patient's ability to survive evacuation to the next level of care. Nontransportable patients are those patients with severe wounds and uncontrollable hemorrhage that may not survive evacuation without immediate resuscitative surgery. These patients are the prime candidates for FST intervention."[7(p1-2)]) The Navy (which also supports the Marine Corps) Role 2 team, the FRSS, is similarly configured and equipped. Air Force Role 2 surgical teams range in size from austere (the MFST, a five-person unit) to robust (Expeditionary Medical Support, or EMEDS, Basic, which is staffed by 25 Air Force medical personnel). Regardless of their size, all FSTs require supporting elements to operate for extended periods of time (Figure 14.5). Some FSTs use parachutes to bring personnel and equipment (including vehicles) to airborne operations.[8] Though the services use different names for their FSTs, their mission capabilities are very similar. We will use an Army FST's specifics to illustrate the capabilities of all.

CAPABILITIES

The Army techniques publication says that an FST's function "is to perform triage/preoperative resuscitation, initial surgery, and postoperative nursing care. Organic personnel set up and break down the shelter system in preparation of operations or unit movement, prepare the patient for surgery, perform essential surgeries for a maximum of 30 patients within 72 hours, and provide postoperative nursing care and stabilization for medical evacuation to the next role of medical care."[6(p3-23)]

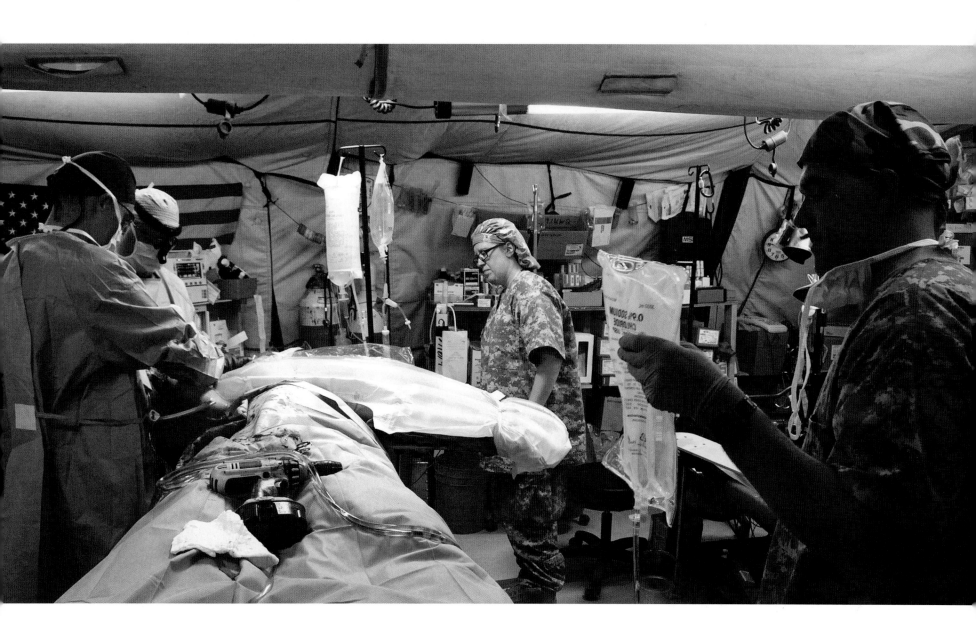

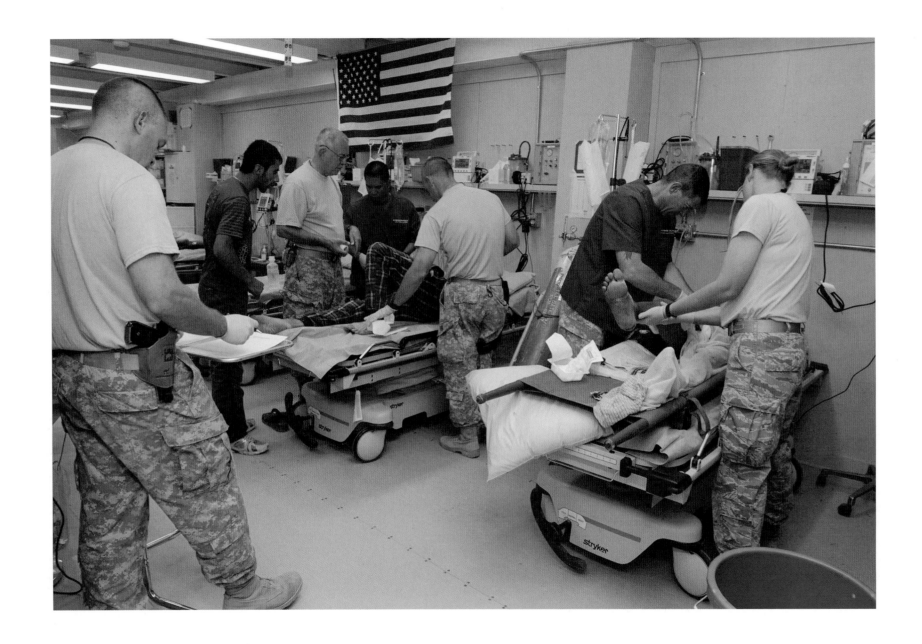

An FST's main task is to immediately resuscitate patients and perform damage control surgery (Chapter 15). The goal is to gain rapid control of internal bleeding, prevent further contamination of the abdomen from wounds, warm the patient as needed, and provide necessary blood products (Chapter 16) to enable the patient to survive transport to the next level of care. Definitive surgical procedures (such as vascular reconstruction, intestinal repairs, and anastomoses) are rarely done at FSTs. Wound closure is generally temporary, recognizing that further procedures, including definitive repair and reconstruction, will take place at the next or even higher levels of care.[9]

Not all patients brought to an FST undergo an operation there. The only ones who do are those who need life- or limb-saving surgery prior to transport to the next level of care. The decision to operate at the FST or defer surgery until later depends on many factors, including patient stability, terrain, weather, combat situation, casualty load, availability of blood and other supplies, and availability of medical evacuation. In war, the traditional meaning of *triage* applies. When resources are finite, as they often are in an FST, surgeons base their decisions on what will do the most good for the largest number of casualties.

FUTURE DIRECTIONS

In Afghanistan and Iraq, FSTs saved many lives. It's tempting to assume they will have similar success in future conflicts. Although we should continue to expect FSTs to provide far-forward surgical intervention to render non-transportable patients sufficiently stable to allow for medical evacuation to a combat support hospital, future battlefields may present different challenges than those encountered in Iraq and Afghanistan (see Chapter 34). For example, in future conflicts where air supremacy is not assured, FSTs may have to provide prolonged field care.

Regardless of future challenges, FSTs will need properly trained personnel who can perform lifesaving procedures in a wide variety of environments. In particular, the military will need well-trained and experienced general surgeons and anesthesia personnel who are skilled at performing damage control surgery and resuscitation (Chapters 15 and 16). Future conflicts may require new skills and capabilities, but they are unlikely to diminish the need for FSTs.

FIGURE 14.5. [*Opposite*] Members of the 934th Forward Surgical Team assess two Afghan patients upon their arrival at Forward Operating Base Sharana, September 9, 2008. Reproduced from: https://www.dvidshub.net/image/323399/934th-fst-waiting-patiently-save-your-life.

Notes

1. Hetz SP. Introduction to military medicine: a brief overview. *Surg Clin North Am.* 2006;86:675–688.
2. Peoples GE, Gerlinger T, Craig R, Burlingame B. The 274th Forward Surgical Team experience during Operation Enduring Freedom. *Mil Med.* 2005;170:451–459.
3. Rush RM, Stockmaster NR, Stinger HK, et al. Supporting the Global War on Terror: a tale of two campaigns featuring the 250th Forward Surgical Team (Airborne). *Am J Surg.* 2005;189:564–570; discussion 570.
4. Eastridge, BJ, Stansbury, LG, Stinger H, Blackbourne L, Holcomb JB. Forward surgical teams provide comparable outcomes to combat support hospitals during support and stabilization operations on the battlefield. *J Trauma.* 2009;66:S48–S50.
5. Nessen SC, Cronk DR, Edens J, et al. US Army two-surgeon teams operating in remote Afghanistan—an evaluation of split-based forward surgical operations. *J Trauma.* 2009;66:S37–47.
6. Headquarters, Department of the Army. *Casualty Care.* Washington, DC: HQDA, 2013. ATP 4-02.5.
7. Headquarters, Department of the Army. *Employment of Forward Surgical Teams.* Washington, DC: HQDA; 2003. FM 4-02.25. (Inactive.)
8. Stinger H, Rush R. The Army forward surgical team: update and lessons learned, 1997-2004. *Mil Med.* 2006;171:269–272.
9. *Emergency War Surgery.* 4th US rev. Fort Sam Houston, TX: Borden Institute; 2013: Chap 12.

Recommended Reading

Freel D, War BJ. Surgical and resuscitation capabilities for the "next war" based on lessons learned from "this war." *US Army Med Dep J.* 2016;Apr-Sep:188–191.

CHAPTER fifteen

Damage Control Surgery

MICHAEL F. ROTONDO, MD; C. WILLIAM SCHWAB, MD; and
BRIAN J. EASTRIDGE, MD

THE CHALLENGE

ACROSS THE CITIES, DESERTS, AND MOUNTAINS of southwest Asia, the battlefield scenario of severe injuries and massive bleeding played out countless times over the last decade and a half. Such injuries generally were caused by explosive devices and high muzzle velocity firearms. The wounded, if able, initiated their own medical care. Medics and corpsman swiftly responded to apply tourniquets and initiate other lifesaving care at the point of injury (Figure 15.1). However, bleeding from noncompressible sources (eg, chest, abdomen, and pelvis) are difficult or impossible to control with the current tools and techniques available in the prehospital or tactical environment. With the "clock ticking" from the moment of injury, it is crucial to get these wounded troops to surgery as soon as possible. That is why the military emphasizes, whenever possible, rapid evacuation from the battlefield to forward surgical capabilities, ideally within the "golden hour" for trauma care.

In addition, the wars in Afghanistan and Iraq sometimes produced mass casualties that threatened to overwhelm a small medical facility's finite resources. In such a circumstance, medical teams triaged casualties for operations, and surgeons had to perform quick but temporary interventions to save as many lives as possible.

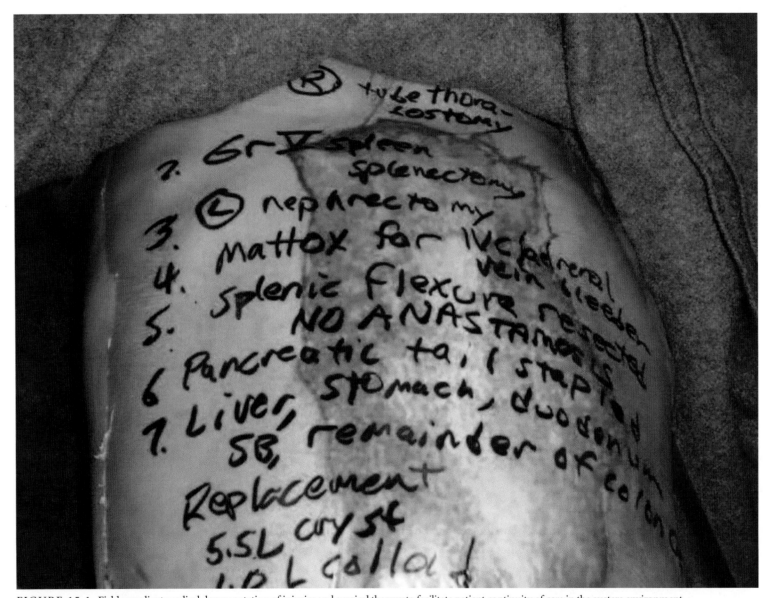

FIGURE 15.1. Field expedient medical documentation of injuries and surgical therapy to facilitate patient continuity of care in the austere environment.
Photograph: Courtesy of the Borden Institute.

VIGNETTE >> A 23-year-old Army Sergeant on foot patrol in a mountainous region of eastern Afghanistan suffered multiple gunshot wounds to the abdomen during a firefight with insurgent forces. An Army medic provided immediate Tactical Combat Casualty Care on the scene and a MEDEVAC (medical evacuation) helicopter flew the soldier to an Army Forward Surgical Team (see Chapter 14) at a nearby forward operating base. Upon arrival, the Sergeant had a dangerously low blood pressure from ongoing bleeding in his abdomen. The medical team quickly placed large-bore intravenous lines and began a massive transfusion of banked blood and plasma. They also issued a base-wide call for donations of fresh whole blood from persons with his blood type (see Chapter 16).

The Forward Surgical Team took the badly injured Sergeant to their operating room, a plywood shack outfitted with two operating room tables, surgical lighting, and surgical instruments. Once he was under anesthesia, they rapidly opened and explored his abdomen, noting multiple gunshot wounds to his liver, spleen, the blood vessels supplying his left kidney, and multiple loops of small intestines. Working quickly to minimize additional blood loss, the surgeons removed the Soldier's shattered spleen and nonsalvageable left kidney and packed his liver injuries to control bleeding. They also removed the injured segments of bowel and closed the open ends with surgical staples. Once the bleeding was controlled, they packed his abdomen with absorbent surgical pads. Instead of closing his abdominal incision, they left it open, opting to cover his entire abdomen with a large adhesive dressing.

Two hours later, a MEDEVAC helicopter team with a critical care nurse and paramedic (see Chapter 23) arrived to fly the Soldier to the US Air Force's Role 3 hospital in Bagram, Afghanistan. There, combat surgeons took the Sergeant back to surgery because he was becoming unstable again and required additional transfusions. They found the bleeding was coming from a damaged artery in his abdominal wall, which they closed off. Because his bowel injuries still were not definitively repaired, they again left the midline abdominal incision open and re-covered it with another occlusive dressing. Resuscitation continued in the intensive care unit (ICU).

The following evening, the patient was flown by C-17 transport, accompanied by an Air Force Critical Care Air Transport Team (CCATT) (see Chapter 25) to the Landstuhl Regional Medical Center in Germany. During surgery the next morning, doctors reconnected the Soldier's previously stapled bowel ends, but were unable to close his abdomen due to bowel swelling. The next morning, he was loaded on another CCATT flight to the United States and eventually to Walter Reed National Military Medical Center (Bethesda, MD). There, his bowel swelling decreased enough for surgeons to close his abdomen. During the 84-hour evacuation from Afghanistan to the United States, this Army Sergeant had four major abdominal operations, and received 21 units of packed red blood cells, nine units of type-specific fresh warm whole blood, and 19 units of plasma (see Chapter 16). After his final operation, he rapidly improved and returned to full duty within six months of his original injuries.

THE INNOVATION

Once wounded service members reached a Forward Surgical Team or combat support hospital, the question was how much surgery should be done versus deferred to a later time. Because these facilities are generally staffed by relatively small teams and have limited holding capability, it soon became apparent that the best approach was not to make every needed repair, but instead to identify and swiftly control life-threatening problems, such as ongoing abdominal bleeding, intestinal perforations, and other dangerous problems. This approach, which had been pioneered by former military surgeons in the civilian world, is known as "damage control" surgery.

Within minutes to hours of completing damage control surgery, casualties are typically evacuated to higher level medical treatment facilities that have increased capabilities, more personnel, greater operating room capacity, more hospital and ICU beds, specialty surgery, and advanced radiographic imaging. Most casualties who undergo damage control surgery are immediately imaged and evaluated by specialty surgeons, then returned to the operating room for further management. These procedures are generally another form of damage control designed to stop internal bleeding and address other immediately life-threatening conditions, followed by ongoing resuscitation and diagnostic evaluation in the ICU. Concurrent with the development of these surgical techniques, the military refined its rotary and fixed-wing evacuation strategies to enable Critical Care Air Transport to higher levels of care far from the war zone. Once a patient is transported to Landstuhl, Germany, or a major military hospital in the United States, teams are better staffed and resourced to focus on definitive repair of injuries, and initiate the process of convalescence and rehabilitation.

THE DAMAGE CONTROL PHILOSOPHY

Naval vessels are constantly at risk of damage from hostile acts or mechanical failures that can compromise their mission. To minimize this possibility, the Navy has long pursued the philosophy of damage control to bolster the "capacity of a ship to absorb damage and maintain mission integrity." Central tenets include suppressing fire, controlling hull breaches (flooding), and preserving the vessel (Figure 15.2).

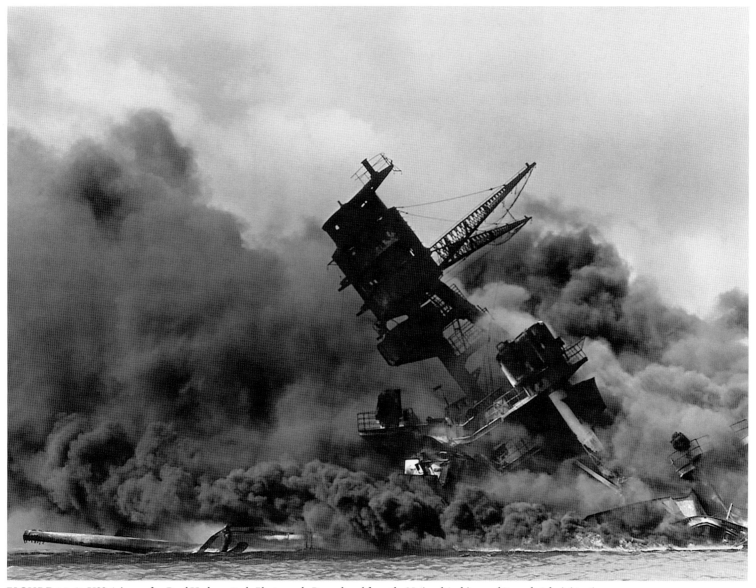

FIGURE 15.2. USS *Arizona* after Pearl Harbor attack. Photograph: Reproduced from the National Archives and Records Administration, Archival Research Catalog, ARC Identifier 195617.

FIGURE 15.3. "Bloody vicious cycle" of hypothermia, acidosis, and coagulopathy, which if not corrected leads to death from hemorrhage after injury.

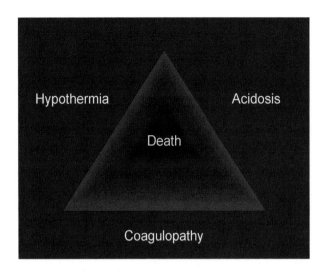

The medical term that emerged from this philosophy, *damage control* surgery, was predicated on similarly simple objectives to save lives. On the battlefield, damage control techniques are valuable to cope with mass casualties and control active bleeding, particularly from injured arms or legs. Severe combat injuries often produce massive hemorrhage, profound consequences of shock (inadequate transport of oxygen to tissues), and insufficient ability to form blood clots (coagulopathy). If bleeding continues, the casualty develops increasingly severe metabolic disturbances, including an inability to regulate body temperature, acidic changes to blood chemistry, and further loss of the body's ability to form blood clots. If these abnormalities are not corrected, a vicious cycle can develop that will lead to death (Figure 15.3).

Damage control surgery involves a brief exploration of the abdomen to find and control major sources of bleeding and control contamination from intestinal contents or external debris driven into the wounds. Meanwhile, the patient receives a balanced mix of blood, plasma, and platelets or fresh whole blood to restore circulating blood volume and correct clotting abnormalities. At this stage, surgeons often leave the abdomen "open" (covered by a large translucent adhesive dressing). This makes it easier to prevent complications related to fluid accumulation and swelling. Resuscitation continues in the ICU to treat shock and other metabolic derangements. Then, new exploratory surgeries can begin in the operating room.

Initially, the damage control philosophy was mainly applied to abdominal injuries. However, as the conflict progressed, doctors had to use the approach to deal with vascular, thoracic, orthopedic, and neurosurgical cases as well. Meanwhile, the concept of "damage control resuscitation"—the administration of a balanced combination of packed red blood cells, plasma, and platelets augmented by proclotting agents such as TXA (tranexamic acid) to reverse the coagulopathy of trauma—replaced lost blood and improved patients' physical condition (see Chapters 16 and 17). The combination of rapidly restoring lost blood, surgically controlling bleeding, and promoting the process of clotting saved many troops who previously would have died from massive hemorrhage.

IMPACT

Use of the damage control approach to control abdominal hemorrhage was first described by Drs. Rotondo and Schwab (the latter a former Navy surgeon). Responding to a surge of urban gun violence in the early 1990s, they devised a three-stage approach to improve survival from penetrating abdominal trauma and introduced the term damage control into the vernacular of civilian trauma surgery.[1] As other civilian doctors refined the technique, and survival rates improved, damage control became a guiding principle in managing critically injured patients. Seasoned trauma surgeons and surgical trainees matured the principles and practiced damage control surgery in the 1990s. Serendipitously, because many of these surgeons were among the first to deploy to Iraq and Afghanistan, they took the principles of damage control surgery with them to the battlefield.

Soon, trauma literature included articles and information suggesting damage control surgery was as effective in war zones as it was in the civilian world.[2,3] Combat areas, however, carried special challenges, including dynamic battlefield environments, austere and hostile surroundings, and the need to continue resuscitation and critical care during medical evacuations spanning great distances.

Over the course of Operation Enduring Freedom and Operation Iraqi Freedom, damage control surgery proved its worth and became the new standard of care. Expanding and refining the concept led to the elaboration and dissemination of several relevant, evidence–based Clinical Practice Guidelines by the Joint Trauma System (see Chapter 8). Metrics tracked to assess the impact of these practice guidelines demonstrated remarkable improvements in outcomes.[4]

The complimentary approaches of *damage control resuscitation* and *damage control surgery* saved innumerable lives in Iraq and Afghanistan. In the early years of Operation Enduring Freedom and

ONE TEAM, ONE FIGHT

Northern Iraq, 2004. An Air Force Special Ops helicopter flew two severely wounded Special Operators—one Army, one Navy—from a battle in northern Iraq to the Army's combat support hospital in Mosul, commanded at the time by Colonel Jim Ficke (Uniformed Services University of the Health Sciences [USU] class of '87). Both operators immediately underwent damage control surgery. Shortly thereafter, they were flown aboard an Army MEDEVAC UH-60 helicopter to Balad Air Force Theater Hospital north of Baghdad. There, Colonel Jack Ingari (USU class of '86) operated on them again. Following this surgery, they were flown on an Air Force C-17 to Landstuhl Regional Medical Center in Germany for additional treatment before being transported back to the United States.

Meanwhile, in southern Iraq, a Marine with severe head and torso injuries as well as burns was flown to the Al Taqaddum Air Base, where he was met by a Navy surgical shock trauma platoon commanded by Captain Bruce Gillingham (USU class of '86). This Marine also underwent immediate damage control surgery. Once his immediate life-threatening injuries were treated, he was flown to Balad in a Navy MEDEVAC C-46 helicopter. At Balad, he went back to the operating room for neurosurgery and additional burn care.

As the Balad team operated on this injured Marine, they contacted Landstuhl, commanded at the time by Colonel Rhonda Cornum (USU class of '86). Colonel Cornum was aware that a Brooke Army Medical Center (BAMC) burn team was at her hospital preparing to accompany another burn patient back to Texas. She asked them to delay their departure so they could also take the inbound Marine.

When the Marine emerged from surgery at Balad, the neurosurgeon who operated on him, as well as the anesthesiologist and a respiratory therapist, rushed him to the airfield and stayed with him throughout the six-hour, 2,100-mile flight to Germany (Chapter 25). At Landstuhl, BAMC's burn team took over and prepared the Marine for the even longer, 5,350-mile flight to San Antonio. Once preparations were complete, the Marine was taken back to Ramstien Air Base, where he, the other burn patient, and the two wounded Special Operators from Mosul were loaded onto a waiting C-17 along with other casualties. Together, these wounded warriors, attended by BAMC's burn team, an Air Force Critical Care Air Transport Team, and an air evacuation crew flew back to the United States.

This precise choreography was possible because the Army, Navy, and Air Force worked as one. Also, it was not unusual for doctors who trained together at USU (Chapter 3) to end up working with each other downrange. Throughout Operations Enduring Freedom and Iraqi Freedom, our military health professionals embodied the phrase "One Team, One Fight."

Brigadier General (Retired) Kory Cornum
Air Mobility Command Surgeon, 2014–2016
Keesler Medical Center Commander, 2010–2014

Brigadier General (Retired) Rhonda Cornum
Commander, Landstuhl Regional Medical Center, 2003–2005
US Army Forces Command Surgeon, 2005–2007
Assistant Surgeon General for Force Projection, 2008
Director, Comprehensive Soldier Fitness, 2009–2012

Operation Iraqi Freedom, only about 40 percent of combat casualties requiring massive transfusions for hemorrhage survived. Refinement of damage control surgical techniques, combined with the development of damage control resuscitation, more than doubled this group's survival rate to 85 percent or better.[5] These advances and other developments pushed the overall combat casualty survival rate to the highest level recorded in the history of warfare.[6]

NEXT STEPS

To sustain and advance military surgery in the interwar interval, we must see that the civilian medical world benefits from what the military has learned. Fostering a strong military–civilian partnership in trauma care will also help prepare young military surgeons for the battlefields of tomorrow. We should use research and development to fill gaps in knowledge and refine damage control principles.

Current recommendations include establishing a joint service standard for predeployment training, sustained support for the Joint Trauma System and the continued development and updating of Clinical Practice Guidelines, greater involvement of military hospitals in civilian trauma systems, improved access to training opportunities for surgeons in the Reserves, leveraging military–civilian trauma training partnerships, augmenting civilian trauma courses with combat trauma-specific content, and the creation of relevant "just-in time" training specific to the deployed environment.[7]

CONCLUSION

Damage control surgery is becoming more important in civilian trauma centers due to the increase in mass shootings and the potential for more frequent acts of domestic and international terrorism. It is also likely that the technique will become more important on future battlefields, where the challenge of providing combat casualty care may be compounded by asymmetric warfare, the requirement for prolonged field care, lack of air supremacy, higher volumes of casualties and more destructive mechanisms of injury (see Chapter 34). For all of these reasons, military and civilian surgeons and all members of trauma teams must be competent in using damage control principles to save patients with life-threatening injuries and respond more effectively to disasters and mass casualty events. One team, one fight.

Notes

1. Rotondo MF, Schwab CW, McGonigal MD, et al. 'Damage control': an approach for improved survival in exsanguinating penetrating abdominal injury. *J Trauma.* 1993;35:375–382, discussion 383–383.
2. Beekley AC, Watts DM. Combat trauma experience with the United States Army 102nd Forward Surgical Team in Afghanistan. *Am J Surg.* 2004;187:652–654.
3. Sambasivan CN, Underwood SJ, Cho S, et al. Comparison of abdominal damage control surgery in combat versus civilian trauma. *J Trauma.* 2010;60(suppl 1):S168–S174.
4. Eastridge BJ, Wade CE, Spott MA, et al. Utilizing a trauma systems approach to benchmark and improve combat casualty care. *J Trauma.* 2010;60(suppl 1):S5–S9.
5. Borgman MS, Spinella PC, Perkins JG, et al. The ration of blood products transfused affects mortality in patients receiving massive transfusions at a combat support hospital. *J Trauma.* 2007;63:805–813.
6. Kotwal RS, Howard JT, Orman JA, et al. The effect of a golden hour policy on the morbidity and mortality of combat casualties. *JAMA Surg.* 2016;151:15–24.
7. Schwab CW. Winds of war: enhancing Civilian and Military partnerships to assure readiness: White Paper. *J Am Coll Surg.* 2015;221:235–254.

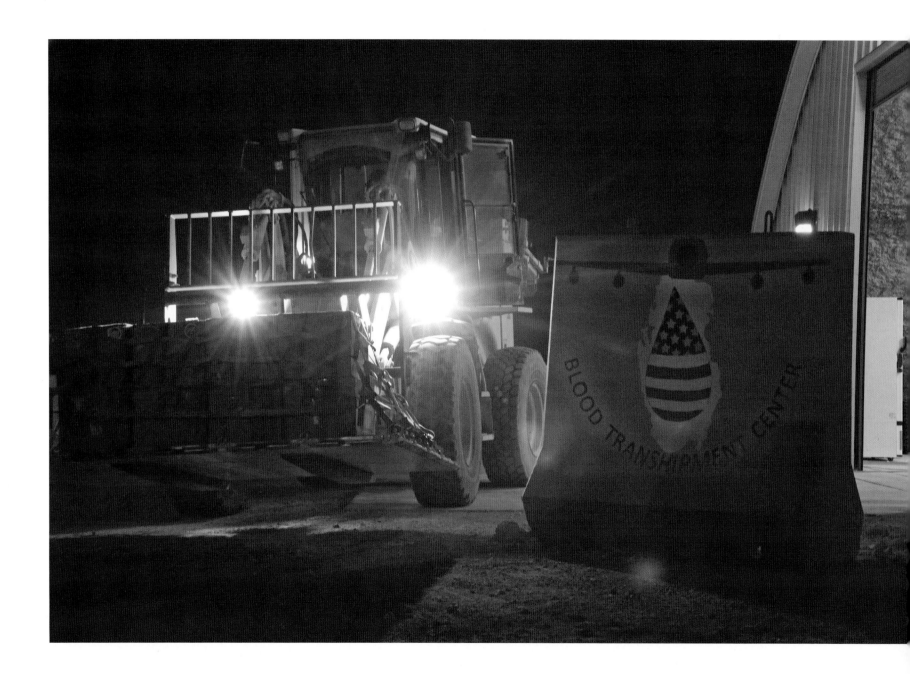

CHAPTER sixteen

Balanced Resuscitation

JEREMY W. CANNON, MD, SM; PETER RHEE, MD, MPH; and
MARTIN A. SCHREIBER, MD

THE PROBLEM

BLOOD IS VITAL FOR LIFE. If too much is lost, irreversible shock ensues and death quickly follows. Preventing death from blood loss requires a coordinated effort to stop the bleeding and restore lost blood volume. On the battlefield, first responders must find and compress visibly bleeding wounds or apply a tourniquet to stop arterial bleeding from badly damaged limbs (Chapters 10–12). At that point, the patient must be quickly transported (Chapter 13) to a forward surgical team or combat surgical hospital for emergency surgery to repair the source of bleeding (Chapters 14 and 15). While surgery is underway, medical teams must restore the patient's blood volume to deliver enough oxygen to preserve vital organ function and support adequate clot formation (Figure 16.1). This may sound straightforward, but determining the best way to resuscitate such patients has dramatically evolved over the past century.

The first human blood transfusion was given in 1818. However, the logistics of collecting and administering blood before it clotted made transfusion very difficult. Viral infections and severe reactions to transfusions made them prohibitively risky for many years.[2] At the same time, the precise cause of shock and the best method of treating it were unknown well into World War II.[2] Edward Churchill, a civilian thoracic surgeon from Harvard serving in the Mediterranean and North African combat zones, was the

FIGURE 16.1. [*Opposite*] US Air Force Senior Airman Celina Garcia, a medical logistics technician with the 379th Expeditionary Medical Group blood transshipment center, drives a 10K forklift in order to move a pallet of blood units at Al Udeid Air Base, Qatar, Jan. 27, 2017. Reproduced from: https://www.dvidshub.net/image/3128419/blood-transhipment-airmen.

first to firmly establish posttraumatic shock with severe blood loss in 1943. Once this cause-and-effect connection was clarified, he concluded that the best approach to treatment involved replacement with whole blood rather than plasma or some other intravenous fluid.[2]

Whole blood transfusions continued until the mid-20th century. Units of whole blood were even shipped from the United States to Vietnam for use in combat casualties. Although some observed that *fresh* whole blood (blood collected on site and immediately transfused) restored clotting function better than stored whole blood, it's not easy to collect and administer fresh whole blood. First, suitable volunteer donors representing all blood types must be available nearby. Second, personnel must be able to quickly test the blood for compatibility and the presence of infectious diseases, and then store it—even if only briefly—in special containers with preservative fluid.

To address these challenges, blood banks in the late 1960s and early 1970s began routinely separating blood into four components—red blood cells, plasma (clotting factors), cryoprecipitate (concentrated clotting factors), and platelets—and storing them separately. Unfortunately for massively bleeding patients, emergently re-creating the right mixture of elements is challenging (Figure 16.2). At worst, doctors focused on giving red blood cells and didn't adequately replace lost platelets and clotting factors. At best, the mix of red cells, platelets, and clotting proteins never restored the patient's blood to the optimum levels found in fresh whole blood.

TRANSFUSION IN THE EARLY 2000S

Throughout the 1980s and 1990s, initial administration of crystalloids (a salt water solution with some minerals) was the preferred method of resuscitation.[1,2] When a trauma patient arrived who had lost a large amount of blood, the first step was to give two liters of crystalloid solution. If the patient still showed signs of shock, red blood cells might be given in relatively small amounts while lab tests were drawn to determine the patient's clotting status and see what else might be needed. If the patient required multiple units of red blood cells (eg, 8–10), or the labs showed that the patient was developing clotting abnormalities or low platelets, these components might be added to the mix in varying amounts. Looking back, it was the wrong approach.

VIGNETTE >> Iraq, 2007: A 28-year-old Soldier was struck in the left chest by a tiny metallic fragment from an explosion. Medics found that his upper chest beneath his collarbone was swollen, and the pulse in his left arm was weaker than the pulse on the right. Based on this worrisome finding, the team quickly flew him to the closest combat support hospital for emergency surgery.

A computed tomography scan confirmed a vascular injury in the Soldier's upper chest, causing blood to collect around the major artery to his arm, just behind the collarbone. A pair of surgeons (trauma and cardiothoracic surgery) quickly took him to the operating room to repair the damaged vessel. Anticipating massive bleeding, they asked the blood bank to prepare for a large-volume transfusion, and they called for an immediate blood drive on the base.

The surgeons started to work as loud speakers announced the patient's blood type throughout the post. Soldiers, Sailors, Airmen, and Marines with that blood type lined up to donate their blood to help save this Soldier's left arm, and ultimately, his life.

While the surgeons worked frantically to expose the badly damaged vessel, blood gushed into suction canisters and onto the floor. After 30 minutes, the Soldier had already lost over half his blood volume. All this time, the anesthetist was pumping in equal amounts of packed red blood cells, plasma, and platelets. Then as warm, freshly collected whole blood arrived from donors on the base, he gave it preferentially.

The surgeons had to open the patient's chest and remove his collarbone to expose the injured artery, which they repaired using a vein from his leg. They got the patient's bleeding under control, and restored blood flow to his left arm. During this part of the procedure, all the blood he lost was replaced by a combination of stored blood products from the blood bank and fresh whole blood collected from donors on base. The transfusion strategy he received provided a balanced mix of red blood cells, platelets, and clotting factors in equal proportions—an approach designed to mimic the composition of the fresh whole blood he subsequently received.[1]

The operation was a success—the patient's left arm was pink and warm, and he had a strong pulse at his wrist. In the recovery area, he woke up with normal brain function. Remarkably, despite losing so much blood so quickly, all of his lab results were normal. The balanced resuscitation combined with rapid surgical control saved this Soldier's arm, and his life.

THE MILITARY CHANGES PRACTICE

In the early stages of the wars in Afghanistan and Iraq, a number of troops suffered severe shock from massive combat injuries. Initially, medical teams dutifully followed the standard approach of starting with two liters of crystalloid before giving blood, and then waiting for lab results to guide use of plasma or platelets. But when this was done, many of the most severely injured casualties developed coagulopathy (ie, diffuse bleeding due to ineffective clotting) and died from massive hemorrhage. But sometimes, instead of giving crystalloid, medical teams went directly to plasma and red blood cells before the labs results came back (Figure 16.2). On some occasions, casualties received warm, fresh whole blood, donated by their fellow Soldiers or Marines only hours or minutes earlier. These casualties seemed to do better and had fewer complications than those managed in the traditional manner. Using research data collected on these different approaches to resuscitation, clinicians' suspicions were proven correct—patients who received fresh whole blood or a balanced mix of ratio plasma and red blood cells (closer to 1:1, meaning one unit of plasma for every unit of red blood cells) survived more often than those who received smaller amounts of plasma using the reactive, lab-based approach (see Figures 16.3 and 16.4).[3,4]

Accordingly, in December 2004 the Department of Defense adopted a clinical practice guideline[5] combining the whole-blood transfusion approach of World War II and the realities of modern blood component therapy. This guideline advocated minimal crystalloid use, plus balanced resuscitation with equal amounts of blood products for the 5 to 10 percent of combat casualties who suffered massive blood loss. When available, platelets were given in equal amounts as well. The guidelines recommended that volunteers immediately donate whole blood, in quickly arranged drives, when a patient appeared likely to need a "massive transfusion" (> 10 units of blood in 24 hours) (Figure 16.3).

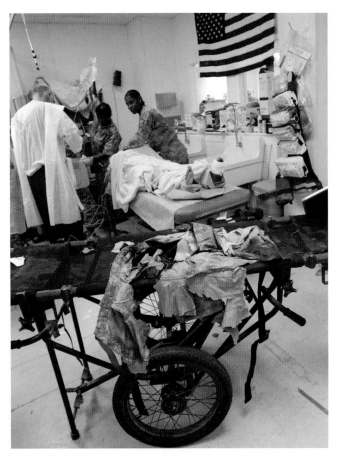

FIGURE 16.2. A dirty litter and ripped clothes of an injured Soldier at the Heath Craig Joint Theatre Hospital, Bagram Airfield, Afghanistan, May 17, 2009. Four US Soldiers and one civilian were seriously wounded by an IED (improvised explosive device) in the Tagab Valley. Balanced resuscitation has dramatically improved the odds that such patients will survive their injuries. Photo by Patrick Barth/Getty Images. Reproduced with permission from: Getty Images.

REFINEMENT AND EVALUATION IN CIVILIAN PATIENTS

This breakthrough strategy transformed the approach to managing severely bleeding patients. Later refinements focused on promptly controlling bleeding and evaluating use of this approach in civilian trauma populations.

Balanced resuscitation is enhanced by early use of hemostatic adjuncts, which are typically topical or intravenous agents that promote clot formation and stop bleeding. Examples include early use of tourniquets (Chapter 10), gauze impregnated with kaolin packed into wounds (Chapter 12), concentrated clotting factors that can be given intravenously (Chapter 16), and administration of tranexamic acid to prevent the abnormal breakdown of clots at bleeding sites (Chapter 17). These therapies represent important advances in treating severely bleeding patients and amplify the effects of a balanced resuscitation strategy. Done together, they save lives (Figure 16.4).

Military physicians returning from Iraq and Afghanistan took the lead in researching the potential application of this approach with civilians. Two landmark clinical studies have shown that for severely bleeding civilian patients, damage control resuscitation (the balanced strategy of using plasma and platelets early along with blood in equal or nearly equal proportions) reduces deaths from hemorrhage.[6,7]

IMPACT

A 2012 study examined the practice patterns of transfusion therapy during combat from 2004 to 2011.[8] It found that over time, a grow-

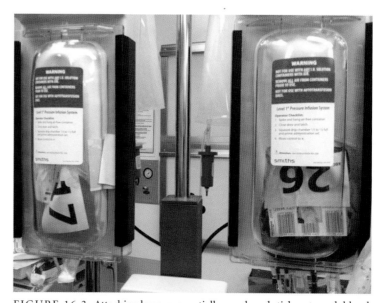

FIGURE 16.3. Attaching large, sequentially numbered stickers to each blood product is one way to track blood product administration during a massive transfusion. This allows all members of the team to see how many units of red blood cells (red) and plasma (yellow) have been given at any given time. A balanced resuscitation can be targeted more easily when an accurate blood product tally is available in real time. Photograph courtesy of Captain Peter Rhee, MD.

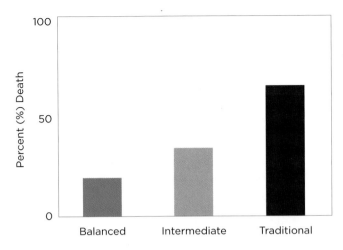

FIGURE 16.4. Results from the landmark study by Borgman et al, which showed a significantly lower death rate in massive transfusion patients who received a balanced resuscitation (19%) as compared to a traditional resuscitation (65%) or even an intermediate approach (34%). Original graph by Jeremy Cannon created from data presented in: Borgman MA, Spinella PC, Perkins JG, et al. The ratio of blood products transfused affects mortality in patients receiving massive transfusions at a combat support hospital. *J Trauma.* 2007;63(4):805-813.

ing proportion of patients received blood-based resuscitations and less crystalloid. Even as injuries grew more severe, survival rates improved, especially among those who required massive transfusions. Relatively high volumes of platelet infusions conferred the greatest survival benefit, while high volumes of plasma were synergistically beneficial.

The potential benefits of a balanced resuscitation strategy can be estimated using previously published results (see Figure 16.4).[3] If all 1,263 massively transfused patients had been managed with a traditional crystalloid and red-cell predominant strategy, about 820 would have died (65 percent mortality). Conversely, if balanced resuscitation had been used from the outset of the war, only 240 would have died (19 percent mortality). Few medical breakthroughs can claim such robust benefits.

THE BOTTOM LINE

These military findings in Afghanistan and Iraq confirm the benefit of a logical approach to transfusion therapy. Patients should either receive fresh whole blood, or a balanced mix of blood products that resembles as much as possible the blood they have shed. Administration of crystalloid, a fluid that does not resemble blood in any way, should be minimized. Resuscitation should begin early, before laboratory results are complete. The ideal resuscitation fluid is fresh whole blood, provided it can be readily collected and screened for transmissible diseases. If this is not possible but blood components are available, they should be administered in balanced proportions using the most recently collected products first. This will help prevent the development of clotting abnormalities or correct abnormalities before they become severe.

Nearly two centuries after the first transfusion, we have learned that the best approach to transfusion is one that restores, as closely as possible, blood that reflects the mix of red blood cells, plasma, and platelets that is found in fresh whole blood. Since transfusion of fresh blood from donors is technically limited and can only provide small amounts, banked blood will remain the mainstay for transfusion therapy. When using banked blood, components should be administered in a balanced way, to ensure that a badly bleeding patient receives platelets and clotting factors in equal proportion to red blood cells. In a remarkably short amount of time, this insight, derived on the battlefields of Afghanistan and Iraq, is already benefitting Americans at home.

Notes

1. Holcomb JB, Jenkins D, Rhee P, et al. Damage control resuscitation: directly addressing the early coagulopathy of trauma. *J Trauma.* 2007;62:307–310.

2. Hoyt DB. Blood and war: lest we forget. *J Am Coll Surg.* 2009;209:681–686.

3. Borgman MA, Spinella PC, Perkins JG, et al. The ratio of blood products transfused affects mortality in patients receiving massive transfusions at a combat support hospital. *J Trauma.* 2007;63:805-813.

4. Spinella PC, Perkins JG, Grathwohl KW, et al. Warm fresh whole blood independently associated with improved survival for patients with combat-related traumatic injuries. *J Trauma.* 2009;66:S69–76.

5. Joint Theater Trauma System clinical practice guideline: damage control resuscitation at level iib/iii treatment facilities. http://www.usaisr.amedd.army.mil/cpgs/Damage%20Control%20Resuscitation%20-%201%20Feb%202013.pdf. Accessed November 25, 2016.

6. Holcomb JB, del Junco DJ, Fox EE, et al. The prospective, observational, multicenter, major trauma transfusion (PROMMTT) study: comparative effectiveness of a time-varying treatment with competing risks. *JAMA Surg.* 2013;148:127–136.

7. Holcomb JB, Tilley BC, Baraniuk S, et al. Transfusion of plasma, platelets, and red blood cells in a 1:1:1 vs a 1:1:2 ration and mortality in patients with severe trauma: the PROPPR randomized clinical trial. *JAMA.* 2015;313:471-482.

8. Pidcoke HF, Aden JK, Mora AG, et al. Ten-year analysis of transfusion in Operation Iraqi Freedom and Operation Enduring Freedom: Increased plasma and platelet use correlates with improved survival. *J Trauma Acute Care Surg.* 2012;73:S445–452.

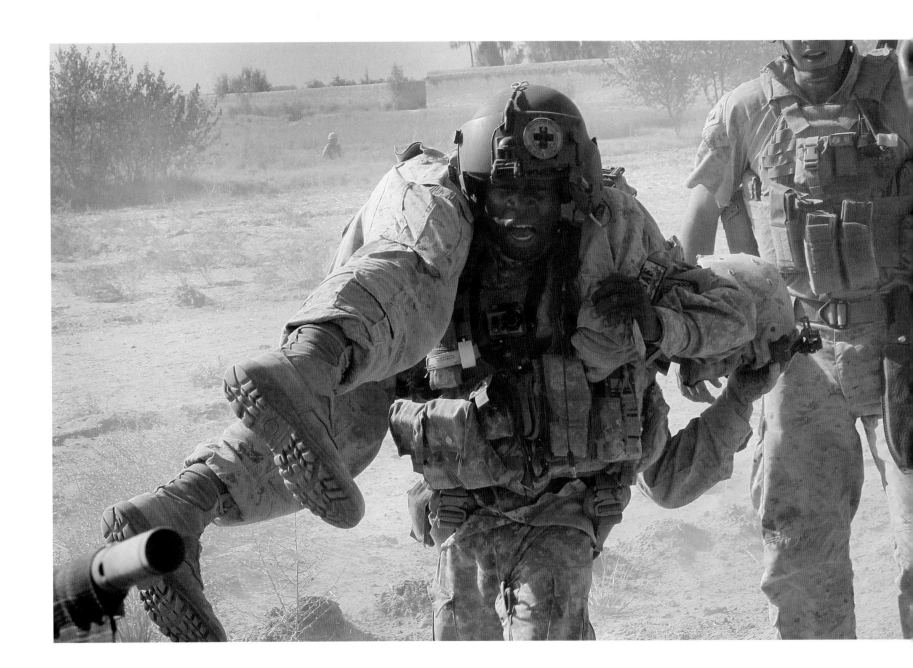

CHAPTER seventeen

Tranexamic Acid

MATTHEW J. MARTIN, MD, and TODD E. RASMUSSEN, MD

THE PROBLEM

BLEEDING IS TYPICAL IN TRAUMA, but the volume and rate of blood loss vary widely. The severity and significance of bleeding depends on the type, degree, and exact location of the injury, and the body's ability to reduce blood loss by activating its natural clotting system. Continued bleeding occurs when an injury is so severe (such as a severed artery) that it overwhelms the body's clotting capacities, or when the body's ability to form strong and stable clots is impaired. This impairment generally occurs in one of two ways: (1) lack of enough blood factors to form a strong and stable clot, or (2) an abnormal increase in blood factors that break down clots as quickly as they form (Figure 17-2).

During Operations Iraqi Freedom and Enduring Freedom, the military made numerous changes to improve the care of wounded service members. One of the most remarkable was a wholesale change in how military doctors approach caring for a patient with severe bleeding, with the initiation of a practice called "balanced resuscitation" (Chapter 16).[1] This strategy involves administering not only packed red blood cells to replace the blood that was lost, but also platelets and special proteins in plasma, called "clotting factors," that combine with platelets to promote clot formation.

FIGURE 17.1. [*Opposite*] US Army flight medic Sergeant Tyrone Jordan of Charlotte, North Carolina, attached to Dustoff Task Force Shadow of the 101st Combat Aviation Brigade, carries Marine Lance Corporal David Hawkins of Parker, Colorado, to a MEDEVAC helicopter after he was wounded by a blast from an improvised explosive device (IED), September 24, 2010, near Marja, Afghanistan. Photo by Scott Olson/Getty Images. Note: Photograph provided for illustrative purposes. These individuals are not the ones described in this chapter. Reproduced with permission from Getty Images.

VIGNETTE >> Afghanistan, 2012: A US Army infantry squad was conducting a dismounted patrol in the Kandahar area when an insurgent detonated an improvised explosive device near four squad members. Two of the Soldiers suffered multiple severe injuries, including loss of both legs, and multiple fragment wounds to their torsos. A combat medic provided immediate aid, placing leg tourniquets to stop the extremity bleeding and arranging for immediate medical evacuation (Figure 17-1). Helicopters carried one Soldier to a nearby forward surgical team (FST), and the other to the closest combat support hospital (CSH). Both arrived in shock from massive blood loss and continued bleeding, and both underwent immediate surgery and received blood products. Unfortunately, both developed major abnormalities of their clotting function, so their bodies broke down blood clots as rapidly as they formed, leading to continued hemorrhage. The Soldier taken to the CSH was treated with tranexamic acid (TXA), a newly deployed drug that reverses clot breakdown and allows the body to form and sustain clots and stop bleeding. The Soldier taken to the FST, where TXA was not yet available, died on the operating table due to uncontrollable bleeding that surgery could not stop.

Although this resuscitation strategy is aimed at early and aggressive correction of abnormalities in the clotting system (termed "coagulopathy"), some patients did not respond fully or quickly enough. Several analyses of battlefield deaths that occurred before as well as after patients reached hospitals found that uncontrollable bleeding caused the vast majority of deaths that might have otherwise been prevented.[2,3] One possible reason is that although balanced resuscitation replaces lost blood, platelets, and clotting factors, it does not counteract the other potential cause of persistent bleeding, such as the rapid breakdown of newly formed blood clots due to an abnormal increase in anti-clotting factors. Therefore, researchers set about finding an effective treatment to stop this abnormal process of clot destruction.

THE INNOVATION

Throughout the history of civilian and military trauma care, doctors and biomedical researchers have looked for an effective treatment to stop excessive bleeding in trauma due to abnormal blood clotting. Over the decades, doctors tried numerous agents, but none proved sufficient. A recent example was recombinant activated factor VII, a drug developed to treat bleeding in hemophiliacs. Initial studies of its use at civilian and military trauma centers seemed promising, but more detailed studies found it had little or no benefit. Moreover, the drug is extremely expensive and caused potentially serious side effects. Doctors pleaded for a drug that could control bleeding, has a low risk of adverse side effects, is easy to store and administer, and is relatively inexpensive so it can be widely used.

At first glance, TXA was an unlikely candidate to become the treatment of choice for bleeding disorders in trauma. Neither newly developed nor bioengineered, it is a decades-old drug that is a synthetic form of a naturally occurring amino acid called lysine. By binding to receptors for lysine on several key components of the body's system for breaking down clots, it inactivates these components and allows the clot to completely form and strengthen. While most of the previously studied products focused on replacing or increasing the formation of new clots, TXA was unique in that it prevented the breakdown of already-formed clots, particularly those that are crucial to stopping traumatic bleeding. Although doctors had successfully used TXA to decrease bleeding during elective operations (primarily orthopedic and cardiothoracic surgery), there were no studies that examined its use in life-threatening trauma.

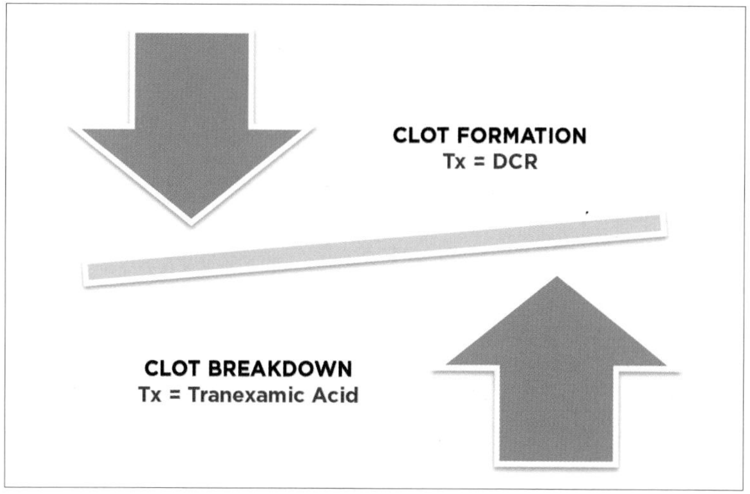

The gold standard of proof for a drug's effectiveness is a randomized clinical trial. In such a research study, patients are randomly assigned to one of two groups: the first group receiving the experimental drug and the second receiving an identical-looking placebo (no drug activity). In Europe, researchers conducted a large multicenter trial that randomized trauma patients to receive either TXA or no TXA in addition to standard resuscitation.[4] The study enrolled 20,000 patients in 40 countries, making it one of the largest randomized trials ever performed in trauma. It found that using TXA reduced the overall risk of death by 9 percent and decreased the risk of death from uncontrolled bleeding by 15 percent. In subsequent analyses, this benefit was mainly evident in patients who were given TXA within three hours of their injury, emphasizing the importance of using the drug early in treatment.

FIGURE 17.2. Graphic showing the two aspects of abnormal coagulation and the primary treatment (Tx) strategies. Decreased clot formation is primarily treated with a damage control resuscitation strategy (DCR), while tranexamic acid focuses on preventing clot breakdown.

IMPACT

TXA gave CSH and FST providers in Iraq and Afghanistan a way to rapidly correct clotting functions to achieve earlier and more sustained control of bleeding from combat wounds (Figure 17.3). It remains the only drug treatment in trauma resuscitation shown to reduce the risk of death in a randomized clinical trial. Based on the European study's promising results, British medical personnel adopted TXA for battlefield use in 2009. Soon thereafter, US and other coalition forward medical teams adopted the drug as well to treat combat casualties—the patients at highest risk for death from bleeding.

FIGURE 17.3. Clot strength and durability can be tested using thromboelastography, which provides a real-time picture of clot formation. As shown in graph A, the width of the graph represents the clot strength, while the x-axis shows clot stability (measured in minutes). Graph B shows a patient forming a strong clot but then immediately breaking this clot down; this process is then reversed after one dose of tranexamic acid (TXA).

FIGURE 17.4. [*Opposite*] Two graphs from the MATTERS 1 study showing the increase in survival (red arrows) between patients who did not receive tranexamic acid (TXA) versus those who did receive TXA. The benefit demonstrated in all patients (left panel) is even more profound among the patients who required a massive blood transfusion (right panel). Reproduced (red arrows added) with permission from: Morrison JJ, Dubose JJ, Rasmussen TE, Midwinter MJ. Military Application of Tranexamic Acid in Trauma Emergency Resuscitation (MATTERs) Study. Arch Surg. 2012;147:113–119.

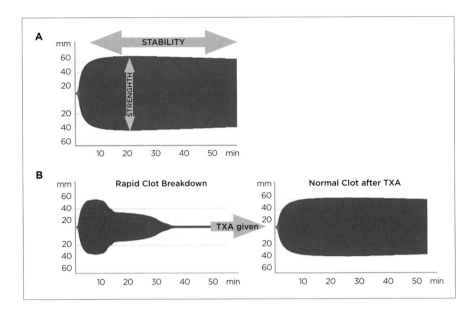

Two later studies examined TXA's impact on combat injuries, called the Military Application of Tranexamic Acid in Trauma Emergency Resuscitation Study (MATTERS) 1 and MATTERS 2.[5,6] These studies examined over 1,000 patients with battlefield injuries requiring multiple blood transfusions, including a large group that received TXA as part of their trauma resuscitation. Both studies found that the risk of death dropped significantly when TXA was used in the initial resuscitation. The research found an even more profound benefit among patients who received massive transfusions of blood products (Figure 17.4). TXA use was linked with a seven-fold higher likelihood of survival among patients with massive hemorrhage.[5] A subsequently analysis (the PED-TRAX study) found a similar survival benefit when TXA was given to severely injured children.[7] Since this research was conducted, additional studies of TXA in civilian trauma have confirmed that it reduces mortality and morbidity. Today, several ongoing studies are looking at its use in the prehospital environment.[8–10]

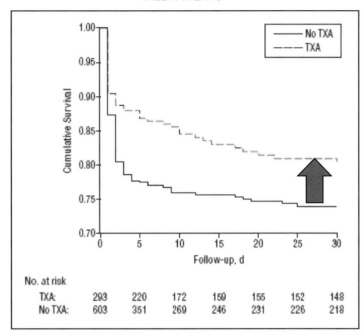

ALL PATIENTS

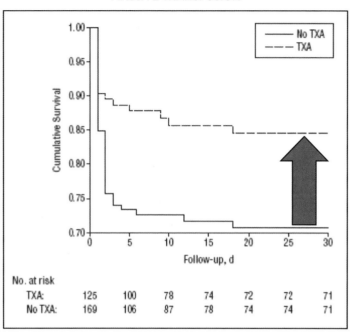

MASSIVE TRANSFUSION

LESSONS LEARNED

TXA is a great example of how medical science can save lives through dogged research and coopera-tion—in this case, the combined efforts of military and civilian health professionals in the United States, Britain, and other European countries. In terms of battlefield care, the identification, study, and implementation of TXA required rapid and real-time analysis of best practices, followed by the drug's incorporation into combat protocols and close monitoring of the resulting effects. Later studies, includ-ing careful analyses of data generated in combat zones, confirmed the medication's effectiveness. The finding that TXA works is good news for untold thousands of military and civilian patients worldwide.

Notes

1. Beekley AC. Damage control resuscitation: a sensible approach to the exsanguinating surgical patient. *Crit Care Med.* 2008; 36:S267–274.

2. Eastridge BJ, Mabry RL, Seguin P, et al. Death on the battlefield (2001–2011): implications for the future of combat casualty care. *J Trauma Acute Care Surg.* 2012;73:S431–437.

3. Martin M, Oh J, Currier H, et al. An analysis of in-hospital deaths at a modern combat support hospital. *J Trauma.* 2009;66:S51–60; discussion S51–60.

4. CRASH 2 trial collaborators, Shakur H, Roberts I, et al. Effects of tranexamic acid on death, vascular occlusive events, and blood transfusion in trauma patients with significant haemorrhage (CRASH-2): a randomised, placebo-controlled trial. *Lancet.* 2010;376:23–32.

5. Morrison JJ, Dubose JJ, Rasmussen TE, Midwinter MJ. Military Application of Tranexamic Acid in Trauma Emergency Resuscitation (MATTERs) Study. *Arch Surg.* 2012;147:113–119.

6. Morrison JJ, Ross JD, Dubose JJ, et al. Association of cryoprecipitate and tranexamic acid with improved survival following wartime injury: findings from the MATTERs II Study. *JAMA Surg.* 2013;148:218–225.

7. Eckert MJ, Wertin TM, Tyner SD, Nelson DW, Izenberg S, Martin MJ. Tranexamic acid administration to pediatric trauma patients in a combat setting: the pediatric trauma and tranexamic acid study (PED-TRAX). *J Trauma Acute Care Surg.* 2014;77:852–858, discussion 858.

8. Ausset S, Glassberg E, Nadler R, et al. Tranexamic acid as part of remote damage-control resuscitation in the prehospital setting: A critical appraisal of the medical literature and available alternatives. *J Trauma Acute Care Surg.* 2015;78:S70–75.

9. Brown JB, Neal MD, Guyette FX, et al. Design of the Study of Tranexamic Acid during Air Medical Prehospital Transport (STAAMP) trial: addressing the knowledge gaps. *Prehosp Emerg Care.* 2015;19:79–86.

10. Cole E, Davenport R, Willett K, Brohi K. Tranexamic acid use in severely injured civilian patients and the effects on outcomes: a prospective cohort study. *Ann Surg.* 2015;261:390–394.

CHAPTER eighteen

Battlefield Pain Control: 19th Century Medicine Meets a 21st Century Conflict

CHESTER C. BUCKENMAIER III, MD, and GUY F. DISNEY

THE PROBLEM

BEFORE THE WARS IN AFGHANISTAN AND IRAQ, managing pain on the battlefield had hardly changed in generations. Until recently, pain was largely seen as a natural symptom of wounds or disease that resolves with appropriate surgical and medical management, healing, and rehabilitation. Today, a more modern understanding of trauma and postsurgical pain recognizes that poorly managed acute pain contributes to the development of debilitating chronic pain and posttraumatic stress.[1] Long after the original wound or disease has resolved, chronic pain can lead to a lifetime of disability.

Since the US Civil War, morphine has been the gold standard for battlefield analgesia. It is one of a class of opioid drugs, which act directly on the brain to treat pain. Historically, doctors considered morphine a safe and effective treatment for many common aches and pains. People could buy it without a prescription (Figure 18.2).

Afghanistan, 2009: West of Babaji in Helmand province, Lieutenant Guy Disney, leading a 16-soldier element of the British Light Dragoons Battle Group (Operation Panchai Palang—Panther's Claw), was tasked with clearing the area of Taliban combatants while also looking for improvised explosive devices

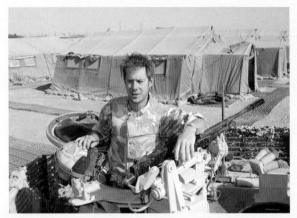

Figure 18.1. Lieutenant Guy Disney in Forward Operating Base, Dwyer, Afghanistan.

(IEDs). The group had intermittently engaged in small arms fire with Taliban forces all day. Late that afternoon, as the column pushed through a tree line, something exploded. Lieutenant Disney (Figure 18.1) initially assumed it was an IED. He reconsidered when he saw smoke coming off the left side of his troop's vehicle. Concluding the blast was caused by a rocket-propelled grenade (RPG), he began formulating the radio report he would make. At that moment, he looked down and noticed that a portion of his right leg was hanging by what appeared to be bootlaces. In fact, they were tendons and sinew attached to his mutilated foot. Then he smelled the pungent aroma of burnt flesh, and felt searing heat and a dull, steadily growing ache.

As Lieutenant Disney formulated his plan for responding to the attack, a nearby soldier administered morphine with an auto-injector from Disney's aid pack. Because the lieutenant was bleeding heavily, another soldier applied a tourniquet to his leg. Lieutenant Disney continued trying to organize his team's response to the attack. Before being evacuated by helicopter, he learned that the RPG had killed one of his men.

As soon as the evacuation helicopter landed at the British combat support hospital (CSH) at Camp Bastion, aides rushed Lieutenant Disney into the triage area. As the trauma surgeon introduced himself, the lieutenant asked if his leg could be saved. The surgeon shook his head no. Lieutenant Disney was not surprised, and tried to make light of his situation with a poor joke about no longer being able to tap dance.

There was pain and fear in the lieutenant's eyes as (then) Colonel Chester Buckenmaier, the hospital's anesthesiologist, stepped forward. He promised Lieutenant Disney that his pain would be controlled when he awoke from surgery. In another time or conflict, this would have been an empty vow, but this CSH's systems and technology had reached the point where the promise could be kept.

Moments later, Lieutenant Disney received a dose of ketamine, an intense analgesic that does not impair blood pressure or breathing, but disconnects the patient from the events around him (see Ketamine for Battlefield Pain Relief). The powerful analgesic relieved him of the anxiety and discomfort of the necessary preparation for surgery, x-ray studies, and movement to the operating room.

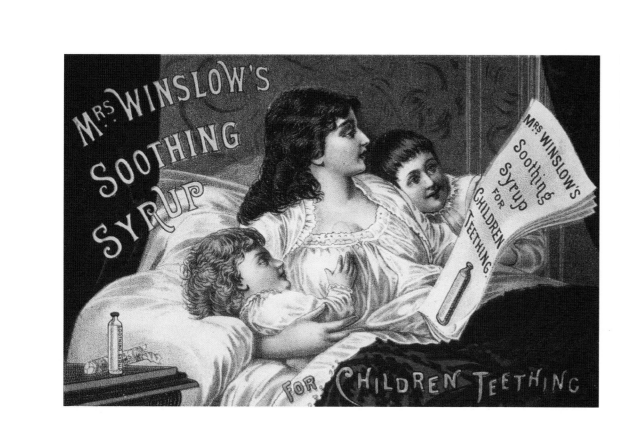

FIGURE 18.2. Advertisement from 1885 on morphine use for teething children. Mrs. Winslow's Soothing Syrup for children teething. Reproduced from National Library of Medicine, https://collections.nlm.nih.gov/catalog/nlm:nlmuid-101402395-img.

Morphine has repeatedly demonstrated its effectiveness in managing severe pain throughout American military history. But recent conflicts exposed the shortcomings of this 200-year-old drug. Large doses of the drug can impair breathing, lower blood pressure, and cause nausea, vomiting, and confusion. In the heat of battle or the confines of a helicopter, these side effects can be difficult to manage and even life-threatening.

Chronic morphine use causes other problems. After the initial surgery, continued reliance on morphine and other opioid medications to manage pain can hinder a Soldier's recovery and rehabilitation. Prolonged use increases the risk for substance abuse.[2] Ironically, ongoing use of opioids can even lower the body's tolerance for pain (opioid-induced hyperalgesia).[3] In short, the opioid "solution" for battlefield pain tended to cause more problems than it solved.

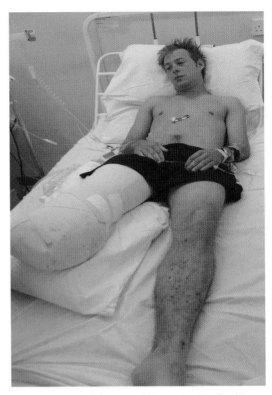

FIGURE 18.3. Lieutenant Disney shortly after his emergency surgery at Camp Bastion, Afghanistan.

THE INNOVATION

Military medical leaders concluded that to improve battlefield pain care, they needed better alternatives. They recognized that these new technologies would require specially trained medical personnel adept at managing pain on the modern battlefield and throughout the evacuation process. To accomplish this, the British surgeon general, Lieutenant General Louis Lillywhite, MD, launched a demonstration mission by inviting Colonel Buckenmaier, the American acute pain physician, to the British Army's CSH at Camp Bastion, Afghanistan, in 2009. This project represented the first deployment of a military medical officer specifically tasked with establishing an acute pain service (APS) at a coalition CSH. In addition to the physician acute pain specialist, the team consisted of nurse pain management champions within each CSH ward. These pain champions were the critical liaisons between the pain service, CSH healthcare providers, and their patients.

Because Lieutenant Disney's injury caused massive blood loss, he required over ten units of blood and blood products during his initial operation. At its conclusion, while he was still under the effects of general anesthesia, Colonel Buckenmaier placed femoral nerve and sciatic nerve block catheters above the patient's shattered leg using ultrasound guidance. This allowed Lieutenant Disney to receive continuous postoperative analgesia (as described in Chapter 22). Both catheters infused ropivacaine, a local anesthetic. This medication, continuously administered at low doses through the nerve block catheters, stopped noxious nerve impulses from the fresh amputation from reaching Lieutenant Disney's brain (Figure 18.3). Additionally, Lieutenant Disney was given intravenous acetaminophen and diclofenac, two non-opioid medications, and was generally pain free after wakening from the general anesthesia. Later that evening, he received a single dose of morphine that reduced his pain but made him nauseous, a common side effect of the medication. Lieutenant Disney also benefitted from the initial dose of ketamine Colonel Buckenmaier had given him when he arrived at the hospital. It's thought that ketamine may limit the creation of aberrant pain pathways in the central nervous system that contribute to later development of chronic pain. This multimodal approach, which uses small amounts of different drugs that work by complementary mechanisms, produces better analgesia with far fewer side effects than giving large doses of a single drug like morphine.

These advances, championed by the APS team, enabled the British CSH to safely implement an advanced, individualized approach to managing acute pain. The APS also provided the needed infrastructure to evaluate new medications and therapies to improve battlefield analgesic practices throughout a patient's evacuation.

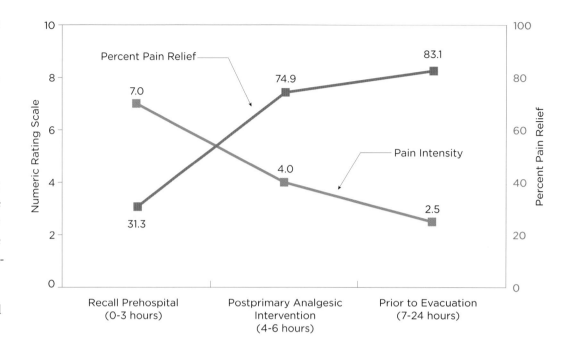

FIGURE 18.4. Mean pain intensity and percent pain relief scores for combat casualties managed by the acute pain service at Camp Bastion, Afghanistan. Reproduced with permission from: Buckenmaier CC 3rd, Mahoney PF, Anton T, Kwon N, Polomano RC. Impact of an acute pain service on pain outcomes with combat-injured soldiers at Camp Bastion, Afghanistan. *Pain Med.* 2012;13(7):924.

The day of Lieutenant Disney's arrival was busy with multiple casualties, so Colonel Buckenmaier was not able to monitor Disney after he was moved to the hospital's recovery ward. Later that day on pain rounds, Colonel Buckenmaier saw Lieutenant Disney sitting upright, talking on the telephone to his mother in the United Kingdom. He appeared free of pain and was calmly telling his mother of the loss of his leg, insisting he was fine and would see her soon. This severely injured man, fresh from the battlefield and operating room, was not ruled by pain. A few hours after he lost his leg in an RPG attack, he was calmly planning for his future, able to visualize his recovery and rehabilitation. This case represents the power and purpose of an APS on a modern battlefield.

IMPACT

During the pilot project at Camp Bastion, the APS managed 71 casualties. To assess the approach's impact, healthcare personnel collected mean pain intensity scores, and percent pain relief scores, three

KETAMINE FOR BATTLEFIELD PAIN RELIEF

Since the Civil War, combat casualties have been treated with morphine. This started to change in 2003, during the invasion of Iraq, when a battalion surgeon with 3rd Battalion, 75th Ranger Regiment, directed his medics to give injured troops fentanyl (a powerful cousin of morphine) lollipops to treat battlefield pain. Although these lollipops were invented to help cancer patients deal with breakthrough pain, they proved to be practical and easy to use under battlefield conditions.

As injuries from improvised explosive devices grew more frequent, we found that the pain of traumatic amputations was extremely difficult to control. Initially, we tried using an even more potent opioid called hydromorphone. Unfortunately, it wasn't much better than fentanyl or morphine.

In 2009, we tried ketamine. Although ketamine is technically an anesthetic, numerous journal articles reported that at sub-anesthetic doses, it is very effective for treating acute pain. Also, unlike morphine and other opioids, ketamine doesn't lower blood pressure or depress breathing—useful qualities on the battlefield.[1] Lacking a better alternative, we implemented a protocol and distributed the drug to our medics.

The following story illustrates ketamine's effects. On October 1, 2010, we were defending a compound surrounded on all sides by the enemy. Our mortar team was trading fire with the enemy. At that moment, one of their mortar rounds exploded inside our compound, injuring 12 members of our unit. I pulled the most severely injured Soldier, Sergeant First Class (SFC) Lance Vogeler, from the open to a semi-covered position and began to treat him. The other medic grabbed Sergeant (SGT) Zak Graner and pulled him into a room. Despite my best efforts, SFC Vogeler died underneath an awning.

After pronouncing SFC Vogeler killed in action, I turned to help my fellow medic treat SGT Graner, who was severely injured with large shrapnel wounds to both legs. We had to put two tourniquets on each of his legs and apply aggressive pressure dressings to control his bleeding. Because SGT Graner was in agonizing pain, I directed the medic to administer 75 mg of ketamine and 1 mg of midazolam (a mild sedative added to reduce any involuntary limb movements).

SGT Graner's pain was immediately controlled. As our assault force continued to exchange fire with the enemy, my fellow medics and I treated other injured members of our force, including the unit commander and our joint terminal air controller as they called in air strikes. Because the firefight delayed the MEDE-VAC helicopter we called for a half hour, we gave SGT Graner an additional 60 mg of ketamine and 1 mg of midazolam. Twenty minutes later, the helicopter picked him up along with our other casualties. Remarkably, after several surgeries and rehabilitation, SGT Graner recovered and deployed with his unit again. Equally remarkably, thanks to ketamine, SGT Graner does not recall anything about the incident after he received his first dose of medication. This additional benefit of ketamine may help reduce the incidence of posttraumatic stress disorder and chronic pain in future conflicts.

Based on successful uses like this one, special operations medics and physician assistants like me swear by this medication. More important, the data back us up.[2,3] Given its ease of use, safety, and battlefield efficacy, ketamine is now recommended as the analgesic of choice for casualties in shock by the Committee on Tactical Combat Casualty Care (Chapter 11),[4] although compliance with TCCC guidelines has room for improvement.[5]

Unfortunately, we continue to face obstacles to the use ketamine to treat battlefield pain because the Food and Drug Administration still classifies it as an anesthetic. Hopefully, that will change one day.

Major Andrew Fisher, MPAS, PA-C
Regimental Physician Assistant, 75th Ranger Regiment

Notes

1. Kotwal RS, et a O'Connor KC, Johnson TR, Mosely DS, Meyer DE, Holcomb JB. A novel pain management strategy for combat casualty care. *Ann Emerg Med*. 2004;44:121–127.
2. Fisher AD, Rippee B, Shehan H, Conklin C, Mabry RL. Prehospital analgesia with ketamine for combat wounds: a case series. *J Spec Ops Med*. 2014;14:11–17.
3. Shackelford SA, Fowler M, Schultz K, et al. Prehospital pain medication use by U.S. forces in Afghanistan. *Mil Med*. 2015;180(3):304–309.
4. Butler FK, Kotwal RS, Buckenmaier CC 3rd, et al. A triple-option analgesia plan for Tactical Combat Casualty Care: TCCC guidelines change 13-04. *J Spec Ops Med*. 2014;14:13–25.
5. Schauer SG, Robinson JB, Mabry RL, Howard JT. Battlefield analgesia: TCCC guidelines are not being followed. *J Spec Ops Med*. 2015;15(1):85-89.

FIGURE 18.5. Means and standard deviations with comparisons of perceptions of an acute pain service (APS) between physicians and nurses. Reproduced with permission from: Polomano RC, Chisholm E, Anton TM, Kwon N, Mahoney PF, Buckenmaier C 3rd. A survey of military health professionals' perceptions of an acute pain service at Camp Bastion, Afghanistan. *Pain Med.* 2012;13(7):931.

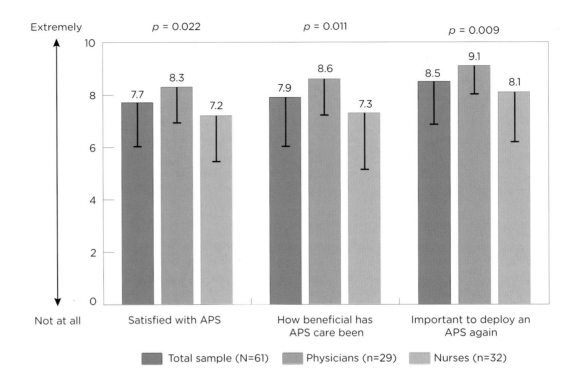

times in the first 24 hours of treatment at the hospital. The data demonstrate significant improvement in pain control over time (Figure 18.4). During the pilot project, the Camp Bastion CSH trauma team members also were surveyed about their perceptions of the value of the APS to overall hospital function. Using a 0 to 10 scale (0 = not at all; 10 = extremely), the camp's physicians and nurses were asked: "How satisfied are you with the APS at Camp Bastion?" "How beneficial has the APS been for your patients at Camp Bastion?" And "How important would an APS be if you had to deploy to a Role 3 facility again?" The survey results are in Figure 18.5. Perhaps most significantly, three out of every four staff members agreed or strongly agreed that "Overall, APS has a significant impact on patient outcome."[4]

There's little doubt that the APS at Camp Bastion's CSH made a difference for Lieutenant Disney. He went on to pursue an extraordinary and active life (Figure18.6), making history as the first amputee to obtain a jockey's license from British horse racing officials. He recently married. He remembers the peripheral nerve blocks as being highly effective at relieving his pain without the severe nausea he associated with the morphine he received during his first hours at the camp's hospital.

CONCLUSION

War is a cruel but efficient instructor in advancing the medical arts. During the last 14 years of conflict, military medicine made substantial advances in managing the pain of acute combat casualties. Based on this experience, more military hospitals are establishing APS systems. The challenge is to learn from this lieutenant's story and countless others, and to ensure that advanced pain care systems are part of CSH facilities and military hospitals in future wars.

Notes

1. Carr DB, Goudas LC. Acute pain. *Lancet.*1999;353:2051–2058.
2. Jeffrey DD, Babeu LA, Nelson LE, Kloc M, Klette K. Prescription drug misuse among US active duty military personnel: a secondary analysis of the 2008 DoD survey of health related behaviors. *Mil Med.* 2013;178:180–195.
3. Mao J. Clinical diagnosis of opioid-induced hyperalgesia. *Reg Anesth Pain Med.* 2015;40:663–664.
4. Polomano RC, Chisolm E, Anton TM, Kwon N, Mahoney PF, Buckenmaier C 3rd. A survey of military health professionals' perceptions of an acute pain service at Camp Bastion, Afghanistan. *Pain Med.* 2012;13:927–936.

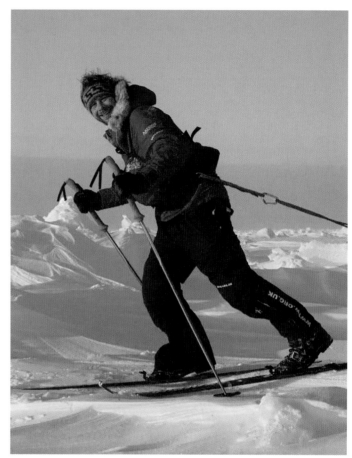

FIGURE 18.6. Guy Disney on a North Pole expedition in 2011.

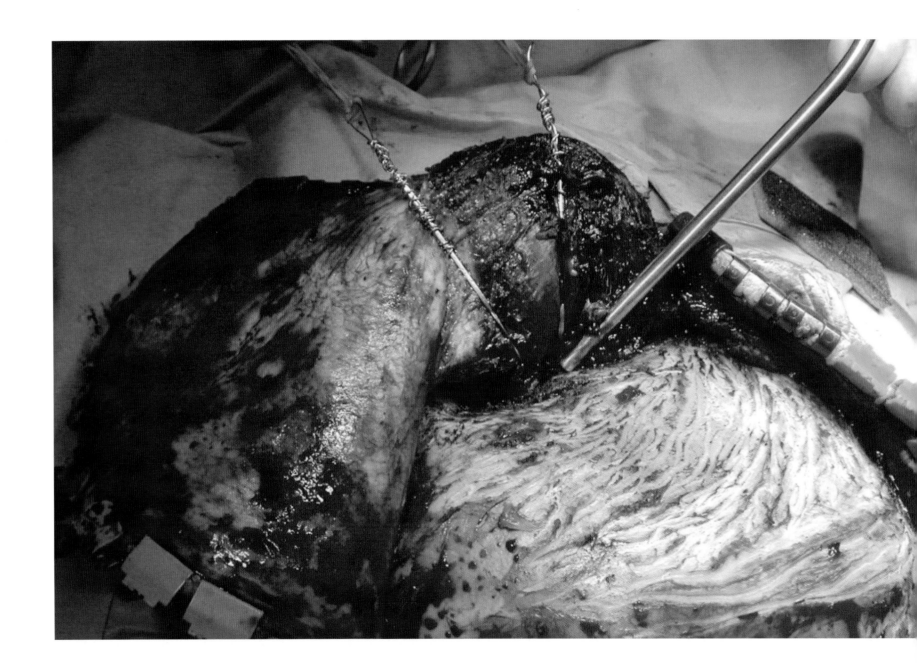

CHAPTER nineteen

Decompressive Craniectomy and Control of Vasospasm

M. BENJAMIN LARKIN, PHARMD; BRIAN CURRY, MD;
ROCCO ARMONDA, MD; and RANDY BELL, MD

THE CHALLENGE

A TRAUMATIC BRAIN INJURY, OR TBI, may be either open (such as when a projectile penetrates the skull or a blow drives skull fragments into the brain), or closed (in which tissue damage occurs without penetration of the skull). Blasts, especially from IEDs, cause most combat-related TBIs today. These can cause devastating injuries to brain tissues and the blood vessels that supply them (Figure 19.3).[1]

Despite more TBIs among military personnel, survival has improved in the modern combat era. This is likely due in part to improved body armor and head protection, better design of armored vehicles (Chapter 9), improved battlefield resuscitation (Chapters 10–12), rapid casualty evacuation (Chapter 13), and the Joint Trauma System (Chapter 8).[1-3] Nevertheless, the burden of TBIs is staggering. It is a major cause of death from trauma, and is one of the most important causes of trauma-related disability among survivors.[4] Although many service members with mild TBI do well, those who sustain a moderate or severe TBI often require extensive rehabilitation, followed by medical discharge from the military. Many TBI patients struggle with reintegration into the civilian world (Chapters 29, 31, and 33). It is especially troubling that injured service members face these challenges during the most productive years of their lives.[5]

FIGURE 19.1. [*Opposite*] Intraoperative photograph of a craniectomy. The scalp has been retracted, revealing the bone of the skull. Next, a large piece of bone will be removed to expose the brain and its coverings, thus reducing the pressure inside the skull.

VIGNETTE >> Iraq, 2004: [Author's note: this story is a composite of many patients treated by the author. The photos are of actual patients.] A 26-year-old American Soldier, severely injured by an improvised explosive device (IED), was found unconscious, with brain tissue coming out of his head. A nearby combat medic inserted a breathing tube into his windpipe to protect his airway, and he was transported by MEDEVAC helicopter to the nearest combat support hospital. There, a computed tomography scan showed severe bleeding and bruising of the front part of his brain, and bone fragments in his brain tissue.

In the operating room, the treating neurosurgeon removed the right half of his skull, opened the dura (a thin but tough layer of tissue that surrounds the brain), scooped out blood clots, and repaired the most visible damage (Figure 19.2). Following modern standards of practice, he did not dig into the brain to remove bone fragments. At the end of the operation, the neurosurgeon placed a thin plastic tube to drain excess cerebrospinal fluid and measure pressure inside the Soldier's skull. The surgeon closed the scalp incision, but left the skull and underlying dura open to give the brain room to swell.

Seven days later, Critical Care Air Transport Teams (CCATs; Chapter 25) flew the Soldier to the Walter Reed Army Medical Center in Washington, DC. At Walter Reed, a computed tomography scan showed additional bleeding in his brain. In addition, an ultrasound study detected signs of decreased blood flow.

When a follow-up angiogram showed vasospasm (constriction of the main blood vessels supplying the brain), the Soldier was treated with a medication that causes blood vessels to relax. To further improve blood flow to his brain, doctors inserted a thin catheter similar to those used to treat heart attack victims into a major blood vessel supplying his brain. Then a small balloon was inflated to open up the vessel. Brain blood flow had improved, but the Soldier remained in a coma. When the procedure was repeated two weeks later, blood flow normalized. A follow-up angiogram demonstrated no further vasospasm. Over the next several days, the Soldier started to respond, and steadily improved after that. At his eight-month follow-up, he was communicative, walking with a cane, and actively participating in rehabilitation (see Chapter 29).

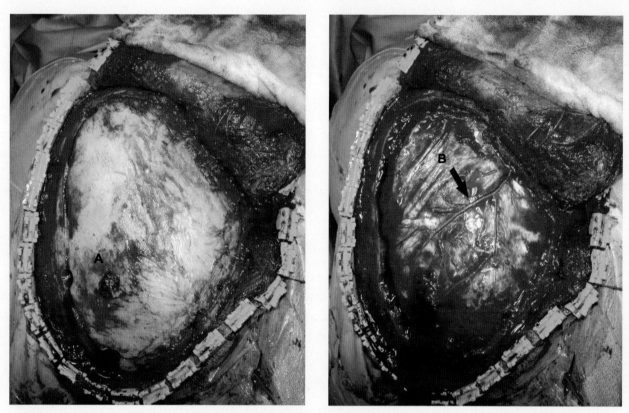

FIGURE 19.2. A trauma flap fashioned by reflecting the scalp and temporalis muscle anteriorly, and a bone flap fashioned using multiple burr holes and a craniotomy footplate high-speed drill attachment (a). Bone removed from the underlying dura mater—note the prominent, middle meningeal artery (arrow) (b). Photos reproduced from: Nessen SC, Lounsbury DE, Hetz SP, eds. *War Surgery in Afghanistan and Iraq: A Series of Cases, 2003-2007*. Washington, DC: Borden Institute; 2008:96-97

For a TBI of any severity, injury is divided into primary and secondary phases. Primary brain injury refers to the immediate tissue damage or destruction resulting from mechanical trauma, whether caused by a blast or a penetrating projectile. Secondary brain injury follows, resulting from processes at the cellular level triggered by the primary brain injury. Because there are no effective therapies for primary brain injury, treatment largely focuses on minimizing factors that can worsen secondary brain injury, a major cause of death and long-term disability.[6]

Many mechanisms contribute to secondary brain injury. Because severe drops in blood pressure and low levels of oxygen can worsen damage, battlefield and emergency care providers try to prevent both complications. During the first few days after injury, uncontrolled brain swelling and spasm of blood vessels supplying the brain become increasingly important.[1,6] Vasospasm can be caused by direct injury to the blood vessels, or from irritation caused by bleeding into the surrounding brain tissue. In either event, vasospasm typically starts about two or three days after injury and lasts ten to fourteen days, although the risk may linger for up to thirty days after injury.[1] In some cases, the vasospasm is severe enough to cause a stroke.

Damaged body tissue tends to swell. But because the skull encases the brain, there is no place for the swelling to go. So pressure inside the skull—intracranial pressure—begins to climb.[6,7] If intracranial pressure gets extremely high, it can not only impair the flow of blood to the brain, it can also actually push brain tissue out of the hole where the brain connects to the spinal cord, leading to death. The immediate goals of treatment following a severe TBI involve minimizing secondary brain injury by optimizing blood flow to brain tissue, preventing vasospasm, and preventing, to the degree possible, brain swelling.

THE INNOVATION

For much of military history, doctors could do little for severely injured TBI patients except prescribe rest and hope they got better. But as our capacity to intervene progressed, we began taking aggressive steps to save service members' lives. Early surgical options included removing large blood clots and severely damaged brain tissue and extracting penetrating fragments that might lead to subsequent infection. Unfortunately, these interventions did little to help severely injured patients. During World War I, the founder of neurosurgery, Dr. Harvey Cushing, described more than 250 patients with penetrating head

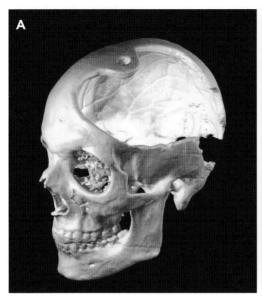

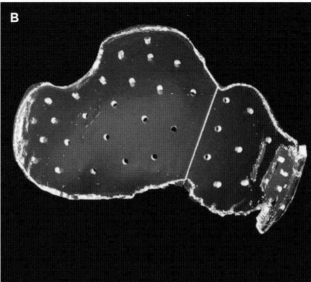

FIGURE 19.3.
(A) Computed tomography 3D reconstruction (left) shows a large skull defect from in-theater decompressive craniectomy after traumatic brain injury. Using mirror imaging from the patient's contralateral skull, a customized polymethyl methacrylate (PMMA) implant is created with computer-aided design (right). (B) 3D craniectomy model with PMMA implant in place. Customized cranioplasty design is further enhanced with faceted attachment brackets based on an individual neurosurgeon's preference and the patient's specific cranial contours. Photographs courtesy of John P. Lichtenberger III, MD; Major, USAF, MC; Assistant Professor, Department of Radiology and Radiological Sciences, Uniformed Services University of the Health Sciences.

injuries who were treated this way.[8] Despite aggressive treatment, mortality still approached 90 percent in severe cases. This more aggressive approach persisted through the Vietnam era, until new data emerged during the Israeli/Lebanon conflict of 2010 indicating that aggressive brain debridement actually worsens outcomes.[3] Accordingly, surgical treatment of penetrating TBI shifted toward minimal debridement unless there is extensive brain tissue damage.[2,3,6,9]

Operations Iraqi Freedom and Enduring Freedom shifted the way neurosurgeons approach the care of patients with severe TBI. In a relatively short period, military neurosurgeons adopted an aggressive approach that consists of far-forward cranial decompression (ie, removing part of the skull to allow the brain to swell without raising intracranial pressure) and rapid evacuation to the United States. via CCAT.[2,3] Studies have demonstrated that this approach can result in higher rates of survival and more patients with severe brain injuries able to benefit from rehabilitation.[2,3] In many cases, bone removed in the first hours after injury may be saved for later replacement. However, technology has progressed to the point that various materials (including titanium and medical grade plastic) can create synthetic skull replacements that can be implanted in some cases (Figure 19.3).

The main purpose of removing part of the skull is to stabilize a patient and prevent uncontrollable increases in intracranial pressure during the 18-hour flight to a US hospital.[2,3,6] Once these patients reach the United States, they are met by an interdisciplinary team adept at critical care management. Efforts at this stage center on preventing secondary brain injury. Options include hypothermia (cooling the brain to prevent further damage); noninvasive monitoring of brain tissue oxygen; non-invasive, careful monitoring of intracranial pressure; assessment of blood vessel injury with noninvasive and invasive imaging; drug treatment to prevent posttraumatic seizures; and, in extreme cases, medication-induced coma to put a damaged brain completely at rest.

IMPACT

In the modern combat era, neurosurgeons have reshaped their approach to patients with severe head injuries, laying the groundwork for future improvements in treating warfighters with these injuries. Thanks to rapid treatment in the field, brain injuries once considered fatal are now regarded as treatable. Effective measures include early neurosurgery to reduce secondary injury and rapid evacuation to the United States. From a military standpoint, early craniectomy (the temporary removal of a portion of the skull) provides an additional margin of safety by helping military doctors and nurses maintain safe intracranial pressure control in hostile settings and during the lengthy transport of severely wounded troops over thousands of miles.

Recognition that blood vessel injury or irritation can extend the severity of TBI has prompted measures to quickly detect and treat vasospasm after a head injury. Once doctors diagnose impaired brain blood flow, they should have a low threshold to intervene with such measures as expanding blood volume, allowing blood pressure to gradually rise (when there is little concern for further intracranial bleeding), and in particularly serious cases, using blood vessel-dilating techniques, such as intracranial balloon angioplasty. While dilating brain blood vessels has not been definitively shown to improve outcomes from brain injury, the technique is relatively safe and appears to reduce the risk of stroke.

CONCLUSION

TBI is one of the greatest challenges facing the military health system and all of medical science. But as the story that opened this chapter illustrates, military surgeons and nurses are saving the lives of service members with brain injuries that were previously regarded as non-survivable. Once-dramatic measures, such as removing part of the skull for weeks at a time to allow the brain to swell, are now commonplace. Hopefully, the day will come when high rates of survival and recovery from severe brain injury are commonplace as well.

Notes

1. Armonda RA, Bell RS, Vo AH, et al. Wartime traumatic cerebral vasospasm: recent review of combat casualties. *Neurosurgery*. 2006;59:1215–1225. doi:10.1227/01.NEU.0000249190.46033.94.

2. Bell RS, Vo AH, Neal CJ, et al. Military traumatic brain and spinal column injury: a 5-year study of the impact blast and other military grade weaponry on the central nervous system. *J Trauma*. 2009;66:S104–111. doi:10.1097/TA.0b013e31819d88c8.

3. Bell RS, Mossop CM, Dirks MS, et al. Early decompressive craniectomy for severe penetrating and closed head injury during wartime. *Neurosurg Focus*. 2010;28:E1. doi:10.3171/2010.2.focus1022.

4. Maas AIR, Stocchetti N, Bullock R. Moderate and severe traumatic brain injury in adults. *Lancet Neurol*. 2008;7:728–741. doi:10.1016/S1474-4422(08)70164-9.

5. Rimel RW, Giordani B, Barth JT, Boll TJ, Jane JA. Disability caused by minor head injury. *Neurosurgery*. 1981;9:221–228.

6. Savitsky E, Eastridge B, Katz D, Cooper R, eds. *Combat Casualty Care: Lessons Learned From OEF and OIF*. Fort Detrick, MD: Borden Insitute; 2012.

7. Narayan RK, Maas AI, Servadei F, et al. Progression of traumatic intracerebral hemorrhage: a prospective observational study. *J Neurotrauma*. 2008;25:629–639. doi:10.1089/neu.2007.0385.

8. Cushing H. A study of a series of wounds involving the brain and its enveloping structures. *Br J Surg*. 1917;5:558–684. doi:10.1002/bjs.1800052004.

9. Guidelines for the management of penetrating brain injury. Antibiotic prophylaxis for penetrating brain injury. *J Trauma*. 2001;51:S34–40.

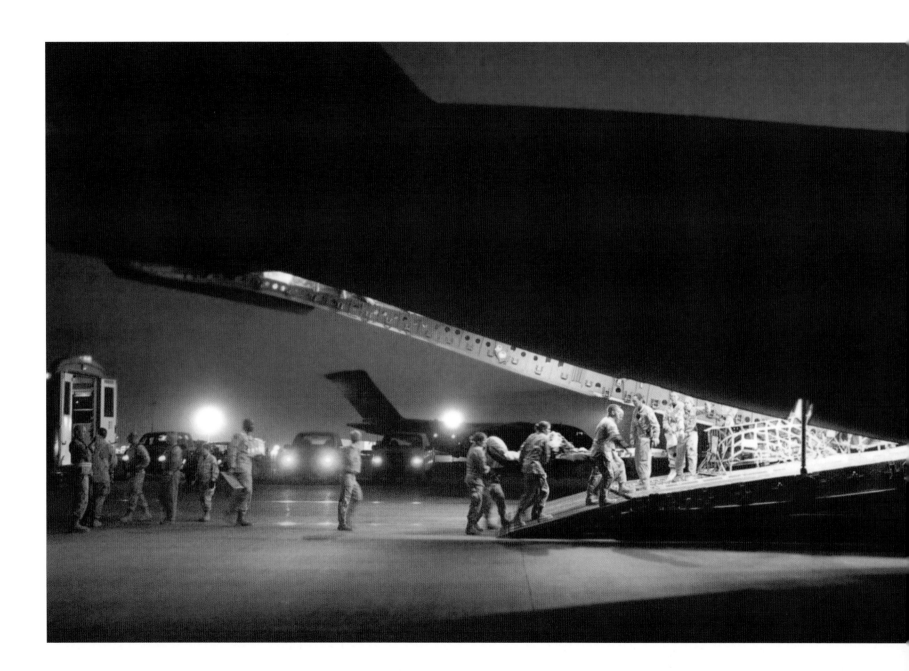

CHAPTER twenty

Advancing Burn Care During Combat

LEOPOLDO C. CANCIO, MD

THE CHALLENGE

THE CASE NOTED IN THE VIGNETTE (PAGE 186) HIGHLIGHTS several important features of burn care during the wars in Iraq and Afghanistan. Burns were documented in 10.7 percent of casualties in the Department of Defense Trauma Registry, reflecting the high incidence of injuries caused by explosions, particularly roadside IEDs. With few exceptions, the most severely burned US service members were treated at the Army Burn Center at Fort Sam Houston. Established in 1949, the Center was significantly downsized at the end of the Cold War. As a result, those planning Operation Iraqi Freedom (OIF) in late 2002 and early 2003 initially considered other options for treating burned service members, including sending them to civilian burn centers near their homes of record. Fortunately, this did not occur. Instead, the Burn Center was appropriately staffed and resourced to treat substantial numbers of military casualties. This created a unique platform to deliver care.

THE INNOVATIONS

Severely burned patients demonstrate a multi-system response to injury, meaning every organ in the body is affected. These changes are proportional to the size and severity of the burns (expressed as a percentage of the body surface area burned). In general, burn patients pass through three phases of care:

FIGURE 20.1. [*Opposite*] Balad, Iraq: Contingency aeromedical staging facility (CASF) team members prepare a critical care patient for Critical Care Air Transport Team (CCATT) transport on a C-17 Globemaster to Landstuhl, Germany, where he will receive further treatment before a subsequent CCATT flight to the United States. Februray 14, 2007. Photo by Master Sergeant Cecilio Ricardo, US Air Forces Central Command Public Affairs. Reproduced from: https://www.dvidshub.net/image/41253/air-force-war.

VIGNETTE >> The US vehicle was engulfed in flames when it was struck by a roadside improvised explosive device (IED). Three Soldiers riding in the vehicle were killed, and the fourth, a 28-year-old US Army noncommissioned officer (NCO), sustained burns to 60 percent of his total body surface area. He was transported by MEDEVAC helicopter to the combat support hospital (CSH) in Baghdad, Iraq. The emergency department team placed a tube into his airway to help him breathe, and inserted catheters into large veins and an artery to replace fluid and monitor his blood pressure. After a computed tomography scan to rule out other injuries, the Soldier was taken to the operating room to cleanse his wounds. Because full-thickness burns threatened to cut off circulation to his extremities, surgeons first performed escharotomies (surgical incisions) to release the tight, swollen, and deeply burned skin (Figure 20.2). Under general anesthesia, the Soldier's blood pressure dropped, so the anesthetist poured in intravenous (IV) fluids and started drugs to support his falling vital signs. Burn shock was setting in. The Soldier would require constant monitoring and fluid replacement for at least two days.

As the Soldier's blood pressure stabilized, the team did a bronchoscopy. This involved passing a thin, flexible fiberoptic scope through his breathing tube to examine the lung's major airways. It was important to determine if the Soldier had smoke inhalation injury (damage to the airways), a complication that is twice as common in combat casualties as in civil-

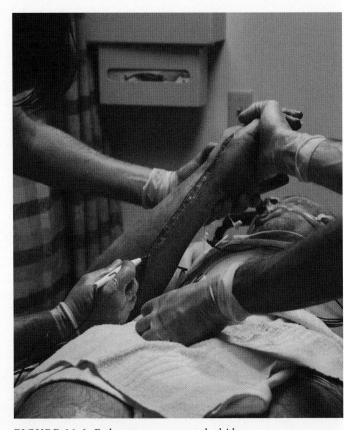

FIGURE 20.2. Escharotomy, an urgent bedside operation performed to relieve tight circumferential burned skin and restore circulation to a burned extremity.

ian patients. The bronchoscope revealed soot, swelling, weeping fluid, and redness in the airways—clear signs of inhalation injury. This presented the team with a critical decision: continue efforts to stabilize the patient in the CSH, or place a potentially unstable patient with burn shock and lung injury on a long Critical Care Air Transport Team flight to Germany? Reasoning that infection of the lungs or burns could set in as soon as a week after injury, the team decided to evacuate the patient to Landstuhl, and from there to San Antonio (see Chapter 25). As they dressed his wounds, they carefully drew a diagram that mapped the full extent of his burns. They also filled out a Burn Resuscitation Flow Sheet to clearly communicate the amount of fluids and medications the Soldier had received to the next team in the evacuation chain. They knew that massive fluid resuscitation can place patients at risk of abdominal compartment syndrome, a condition that causes such severe swelling of the abdomen that vital organs cease to function. This condition is about 90 percent lethal. Fortunately, careful tracking and adjustment of fluids helped prevent this.

CSH personnel placed the injured Soldier on a customized NATO litter able to secure life support equipment for transport—a mechanical ventilator, IV infusion pumps, a vital signs monitor, and a suction machine (Figure 20.3). The surgical team in Baghdad contacted the US Army Burn Center (part of the US Army Institute of Surgical Research) at Fort Sam Houston, Texas, the only burn center operated by the US Department of Defense. In response, the Center dispatched a special Burn Flight Team consisting of a burn surgeon, critical care nurse, respiratory therapist, licensed vocational nurse, and senior medic to

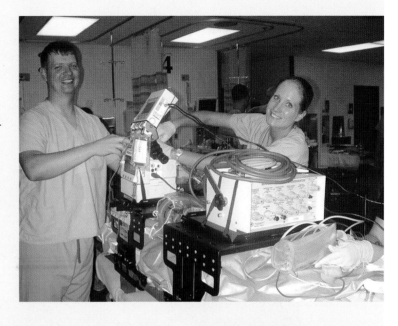

FIGURE 20.3. Preparing a burn patient for transport by attaching critical care equipment to platforms atop a NATO litter. Photograph courtesy of the US Army Institute of Surgical Research.

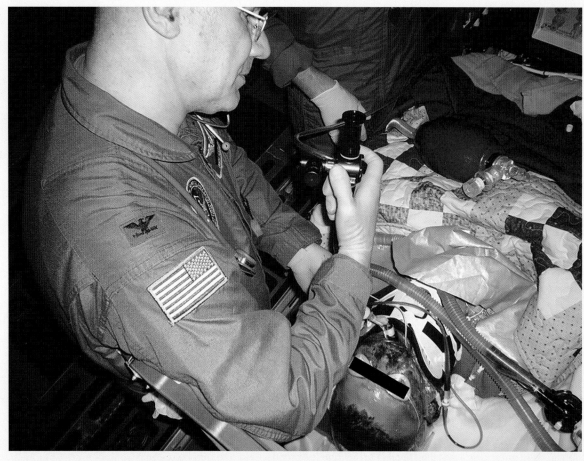

FIGURE 20.4. Colonel David Barillo, US Army Burn Flight Team surgeon, uses a fiber optic scope to examine the airways of a combat casualty with burns and smoke inhalation injury being flown from Landstuhl, Germany, to Fort Sam Houston, Texas. Photography courtesy of C.K. Thompson, PA-C.

Landstuhl to meet the patient and provide care during the second leg of his transcontinental evacuation (Figure 20.1).

In Germany, the Burn Flight Team assumed responsibility for the Soldier's care, making sure he was stable enough to survive a 12-hour trans-Atlantic flight. The first day of fluid resuscitation gave him 19 liters (roughly 5 gallons) of IV salt solution. As a result, his facial features and body were largely swollen beyond recognition. Fortunately, his burn shock responded to this treatment, so providers could begin to wean down his IV fluids and blood pressure medications. Since the patient had severe airway damage and compromised breathing from the inhalation injury, the team placed him on a special ventilator to help keep his airways clear of debris and to maintain adequate oxygen levels at altitude. The next day, they departed Germany by C-17 aircraft (Figure 20.5).

Arriving at the Army Burn Center 3-1/2 days after his injury, this Soldier was lucky to be alive, but his arduous journey was just beginning. As long as full-thickness burns remained, he would be at high risk for infection, inflammation, and multi-system organ failure. The Burn Center had to weigh the risks and benefits of early, massive excision of the dead tissue, versus a more staged, gradual approach to healing his skin. Since the Soldier was physically fit, they opted for high-risk surgery. They removed all of the destroyed skin tissue during a single operation, except for his head, neck, and hands. They used a "sandwich" technique to combine widely meshed skin from the patient (autograft) with skin from a deceased organ donor (allograft). In this manner,

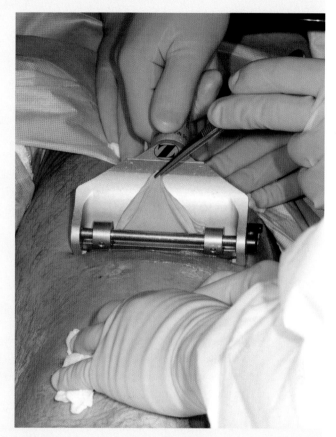

FIGURE 20.5. Harvesting a split-thickness skin graft using an air-powered dermatome.

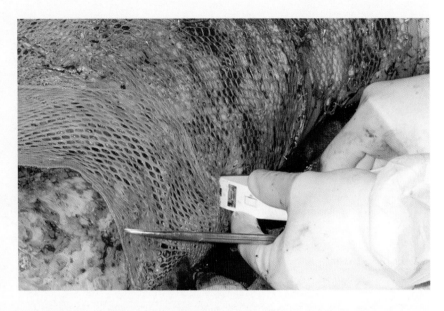

FIGURE 20.6. Stapling a meshed, expanded, split-thickness skin graft to an excised burn wound.

they covered all excised areas with new skin (Figures 20.4 through 20.6).

At least once a week (sometimes twice), the patient was brought back to the operating room for more surgery until his wounds were completely healed. This required ten major operations and three months in the burn intensive care unit (ICU). Meanwhile, a multi-disciplinary team had to carefully manage every other aspect of the Soldier's physical and mental health. Surgeons, medical internists, critical care nurses, respiratory therapists, physical and occupational therapists, social workers, and dieticians participated daily in rounds to address these issues in exquisite detail.

Not surprisingly, the Soldier's course was challenging. His inhalation injury led to several bouts of pneumonia caused by virulent bacteria. During one episode he developed acute kidney failure and required treatment similar to dialysis. Fortunately, his kidneys recovered. Eventually, rehabilitation—which had started the day he entered the ICU—became his top therapy goal. Four months after arriving in San Antonio, he was discharged from the hospital, but he made near-daily visits to the Burn Outpatient Clinic for several months. Posttraumatic stress disorder, body-image issues, and feelings of guilt about the loss of fellow soldiers were prominent in both his inpatient and outpatient psychotherapy (Chapters 30–33). Eventually the Soldier was medically retired. Today, he is a teacher.

(1) resuscitation, (2) surgery and critical care, and (3) rehabilitation and reconstruction. In reality, these phases overlap, usually with rehabilitation beginning on admission. If we wait for all the surgeries to be completed before starting rehabilitation, it is very difficult to overcome scar contractures and deconditioning.

During the resuscitation phase, the focus of the first 48 hours is on providing enough IV fluids to replace the massive loss of plasma from damaged small blood vessels. Formulas for this process are only guidelines, so clinicians must carefully adjust the replacement rate at least hourly according to the patient's response. Urine output within targeted amounts and timeframes is the main sign of a good response. Inattention to this detail can occur anywhere, but is a special risk during aeromedical evacuation. Infusion of too much fluid can lead to abdominal or extremity compartment syndromes, especially when the amount of fluids infused exceeds 250 mL/kg during the first 24 hours. To assist clinicians, military burn specialists devised clinical practice guidelines, a burn resuscitation flow sheet, and an innovative decision support system to help clinicians with burn resuscitation (the software package is now commercially available as Burn Navigator [Arcos Medical Inc., Houston, TX]).[1]

During the surgical phase of care, areas of full-thickness (third-degree) and deep partial-thickness (second-degree) burns are removed, and the exposed wounds are covered with skin grafts. Patients with small burns can be treated with autografts harvested from unburned sites on their body. These donor sites typically heal within 12 to 14 days, and can provide skin grafts again. By meshing the skin graft, burn doctors can expand its size to cover a larger area (see Figure 20.6). The grafted skin grows into the spaces in the mesh as it heals. If the total area of the burn exceeds about 40 percent of the body, doctors typically add skin from an organ donor (allograft). Allograft skin is used as a temporary covering (a "biological dressing") to protect the wound while the patient's own donor sites heal.

In many instances, skin harvested from the patient's body and skin from an organ donor can be combined in the form of a "sandwich." First, the autograft (the patient's own skin) is meshed with large "holes" to maximize the area it can cover. This graft is placed directly on top of the clean, recently excised wound. Then, the allograft (skin from a donor) is placed on top. The allograft protects the underlying wound while the patient's autograft gradually becomes vascularized and grows into the spaces in the mesh. More experimental approaches to closing wounds from massive burns include lab-grown skin cells or artificial tissue matrix. Regardless of the technology used, the key to survival is to bring about rapid and effective wound healing. Which patients will survive (and which may not) can be distinguished as soon as 21 days after injury, based on their rate of healing.[2]

For patients with particularly large burns, the surgical phase and the critical care phase overlap. A typical burn patient spends about one day in the ICU for every percentage point the body is burned. During this phase, infections of the blood, lungs, or wounds are the main threat to survival.[3] Lung support is a primary goal. Burn patients with inhalation injury face a higher risk of dying. Inhalation injury is more common when a patient is burned inside an enclosed space such as a building, vehicle, or ship. These structures can trap heat, fumes, and soot that are then drawn into the patient's lungs. Inhalation injury is also more common in patients with large body surface area burns. Due to the mechanism of injury, combat casualties sustain inhalation injury at twice the rate of civilians.[4] Mechanical ventilation is frequently required to support patients with inhalation injury. Respiratory therapists play a vital role in the burn ICU, not only by managing the settings of complex ventilators and frequently suctioning fluid from damaged airways, but also by aggressively weaning and extubating patients as soon as they can breathe without assistance.[5]

Acute kidney failure from various causes is another dreaded complication. Army studies have produced improved methods of kidney replacement therapy (similar to dialysis) that is delivered by burn ICU nurses under the guidance of burn physicians.[6]

The rehabilitation and reconstruction phase begins in the ICU and continues long after discharge. In many ways, rehabilitation represents a frontier for burn research. Studies are examining the amount of rehabilitation required by critically ill burn patients, and the effect that rehabilitation has on long-term outcomes. The military's goals during OIF and Operation Enduring Freedom (OEF) were to maximize rates of recovery and return-to-duty among injured service members, and, for those leaving the military, to optimize their rehabilitation before they transitioned to civilian life and care in the Veterans Administration system. This required a much greater commitment to inpatient and outpatient rehabilitation than in previous conflicts (Chapter 31). The effort was worth it. During OIF and OEF, two out of every three burn patients treated in this manner returned to duty.[7]

Surgeons try to postpone reconstructive surgery as long as possible, since the pro-inflammatory response to injury, which increases the tendency to form aggressive scar contractures, begins to abate a year after injury. Some patients need earlier reconstructive surgery if contractures limit their ability to perform routine activities or place critical body parts at risk. For instance, eyelid contractures can expose the corneas, endangering sight. To address these issues, the Army Burn Center hired a full-time plastic and reconstructive surgeon.

Recognizing the value of prevention, burn doctors actively promoted strategies to keep patients from requiring their services. Hand burns are particularly devastating because they often lead to lifelong disability. Prevention was advanced by educating service members about the vital importance of wearing proper hand protection (such as Nomex [DuPont, Wilmington, DE] gloves) when involved in convoy duty and other high-risk activities (see Chapter 9).

When is a burn injury over? Severely burned patients such as the 28-year-old NCO described in the vignette do not return to life "as before." Like many injured combat veterans, they adapt to a "new normal." Severe burns require a lifelong commitment to care, rehabilitation, and recovery.

IMPACT

From 2003 to 2013, 903 wounded warriors with burns were admitted to the Army Burn Center from overseas contingency operations. Of these, 725 were from OIF, 167 from OEF, and 11 from Operation New Dawn. The average burn size was 16 percent ± 19 percent total body surface area; the average full-thickness burn size was 10 percent ± 18 percent, and 16 percent of patients had concurrent inhalation injuries. The leading cause was IED explosions, which generated nearly half of all cases.[8] The Army Burn Flight Team transported the highest risk patients, a total of 305. The overall mortality rate was 5.8 percent—very low, given the severity and complexity of these cases. Moreover, the preservation of the Army Burn Center ensured that the difficult transition from inpatient to outpatient care, and the subsequent months of outpatient treatment and rehabilitation, were handled in a uniquely military environment. Advantages of so doing included psychological support attentive to the sequelae of combat, maintenance of the strong social bond among injured warfighters, attention to the needs of military families, and a focus on recovery of function rather than on disability.

TABLE 20.1. Recent Advances in Burn Care Developed by the US Military

- Rapid deployment of Burn Flight Teams.

- Faster evacuation of eligible patients to the Army Burn Center.

- Early massive excision of burn wounds.

- Use of advanced ventilators (high-frequency percussive ventilation) to treat inhalation injury.[1]

- Use of continuous renal replacement therapy to treat acute kidney injury.[2]

- Development and commercialization of Burn Navigator (Arcos Medical Inc, Houston, TX) for fluid resuscitation.[3]

- Initiation of early and aggressive physical and occupational therapy in the intensive care unit.

- Long-term outpatient follow-up of burn survivors, including provision of reconstructive surgery.

Sources:
1. Chung KK, Wolf SE, Renz EM, et al. High-frequency percussive ventilation and low tidal volume ventilation in burns: a randomized controlled trial. *Crit Care Med.* 2010;38(10):1970–1977.
2. Chung KK, Lundy JB, Matson JR, et al. Continuous venovenous hemofiltration in severely burned patients with acute kidney injury: a cohort study. *Crit Care.* 2009;13(3):R62.
3. Salinas J, Chung KK, Mann EA, et al. Computerized decision support system improves fluid resuscitation following severe burns: an original study. *Crit Care Med.* 2011;39(9):2031–2038.

NOTABLE ADVANCES

Between the Vietnam War and the conclusion of OEF and OIF, the Army Burn Center championed numerous advances in burn and surgical critical care. A few of these are summarized in Table 20.1. The high level of care provided to severely burned service members during OEF and OIF would not have been possible if the Burn Center had not maintained a core level of commitment to excellence during the difficult interwar years, and if policymakers had not reinforced its staffing and resources at war's onset.

CONCLUSION

It is easy to get distracted by the high-tech nature of burn critical care. Skillful use of technology is an important aspect of burn treatment, but it's not the essence. The core aspect of successful burn care is teamwork, professionalism, and compassion. The remarkable care provided to wounded warriors throughout OEF and OIF, and continuing to this day, is the product of dedicated physicians, nurses, and therapists working together as a cohesive multidisciplinary team.

Notes

1. Salinas J, Chung KK, Mann EA, et al. Computerized decision support system improves fluid resuscitation following severe burns: an original study. *Crit Care Med.* 2011;39(9):2031–2038.
2. Nitzschke SL, Aden JK, Serio-Melvin ML, et al. Wound healing trajectories in burn patients and their impact on mortality. *J Burn Care Res.* 2014;35:474–479.
3. Gomez R, Murray CK, Hospenthal DR, et al. Causes of mortality by autopsy findings of combat casualties and civilian patients admitted to a burn unit. *J Am Coll Surg.* 2009;208(3):348–354.
4. Wolf SE, Kauvar DS, Wade CE, et al. Comparison between civilian burns and combat burns from Operation Iraqi Freedom and Operation Enduring Freedom. *Ann Surg.* 2006;243(6):786–792.
5. Chung KK, Wolf SE, Renz EM, et al. High-frequency percussive ventilation and low tidal volume ventilation in burns: a randomized controlled trial. *Crit Care Med.* 2010;38(10):1970–1977.
6. Chung KK, Lundy JB, Matson JR, et al. Continuous venovenous hemofiltration in severely burned patients with acute kidney injury: a cohort study. *Crit Care.* 2009;13(3):R62.
7. Chapman TT, Richard RL, Hedman TL, et al. Military return to duty and civilian return to work factors following burns with focus on the hand and literature review. *J Burn Care Res.* 2008;29:756–762.
8. Kauvar DS, Wolf SE, Wade CE, Cancio LC, Renz EM, Holcomb JB. Burns sustained in combat explosions in Operations Iraqi and Enduring Freedom (OIF/OEF explosion burns). *Burns.* 2006;32(7):853–857.

Note: The author is a co-inventor of Burn Navigator (Arcos Medical, Inc, Houston, TX). He has assigned his rights to the Army.

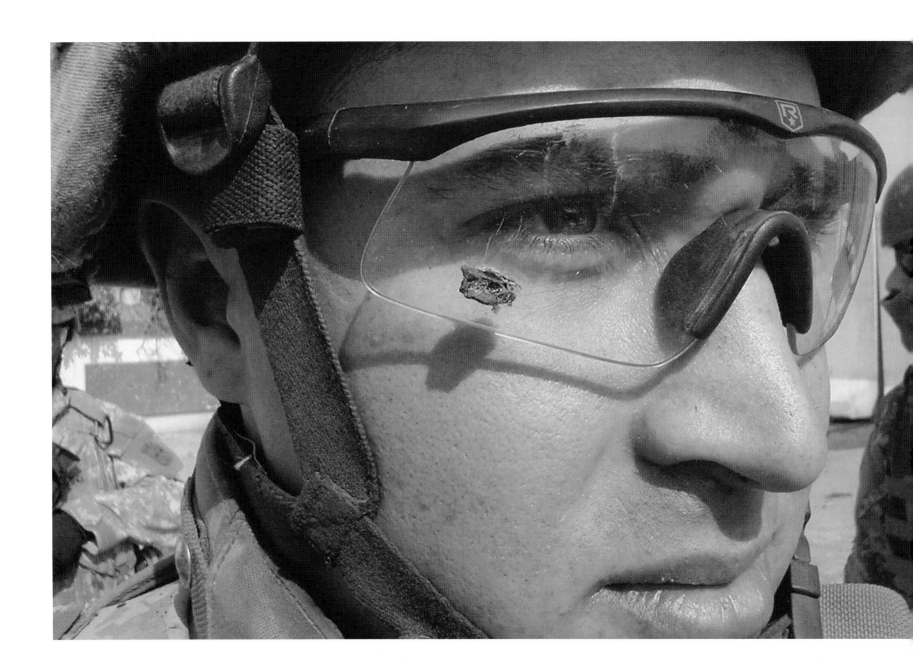

CHAPTER twenty-one

Combat Ocular Trauma

MARCUS H. COLYER, MD, and KEVIN M. JACKSON, OD, MPH

THE CHALLENGE

T HANKS TO MODERN BODY ARMOR AND KEVLAR (Du Pont, Wilmington, DE) helmets, more troops survive combat injuries that would have previously been fatal. However, body armor does not protect the face and neck.[2,3] Combat eye protection has been available for decades,[4] but military personnel often fail to use it. Because ambushes and improvised explosive devices are common methods of attack in Iraq and Afghanistan,[5] failure to consistently wear eye protection results in eye injuries that otherwise might have been avoided (Figure 21-1). Although dramatic advances in ophthalmic surgery enable the military health system to repair and rehabilitate eyes that would have been lost in prior wars, the complexity of these injuries requires a prolonged, multidisciplinary approach to achieve good results. Even then, some eyes cannot be saved, and many more cannot be restored to optimal function.

Treating vision-threatening ocular injuries requires provision of the right care at the right time. Immediately after an injury, self-aid and buddy aid for ophthalmic wounds requires recognizing the signs of an open globe injury, protecting the damaged globe with a rigid eye shield, initiating antibiotics early, and immediately referring the patient to an ophthalmic surgeon for care.[6] Typically, life- and limb-saving surgeries take priority over eye surgery, unless both eyes are involved. Still, it's critical to recog-

FIGURE 21.1. [*Opposite*] 1st Lieutenant Anthony Aguilar wears the ballistic protective eyewear that stopped a bomb-fragment from potentially damaging his right eye when an improvised explosive device detonated near his Stryker armored vehicle while on patrol in Mosul, Iraq. June 2, 2006. US Army photo, 138th Public Affairs Detachment. Reproduced from: https://www.dvidshub.net/image/22317/eye-protection.

VIGNETTE >> Afghanistan, 2010: A 20-year-old Army specialist riding in an MRAP (mine-resistant ambush-protected vehicle) sustained severe injuries to his left arm, left leg, and right eye when a rocket-propelled grenade penetrated the side of the vehicle and struck an ammunition canister beside him. He was not wearing his combat eye protection at the time, because he didn't think he needed it inside an MRAP. He was brought to a nearby forward operating base with tourniquets on his injured arm and leg. The evaluating physician noted that he had a corneal laceration and blood in the anterior chamber of his right eye, and documented his visual acuity as "dim and blurry." Because he still had arterial bleeding from a large gash in his left wrist, he was rushed to surgery to stabilize his arm and leg injuries.

Nine hours later, the specialist arrived at the Role 3 combat support hospital at Bagram Air Base. In addition to ongoing care for his multiple orthopedic injuries, he received a detailed examination that revealed small foreign bodies peppering the right side of his face. Microscopic examination of his right eye revealed a T-shaped corneal laceration extending across the width of the eye, with the internal layer of the eye protruding through the wound. The anterior chamber (the area in front of his iris) was abnormally deflated, and the lens was missing. A computed tomography (CT) scan of his head and face revealed a foreign body lodged in the internal wall of the right eye.

Based on the worrisome scan and exam findings, the specialist underwent surgical exploration to repair his damaged right eye. The ophthalmologist carefully inspected his eye, removed the surface layers and stripped out inflammatory tissue. The lens was missing, but the structures that usually hold it remained intact. Surgeons repaired the large corneal laceration using nine hair-thin corneal sutures. They restored the eye's internal structures to their normal positions, and verified that no wounds were leaking. After surgery, they started the patient on powerful broad-spectrum antibiotics in pill and drop forms, and gave steroid eye drops to reduce inflammation. Shortly thereafter, he was flown by Critical Care Air Transport Team (CCATT) to Landstuhl Regional Medical Center in Germany. After two days of observation, he was flown to Andrews Air Force Base aboard a second CCATT flight.

After ground transport to Walter Reed National Military Medical Center, a high-resolution CT scan of the eye socket localized several foreign bodies. The Soldier's vision was limited to "light perception" in the right eye and 20/25 in his left eye (nearly perfect). Eye pressure was low in the right eye and normal in the left. A microscopic exam of the right eye revealed a sealed corneal laceration, absent lens, and extensive hemorrhage. Small debris was visible on ophthalmic ultrasound, and two small foreign bodies were visible just below the muscle that controls side movements of the eye. Because the patient also needed orthopedic surgery, the ophthalmology service scheduled his definitive repair for 13 days post-injury.

The subsequent eye surgery was performed using an endoscope, a special camera placed inside the globe of the Soldier's eye. Through this scope, the eye surgeons located and removed several foreign bodies, and repaired the eye's internal structures, including a retinal tear with bleeding. To keep the retina from peeling off the back of the eye, doctors injected a special gas into the globe of the eye to hold it in place. This was particularly important because the patient's orthopedic injuries prevented him from maintaining the preferred position after surgery.

After the operation, the patient developed high pressure in the eye. Eye drops and oral medications helped, but he eventually required another surgery to permanently lower the pressure. Three months after his original injury, he developed scar tissue with swelling in the macula, the most important part of the retina, which enables detailed sight. He underwent more surgery to gently peel the scar tissue off the macula, and 10 months after his injury, he had a corneal transplant. Two months after this surgery, his vision was 20/80 once he was fitted with a custom-designed +10.00 scleral contact lens.

In total, this patient underwent six surgeries on the right eye to restore him to functional vision. He also required 30 operations to salvage the function of his left arm. In addition, he required intensive rehabilitation to avoid side effects commonly associated with head and eye injuries, such as excessive light sensitivity, problems with visual perception issues, and severe headaches due to the eyes' reduced ability to work together.[1]

nize ocular injuries and deliver the patient to a qualified ophthalmic provider as soon as possible. The provider must assess the integrity of the eye and quickly close any open wounds. Then the patient can be safely returned home for more definitive treatment and, eventually, long-term rehabilitation.

THE INNOVATION: EYE ARMOR

Prevention is by far the best way to reduce loss of vision. Regular eye glasses, including wrap-around sunglasses, vary widely in the degree of protection they provide. Most sports glasses are inadequate for battlefield use because they do not have a high enough impact rating to provide adequate protection from ballistic fragments. In response, the military funded government research to develop battlefield eye protection. The products researchers produced were highly protective but so visually unappealing that few warfighters would wear them. At that point, the military took a different tack: setting a high standard, drawing on the performance data used to create the prototypes, for industry. When commercial vendors came forward with products that met that standard, the military allowed its warfighters to choose their protective eyewear based on their personal preference. Most opted for models that feature high impact polycarbonate lenses set in attractive, wrap-style frames.

IMPACT

Studies among deployed service members determined that use of approved eye armor reduces the frequency of eye injuries by 84 percent. Eye-penetrating injuries (the most common cause of blindness in deployed service members) were reduced by 86 percent.[7,8] Similar rates of protection have been noted in civilian populations at risk for eye injury. Unfortunately, the protection occurs only when warfighters consistently wear the protective gear.

Over the course of Operations Enduring Freedom and Iraqi Freedom, the military made great strides in promoting the use of eye protection. In 2004, the Army and Marine Corps picked a commercial product and directed its deploying combatants to use it. Unfortunately, compliance with the order was sporadic. By 2008, all services deploying service members required personnel in war zones to use eye protection. Compliance with the order improved when the services expanded the range of choices.

Today, service members can pick the qualified eye armor they want, including well-known, stylish brands. This substantially increased rates of use among deployed personnel and reduced the severity of eye injuries.[9]

CONCLUSION

Sometimes, the most effective measure to address an important cause of injury is the simplest. Complex ophthalmic surgery can restore a remarkable degree of function to severely injured warfighters with penetrating injuries to the eye. However, it is extremely costly and the outcomes are often less than perfect. The most effective countermeasure, by far, is consistent use of eye armor.

As is true with other lessons from war, this observation applies with equal relevance to civilian populations. In the United States, more than 1.9 million Americans per year injure their eyes and require medical attention.[10] By stressing the importance of preventing penetrating eye injuries, and making eye armor available in fashionable designs, the US military increased compliance and reduced the incidence of severe eye injuries.

Notes

1. Greenwald BD, Kapoor N, Singh AD. Visual impairments in the first year after traumatic brain injury. *Brain Inj.* 2012;26:1338–1359.
2. Breeze J, Gibbons AJ, Shieff C, Banfield G, Bryant DG, Midwinter MJ. Combat-related craniofacial and cervical injuries: a 5-year review from the British military. *J Trauma.* 2011;71:108–113.
3. Hilber D, Mitchener TA, Stout J, Hatch B, Canham-Chervak M. Eye injury surveillance in the U.S. Department of Defense, 1996-2005. *Am J Prev Med.* 2010;38:S78-85.
4. La Piana FG WT. The development of eye armor for the American infantryman. *Ophthalmol Clin North Am.* 1999;12:421–434.
5. Vlasov A, Ryan DS, Ludlow S, Weichel ED, Colyer MH. Causes of combat ocular trauma-related blindness from Operation Iraqi Freedom and Enduring Freedom. *J Trauma Acute Care Surg* 2015;79:S210–215.

6. CoTCCC. Tactical Combat Casualty Care guidelines for medical personnel. http://www.usaisr. amedd.army.mil/pdfs/TCCC_Guidelines_for_Medical_Personnel_151111.pdf. Accessed December 23, 2016.

7. Parker P, Mossadegh S, McCrory C. A comparison of the IED-related eye injury rate in ANSF and ISAF forces at the UK R3 Hospital, Camp Bastion, 2013. *J R Army Med Corps.* 2014;160:73–74.

8. Hilber DJ. An update of combat eye protection effectiveness and eye injury incidence in recent conflicts. *VC&R Quarterly.* 2015;7(2):7–8.

9. Thomas R, McManus JG, Johnson A, Mayer P, Wade C, Holcomb JB. Ocular injury reduction from ocular protection use in current combat operations. *J Trauma.* Apr 2009;66:S99–103.

10. McGwin G, Jr, Xie A, Owsley C. Rate of eye injury in the United States. *Arch Ophthalmol.* 2005;123:970–976.

Recommended Reading

Auvil JR. Evolution of military combat eye protection. *US Army Med Dep J.* 2016;Apr-Sep:135–139.

Acknowledgements

The authors would like to thank Colonel (Retired) David Hilber OD, MBA, for reference material for this chapter and his leadership at the Tri-Service Vision Conservation and Readiness Program at the US Army Public Health Command.

CHAPTER twenty-two

Controlling Pain with "Soldier-Friendly" Regional Anesthesia

CHESTER C. BUCKENMAIER III, MD, and BRIAN WILHELM

FIRST USE OF REGIONAL ANESTHESIA IN WAR

LIEUTENANT COLONEL BUCKENMAIER AND SPECIALIST WILHELM met for the first time in a combat support hospital's trauma receiving area (see vignette, page 204). A quick examination revealed that much of Specialist Wilhelm's left calf was missing (Figure 22.1). Despite receiving a total of 18 mg of morphine in incremental doses during his medical evacuation, he complained of "10 out of 10" pain—the worst imaginable pain on a verbal analog scale. Lieutenant Colonel Buckenmaier explained how a continuous peripheral nerve block (CPNB) works, and offered to use the technique to ease Specialist Wilhelm's pain. Specialist Wilhelm briefly listened with tolerance, then held up his hand and stated that if something could be done to ease the pain, the anesthesiologist should get on with it. Energized by the request, Buckenmaier proceeded with the first use of CPNB on a modern battlefield. The orthopedic surgeon, Lieutenant Colonel Kimberly Kessler, graciously allowed the 30 minutes he required to set up and perform the nerve block procedure in the operating room.

Today, peripheral nerve blocks are done primarily under ultrasound guidance. But in 2003, that technology had not yet been integrated into the practice of regional anesthesia. At the time, doctors placed most nerve blocks with the guidance of peripheral nerve stimulation.

VIGNETTE >> Iraq, 2013: Specialist Brian Wilhelm (one of this chapter's authors) was driving the rear vehicle of a 4th Infantry Division convoy tasked with resupplying forward operating bases. As the column of vehicles approached the Tigris River, enemy forces ambushed it from a grove of trees abutting the river. A rocket-propelled grenade hit the rear vehicle, passed through the firewall and tore a gaping hole in Specialist Wilhelm's left calf. Not realizing he'd been hit, Wilhelm grabbed his rifle and exited the vehicle to return fire. He realized the severity of his injury when he nearly fell, breaking his fall with his M16 rifle's buttstock. A nearby Soldier attempted to fashion a makeshift tourniquet from cloth remnants of Specialist Wilhelm's pant leg, and tried to tighten it with a small stick. (Note: the manufactured tourniquets all Soldiers now carry were not yet available; see Chapter 10). The stick broke, so the vehicle's gunner applied a second tourniquet using Specialist Wilhelm's cravat, tightened by a crowbar. As the firefight raged, Specialist Wilhelm engaged the enemy with his M16.

Thirty minutes later, arriving reinforcements carried Specialist Wilhelm to a nearby medical evacuation helicopter (Figure 22.2). Less than an hour after his injury, he entered the trauma receiving area of the 21st Combat Support Hospital, Camp Anaconda, Balad, Iraq (Figure 22.3).

A Novel Approach to an Ancient Problem: Battlefield Pain

Less than 72 hours before Specialist Wilhelm was injured, Lieutenant Colonel Chester "Trip" Buckenmaier, an Army anesthesiologist, arrived in Iraq. He had recently become the first military medical officer to complete a fellowship in regional anesthesiology at Duke University. The support for his training came from Colonel John "Jack" Chiles, then chief of anesthesiology at Walter Reed Army Medical Center and the anesthesiology consultant to the Army surgeon general. Colonel Chiles believed that recent advancements in needle technology and nerve localization using peripheral nerve stimulation could enable the precise use of regional anesthesia on the battlefield. When he heard Army Surgeon General James Peake lament shortcomings in controlling the pain of casualties arriving at Landstuhl Regional Medical Center, Germany, Colonel Chiles saw his opportunity. He recommended deploying his new fellowship-trained anesthesiologist to Iraq to determine if regional anesthesia and administration of continuous peripheral nerve blocks could help improve pain control for casualties being evacuating back to Germany and the United States. Everything Lieutenant Colonel Buckenmaier required to provide advanced regional anesthesia fit into a single duffle bag.

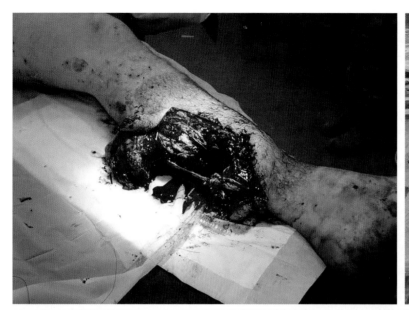

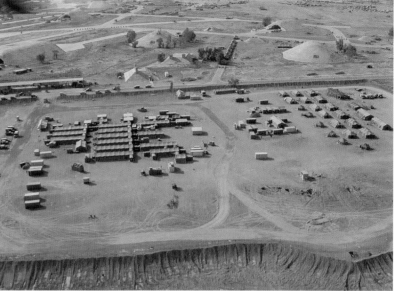

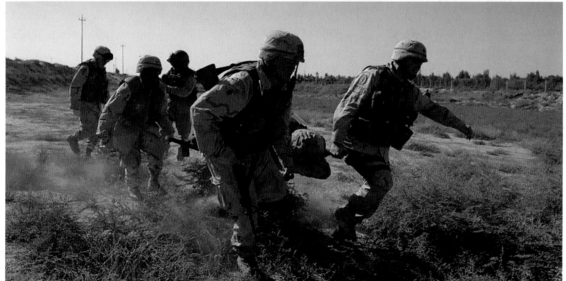

FIGURE 22.1. [*Top Left*]
Specialist Wilhelm's injured left calf.
The extensive damage is the result of
being struck by a rocket-propelled
grenade.

FIGURE 22.2. [*Bottom*]
With a left leg tourniquet fashioned
from a cravat and vehicle crowbar,
Specialist Wilhelm is removed from
the battle to an evacuation helicopter.

FIGURE 22.3. [*Top Right*]
21st Combat Support Hospital,
Camp Anaconda, Balad, Iraq, 2003.
Hospital tents are left of the central
road, with hospital personnel quarters
and support tents to their left.

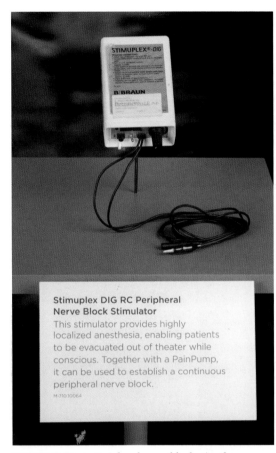

FIGURE 22.4. Peripheral nerve block stimulator used in the first continuous peripheral nerve block on a wounded American soldier in 2003. Object is on display in the Innovations in Military Medicine exhibit gallery as of August 2015. National Museum of Health and Medicine photo by Matthew Breitbart/ Released.

A peripheral nerve stimulator (Figure 22.4) is a box that generates a small electric current through a thin, insulated needle. The operator inserts the needle, based on knowledge of nerve location, and then uses the stimulator to precisely position the needle next to the target nerve. When muscles twitch in the distribution of the nerve, the operator knows the needle is correctly placed.

Significantly, peripheral nerve stimulation and nerve blocks are useful even in patients with traumatic amputations of limbs because they can still perceive motor stimulation of the missing hand or foot. This is termed "phantom stimulation"[1] and was used to great effect by Dr. Buckenmaier while deployed in Iraq. Modern ultrasound technology, which allows real time observation of target nerves, has largely eliminated the need for phantom stimulation today.

After precisely placing two stimulating needles next to the major nerves that carry impulses to and from Specialist Wilhelm's damaged leg, Dr. Buckenmaier injected a concentrated local anesthetic. The drug acts to block noxious pain impulses from traveling up the nerve to reach the brain. Within seconds, Specialist Wilhelm's pain began to rapidly subside. At that point, Dr. Buckenmaier replaced the needles with thin, plastic catheters connected to infusion pumps. This allowed him to administer a continuous infusion of local anesthetic to control the pain (Figure 22.5).

With the nerve block catheters in place, the surgical team began to prepare Specialist Wilhelm for surgery. As they lifted his injured leg for cleaning, the badly damaged shin bone snapped in two, his foot striking the table at an unnatural angle. Specialist Wilhelm, still conscious, asked what had happened. His pain relief was so complete that he didn't realize that the sound was caused by his foot striking the table. With little more than light sedation, he slept soundly as Dr. Kessler repaired the broken shin bone and dressed his wound.

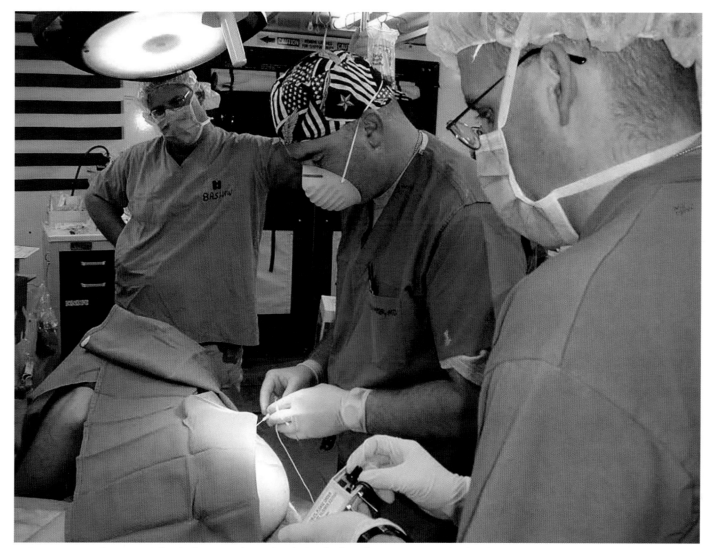

FIGURE 22.5. Lieutenant Colonel Chester Buckenmaier placing the first of two continuous peripheral nerve block (CPNB) catheters (lumbar plexus) using a peripheral nerve block stimulator and insulated needle at the 21st Combat Support Hospital, Balad, Iraq. This was the first CPNB catheter placed in a wounded American Soldier on a modern battlefield.

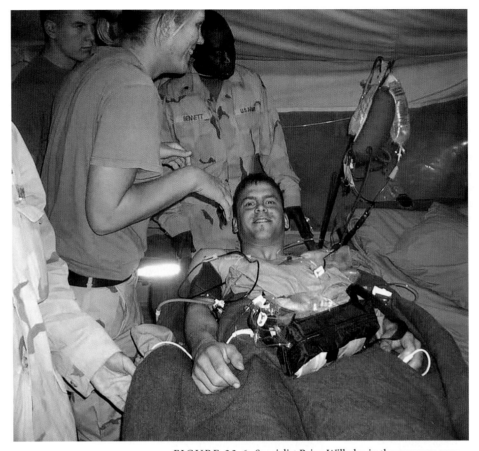

FIGURE 22.6. Specialist Brian Wilhelm in the recovery area moments after surgery on his injured left leg, after receiving the first continuous peripheral nerve block in an American combat support hospital. The infusion pumps for the catheters are in the blue bag on his lap.

IMPACT

After the operation, Specialist Wilhelm entered the recovery area alert, awake, and comfortable. Many of his unit comrades visited him, and the mood was surprisingly upbeat as they laughed off the stress of the battle and his injury (Figure 22.6). For Lieutenant Colonel Buckenmaier, standing quietly in the back of the tent, the scene validated the vision of Colonel Chiles, the support of Lieutenant General Peake, and years of personal effort.

The CPNB catheters Dr. Buckenmeier placed in the operating room of the 21st Combat Support Hospital in Balad enabled military healthcare providers to control Specialist Wilhelm's pain for the next 16 days. They were used during his evacuation flight to Germany and from there to the United States, dramatically reducing his need for opioid medication during the long flights. Subsequently, the nerve block catheters provided a means to quickly achieve a surgical level of pain control during four subsequent operations, as doctors tried to save his shattered leg. Between these operations, continuous infusion of local anesthetic controlled Specialist Wilhelm's pain without the nausea, dizziness, constipation, and respiratory depression that are common side effects of morphine and other opiate-based pain medicines.

Unfortunately, the surgeons couldn't save Specialist Wilhelm's leg. One month after his injury, he walked out of the hospital with a prosthetic leg. His function was so good that he remained on active duty. He never developed symptoms of phantom limb pain or chronic regional pain syndrome, complications that frequently happen after traumatic limb loss.[2] Recent research into troops with traumatic amputations has confirmed that applying continuous peripheral nerve blocks shortly after injury reduces the incidence of neuropathic (nerve damage) pain during recovery.[3]

THE TRANSFORMATION OF BATTLEFIELD PAIN CONTROL

Based on this success, many more casualties received CPNB as part of their initial care. The advance did more than benefit these patients— it sparked a revolution in the US military's approach to battlefield pain management. The development led to the routine use of CPNB catheters, epidural catheters on evacuation flights, the first deployed pain infusion pump system, and hospital and even prehospital use of ketamine (an intense analgesic that works by disconnecting the injured warfighter from the experience of severe pain). Shortly thereafter, the Army detailed now Colonel Buckenmaier to a British combat support hospital to establish an acute pain service (see Chapter 22). Perhaps most importantly, Specialist Wilhelm's experience demonstrated that the military health system can provide effective pain relief to casualties, but only if it develops trained providers, appropriate equipment, and tri-service doctrine to allow the safe application of advanced acute pain management on the battlefield, in combat support hospitals, and during the evacuation home.[4]

Based on early successes like this one, the Army established its first Acute Pain and Regional Anesthesia fellowship program in 2003 and graduated its first Pain Fellow the following year. Graduates of this program are specifically trained to lead acute pain services that provide advanced pain care in our nation's military hospitals and deployed settings. The effort also produced the first military textbook devoted to casualty pain management, *Military Advanced Regional Anesthesia and Analgesia Handbook*.[5]

Today, Specialist Wilhelm (Figure 22.7) is married and has a two-year-old daughter. He recently completed a Master of Science degree and works as a technical consultant for a major pharmaceutical company. In the course of writing this chapter, Colonel (ret) Buckenmaier asked his former patient,

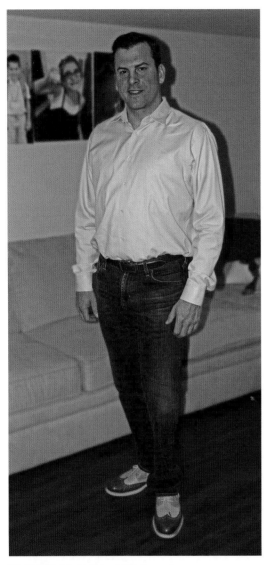

FIGURE 22.7. Brian Wilhelm today.

"What value did you place on the local anesthetic infused through the catheters?" Specialist Wilhelm replied, "I think this one answers itself. Twelve years later, we are still in communication. You changed my life." For a military physician, this is the highest compliment, and a fitting epilogue.

Notes

1. Klein SM, Eck J, Nielsen K, Steele SM. Anesthetizing the phantom: peripheral nerve stimulation of a nonexistent extremity. *Anesthesiology.* 2004;100:736–737.
2. Buckenmaier CC, McKnight Gm, Winkley JV, et al. Continuous peripheral nerve block for battlefield and evacuation. *Reg Anesth Pain Med.* 2005;30:202–205.
3. Buchheit T, Van de Ven T, John Hsia HL, et al. Pain phenotypes and associated clinical risk factors following traumatic amputation: results from Veterans Integrated Pain Evaluation Research (VIPER). *Pain Med.* 2016;17:149–161.
4. Buckenmaier CC, Brandon-Edwards H, Borden D, Wright J. Treating pain on the battlefield: a warrior's perspective. *Curr Pain Headache Rep.* 2010;14:1–7.
5. Buckenmaier C, Bleckner L. *Military Advanced Regional Anesthesia and Analgesia Handbook.* Washington, DC: Borden Institute; 2009. http://www.dvcipm.org/clinical-resources/dvcipm-maraa-book-project. Accessed December 16, 2016.

Recommended Reading

Croll SM, Griffith SR. Acute and chronic pain on the battlefield: lessons learned from the point of injury to the United States. *US Army Med Dep J.* 2016;Apr-Sep:102–105.

CHAPTER twenty-three

Helicopter Evacuation with En Route Critical Care Nurses

MARLA J. DE JONG, PHD; JAMES J. GERACCI, MD; and KIMBERLIE BIEVER, AN

THE CHALLENGE

FROM THE FIRST DAYS OF THE WARS IN IRAQ AND AFGHANISTAN, where combat medical care was complicated by tactical challenges, difficult terrain, and austere environments, the concept of "time to required lifesaving medical capability" drove the military health system to push advanced medical capabilities far-forward onto the battlefield. As a result, non-medic first responders (self-aid and buddy care), Army medics, Navy corpsmen, and Air Force pararescue personnel learned to apply tourniquets and hemostatic dressings, insert IV and intraosseous lines, perform needle decompression, and accomplish emergency airway maneuvers to save lives at the point of injury, often under fire (Chapter 11 and 36). MEDEVAC helicopters quickly rushed the most critically injured to the nearest forward surgical team (FST) or combat support hospital (CSH) for balanced resuscitation and damage control surgery to save critically injured warfighters who would have died in prior conflicts.

The remarkable advances in point-of-injury care and far-forward surgery created a capability gap: the need to provide expert en route care to critically injured patients during the subsequent flights to Role 3 CSHs and, ultimately, to Role 4 hospitals in Germany and the United States. The problem was acute because the MEDEVAC helicopters sent to handle these calls were neither equipped nor staffed to provide ongoing critical care, and the thinly-staffed FSTs could not easily spare a team member

VIGNETTE >> A 28-year-old Soldier conducting convoy operations was severely wounded in a firefight, sustaining multiple gunshot wounds to his upper and lower body. To stop him from bleeding to death, the combat medic on scene applied tourniquets to both legs and summoned a medical evacuation (MEDEVAC) helicopter. Twenty minutes later, the helicopter transported the Soldier to a nearby far-forward surgical team (FST; Chapter 14). Due to the severity of the patient's injuries, the medical team immediately administered balanced blood products (Chapter 16), intubated him to protect his airway, and took him directly to surgery. The surgeon was able to locate and close several badly damaged blood vessels, pack other sources of bleeding in his abdomen, and restore blood flow to his lower extremities. After this damage control surgery (Chapter 15) was completed, the same MEDEVAC team flew the patient to a Role 3 theater hospital 80 miles away for more definitive surgery. During the second flight, he was heavily sedated, mechanically ventilated, and received additional units of blood and intravenous (IV) medications to keep him alive. The flight crew consisted of two MEDEVAC pilots, a crew chief, a flight paramedic, and an en route critical care nurse. The team's knowledge, skill, and clinical experience assured that the critically injured Soldier received expert care throughout both flights.

to accompany the patient. As noted elsewhere in this book, the Army's stance at the time contrasted with the more aggressive approach taken by civilian aeromedical emergency medical services, which staffed their helicopters with critical care-trained flight nurses and paramedics (Chapter 13).

THE INNOVATION

In 2006, based on feedback from the field, operational data from Afghanistan (Chapter 8), and strong advice from Army, Navy, and Air Force en route care experts, the services began to staff selected MEDEVAC helicopters with en route critical care nurses and paramedics to ensure a consistent level of care during transport to theater hospitals.[1] To ensure an adequate supply of qualified personnel, Brigadier General William Bester directed educators at the US Army School of Aviation Medicine at Fort Rucker, Alabama, to develop the Joint Enroute Care Course (JECC).[2,3] This 10-day course was designed to prepare critical care nurses, physicians, physician assistants, and medics to provide tactical combat casualty care (Chapter 11) and en route critical care to severely injured patients being evacuated by helicopter.

Soon thereafter, Air Force Brigadier General Bart Iddins directed trauma and en route care experts at the US Air Force School of Aerospace Medicine at Wright-Patterson Air Force Base to create the Tactical Critical Care Evacuation Team (TCCET) course (see "Tactical Critical Care Evacuation from the Point of Injury"). This course taught emergency and critical care nurses, certified

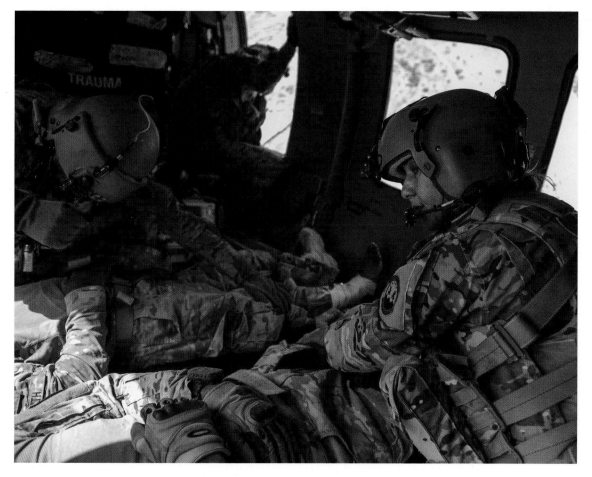

FIGURE 23.1. US Air Force Major Sandra Nestor, tactical critical care evacuation team nurse, provides patient care en route to Forward Operating Base Orgun East in eastern Afghanistan, May 15, 2013. US Air Force photo by Staff Sergeant Marleah Miller. Reproduced from: https://www.dvidshub.net/image/968854/er-black-hawk-helicopter-air-force-nurse-returns-army.

registered nurse anesthetists, and emergency and critical care physicians how to aggressively resuscitate combat casualties at the point of injury and throughout MEDEVAC transport to FSTs and CSHs. Both courses—the Army's JECC and the Air Force's TCCET—taught important concepts and practical skills to enable military healthcare providers to deliver expert critical care to complex postoperative patients being transferred by helicopter or fixed-wing aircraft to higher levels of care.

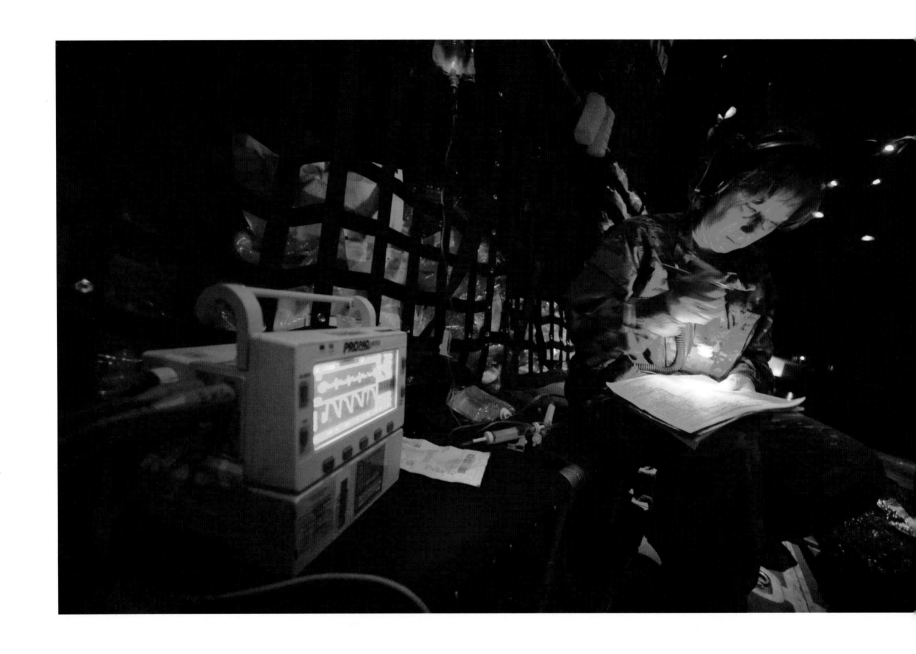

In addition to receiving focused training in the delivery of en route critical care, military nurses tasked with supporting rotary-wing MEDEVAC flights took additional coursework, including Advanced Trauma Care for Nurses, Advanced Trauma Life Support, and Emergency War Surgery. These courses assured that the nurses who deployed to Afghanistan and Iraq were well prepared to provide care at the intensive care unit (ICU) level to severely injured warfighters in austere and often dangerous combat environments (Figure 23-1).

The addition of highly trained nurses to MEDEVAC teams immediately bolstered the level of care provided to injured warfighters during transport. It also allowed advanced resuscitation to begin before casualties reached an FST or CSH. This bridged an important gap in critical care between the point of injury and initial surgical care, and ensured that patients were well cared for during subsequent movement from FSTs and smaller Role 3 CSHs to larger Role 3 hospitals, such as the Air Force Theater Hospital in Balad, Iraq, or Craig Joint Theater Hospital at Bagram Airfield, Afghanistan.

EN ROUTE CRITICAL CARE NURSING TODAY

A decade has passed since critical care nurses first began transporting patients, and later were embedded in Army MEDEVAC units throughout Iraq and Afghanistan. Then and now, these nurses and their accompanying flight medics aggressively resuscitate casualties during evacuation from the battlefield and on subsequent inter-facility flights between Role 2 and Role 3 facilities. During these flights, critical care nurses prioritize, direct, and deliver advanced interventions, including infusion of blood products, administration of IV analgesics, and management of mechanical ventilators and other IV medications in accordance with established clinical guidelines. They also operate and troubleshoot sophisticated transport equipment such as mechanical ventilators and intravenous pumps, and make independent medical decisions during extended transports. All of these activities are performed in challenging environmental conditions, with loud aircraft noise and vibration, low light or black-out conditions, and extreme fluctuations in cabin temperature (Figure 23.2).

In addition to staffing selected MEDEVAC helicopters, critical care nurses have served as key members of Critical Care Air Transport Teams (CCATTs) since the mid-1990s.[4] CCATTs provide continuous "critical care in the air" during intercontinental flights by performing sophisticated interventions such

FIGURE 23.2. [*Opposite*] A US Air Force flight nurse with the 651st Expeditionary Aeromedical Evacuation Squadron ensures an Afghan local national burn patient remains in stable condition, Forward Operating Base Tarin Kowt, Afghanistan, April 9, 2012. Reproduced from: https://www.dvidshub.net/image/557614/afghanistan-air-medical-evacuation-team.

as damage control resuscitation, advanced airway management, mechanical ventilation, administration of blood products and intravenous medications, advanced pain management, sedation, intracranial pressure monitoring, and frequent laboratory analysis (Chapter 25).[5] Depending on the distance flown, a CCATT mission may last 16 hours or longer.[6]

SPECIALTY TEAMS

Some causalities transported from Iraq and Afghanistan required even more specialized ICU care. Severely burned casualties were often accompanied by an Army Burn Flight Team, which included a burn critical care nurse, so they could receive burn-specific care such as advanced airway management, mechanical ventilation, burn care, complex pain and fluid management, and invasive monitoring.[7] Similarly, an Acute Lung Rescue Team delivered specialized interventions such as advanced mechanical ventilation, extracorporeal membrane oxygenation (ECMO), vasoactive and cardioactive medications, sedation, invasive monitoring, and laboratory analysis for patients with severe acute lung injury (Figure 23.3).[8] When needed, these teams provided exceptional care throughout lengthy flights to Landstuhl Regional Medical Center in Germany.

IMPACT

Despite initial concerns about the feasibility of providing ICU-level care in dark, noisy, cramped, high-vibration environments, and under the physiologic stress of flight, especially the heavy physical and mental demands of providing critical care during extremely long flights, military critical care nurses repeatedly demonstrated their ability to meet the challenge.[9] Today, it's clear that critical care nurses, through their support of MEDEVAC, tactical evacuation, and critical care air transport flights, materially contributed to the exceptionally low case-fatality rates among combat casualties in Iraq and Afghanistan (Figure 23.4).

LOOKING AHEAD

To make sure we retain the lessons learned in Iraq an Afghanistan and apply them in future wars, it is essential that we codify these insights into doctrine. At the present time, military leaders are writing new

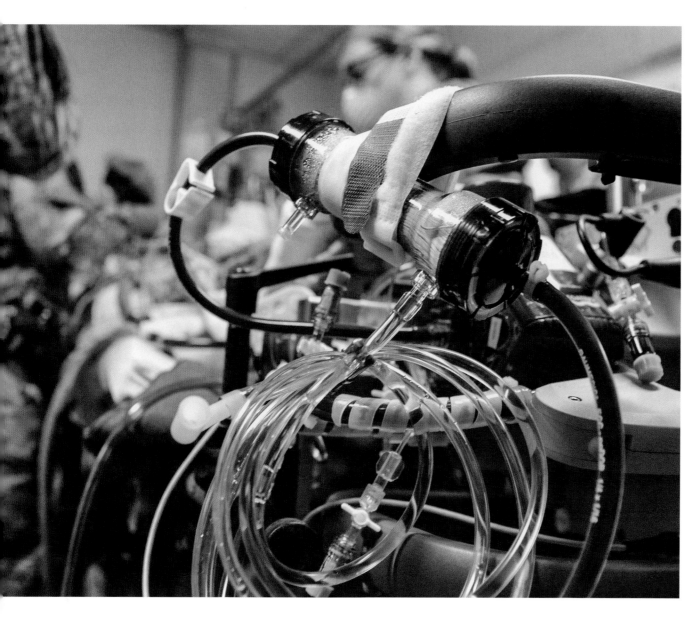

FIGURE 23.3. A 455th Expeditionary Medical Group team combines efforts with the extracorporeal membrane oxygenation (ECMO) team to save the life of a NATO ally at the Craig Joint Theater Hospital at Bagram Air Field, Afghanistan, on February 18, 2016. The patient was airlifted to Landstuhl Regional Medical Center, Germany, where he will receive 7 to 14 days of additional ECMO treatment. US Air Force photo by Technical Sergeant Nicholas Rau. Reproduced from: https://www.dvidshub.net/image/2410003/desperate-ecmo-treatment-used-bagram-breathe-life-into-nato-ally.

TACTICAL CRITICAL CARE EVACUATION FROM THE POINT OF INJURY

My first direct participation in a point-of-injury casualty evacuation mission was during Operation Provide Comfort (initiated by the United States and other coalition nations to protect and assist Kurds fleeing their homes in northern Iraq following the Gulf War). In January 1993, while serving as a flight surgeon assigned to the 352nd Special Operations Group, I was tasked to augment two pararescuemen (PJs) on an urgent casualty evacuation mission into northern Iraq involving a coalition Soldier who was thought to be near death due to acute pneumonia. The mission launched on two MH-53J Pave Low helicopters supported by MC-130P Combat Shadow aircraft (for in-flight refueling). We successfully evacuated the Soldier to an intermediate staging base. Although this casualty did not require in-flight clinical decision-making or clinical interventions beyond a PJ's scope of practice, there were other missions during my tenure with Air Force Special Operations Command (AFSOC) when high-level clinical decision-making and interventions were called for. As a result, AFSOC and other US Special Operations Command components developed special medical teams that could be scaled up and configured to meet different mission requirements, including en route resuscitation of critically injured casualties. Unfortunately, this innovative approach was not embraced as doctrine by US conventional forces.

However, as casualty data accumulated from combat operations in Afghanistan and Iraq, visionary thinkers like Air Force Lieutenant General P.K. Carlton began advocating expansion of the Special Ops approach to bolster the capabilities of MEDEVAC units supporting our conventional forces. The need for advanced resuscitation capabilities to help severely injured casualties survive transport from the point of injury to the closest forward surgical team became clear to me during my 15-month tour of duty (2007–2008) as the commander of Task Force MED (TF MED), the medical support brigade assigned to Combined Joint Task Force 82 in Afghanistan.

To achieve the needed capability, we leveraged TF MED assets to create what would later be called "Tactical Critical Care Evacuation Teams" (TCCETs). Unlike CCAT teams, which provide critical care during long-distance inter-facility flights (Chapter 25), TCCETs deliver lifesaving prehospital care from the battlefield to forward surgical care (Chapter 14). To avoid taking "out of hide" the resources required to sustain this capability, we submitted a formal request for forces (RFF) to secure the needed personnel. Although Colonel (later Lieutenant General) Douglas Robb, US Central Command surgeon, strongly supported our RFF, it was not filled because others considered putting highly skilled providers on these MEDEVAC flights controversial and unnecessary. This led to a multi-year struggle driven by medical personnel at Headquarters, Air Mobility Command, that culminated with the formal establishment, deployment, and life-saving impact of TCCETs.

Each three-person TCCET was, and still is, comprised of a specialty-trained emergency medicine or critical care physician and two certified registered nurse anesthetists (an emergency medicine nurse or critical care nurse can be substituted for one of the nurse anesthetists). Subsequently, the TCCET evolved to incorporate an "enhanced" component (TCCET-E) that adds a surgeon able to perform in-extremis damage control surgery during casualty evacuation (Chapter 1). The TCCET-E is used in particularly challenging tactical environments including anti-access, area denial, and joint forcible entry operation scenarios. It has also recently been used to support President of the United States travel missions.

Bart Iddins, Major General, US Air Force, Medical Corps, CFS

Commander, 59th Medical Wing

San Antonio, Texas

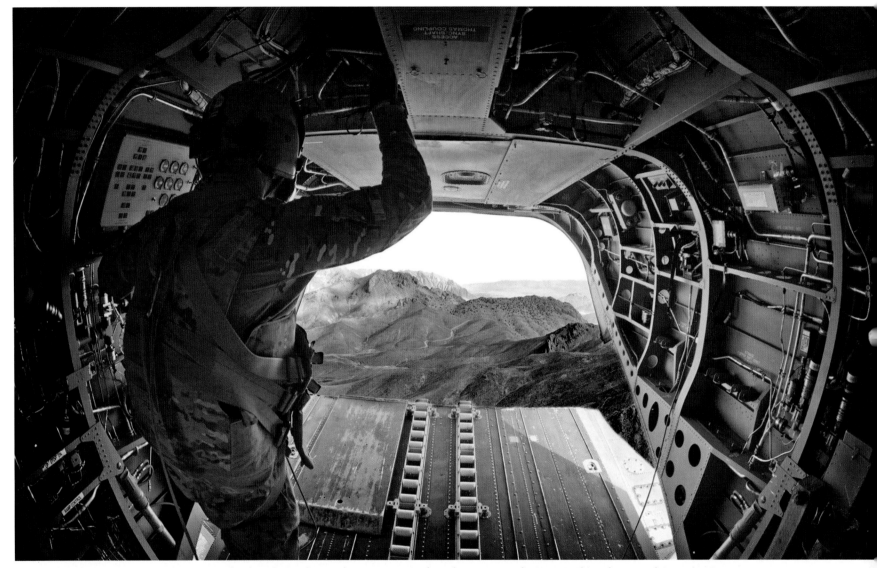

FIGURE 23.4. US Army crew chief and mechanic observes for enemy activity from the rear ramp of a CH-47F Chinook, Forward Operating Base Shank, Afghanistan, August 13, 2012. Photo by Sergeant 1st Class Eric Pahon, 82nd Combat Aviation Brigade. Reproduced from: https://www.dvidshub.net/image/648415/task-force-corsair-chinooks-soar-over-regional-command-east.

policies, developing new training curricula, and devising new technologies to further improve en route care. Projects are underway to create better ways to monitor patients, document care, transmit clinical data, and even remotely monitor patients during transport. Biomedical engineers are devising critical care equipment that will be able to make minute-to-minute adjustments in oxygen, intravenous fluid, medications, temperature, and other settings based on the patient's status. Innovations like these will help future critical care nurses efficiently transport multiple critically ill and injured patients and ensure their safety.

Notes

1. Blackbourne LH, Baer DG, Eastridge BJ, et al. Military medical revolution: deployed hospital and en route care. *J Trauma Acute Care Surg.* 2012;73:S378–S387.

2. Davis RS, Connelly LK. Nursing and en route care: history in time of war. *US Army Med Dep J.* 2011;Oct-Dec:45-50.

3. Hudson TL, Morton R. Critical care transport in a combat environment: building tactical trauma transport teams before and during deployment. *Crit Care Nurse.* 2010;30:57–66.

4. Beninati W, Meyer MT, Carter TE. The critical care air transport program. *Crit Care Med.* 2008:36:S370–376.

5. Mason PE, Eadie JS, Holder AD. Prospective observational study of United States (US) Air Force Critical Care Air Transport team operations in Iraq. *J Emerg Med.* 2011;41:8–13.

6. Ingalls N, Zonies D, Bailey JA, et al. A review of the first 10 years of critical care aeromedical transport during Operation Iraqi Freedom and Operation Enduring Freedom: the importance of evacuation timing. *JAMA Surg.* 2014;149:807–813.

7. Renz EM, Cancio LC, Barillo DJ, et al. Long range transport of war-related burn casualties. *J Trauma.* 2008;64:S136–144.

8. Fang R, Allan PF, Womble SG, et al. Closing the "care in the air" capability gap for severe lung injury: the Landstuhl Acute Lung Rescue Team and extracorporeal lung support. *J Trauma.* 2011;71:S91–97.

9. Butler FK Jr, Blackbourne LH. Battlefield trauma care then and now: a decade of Tactical Combat Casualty Care. *J Trauma Acute Care Surg.* 2012;73:S395–S402.

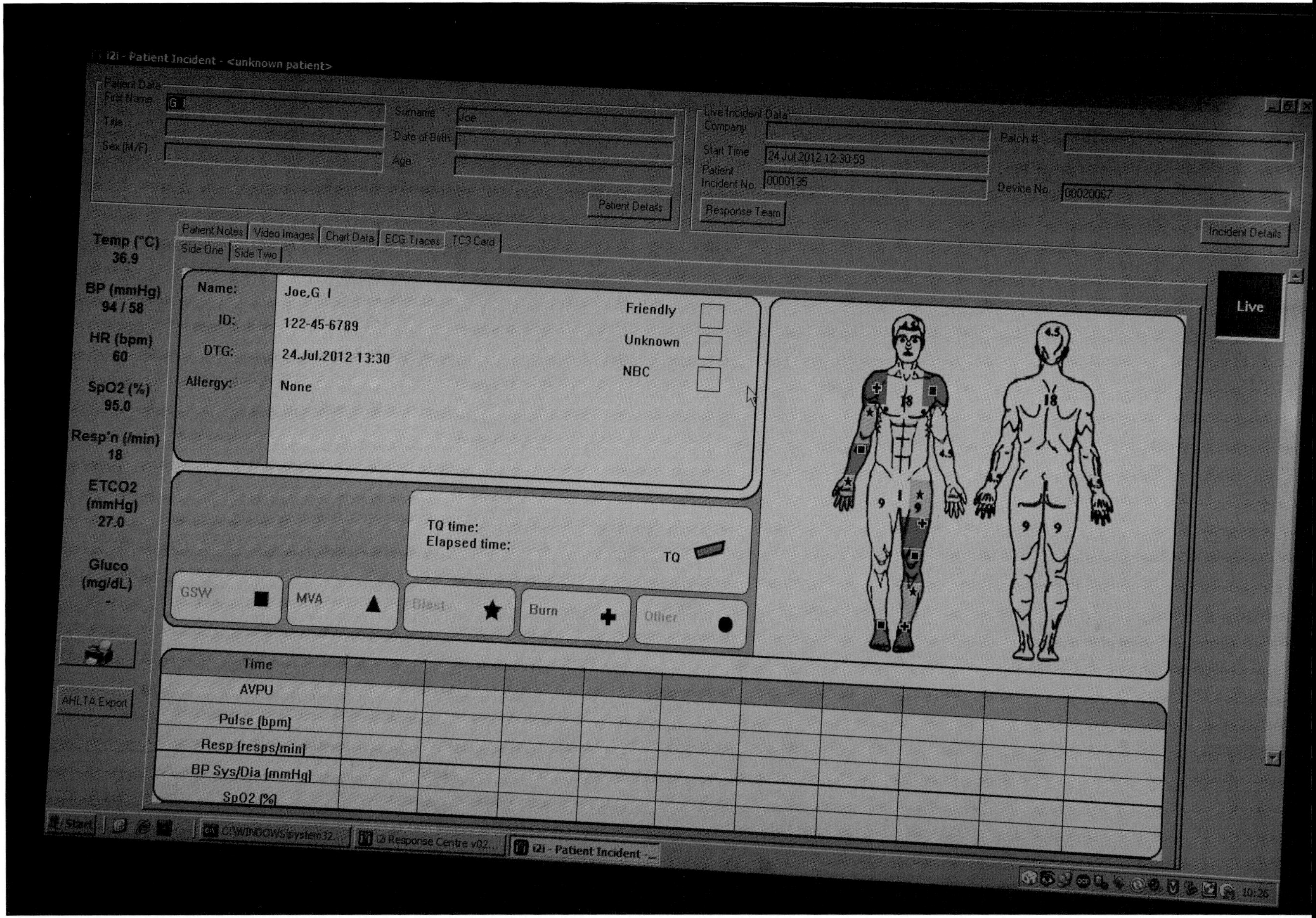
i2i - Patient Incident - <unknown patient>
Patient Data
First Name
Title
Sex (M/F)
Surname
Joe
Date of Birth
Age
Patient Details
Live Incident Data
Company
Start Time
24 Jul 2012 12:30:59
Patient Incident No.
0000135
Patch #
Device No.
00020057
Response Team
Incident Details
Temp (°C)
36.9
BP (mmHg)
94 / 58
HR (bpm)
60
SpO2 (%)
95.0
Resp'n (/min)
18
ETCO2 (mmHg)
27.0
Gluco (mg/dL)
-
AHLTA Export
Patient Notes
Video Images
Chart Data
ECG Traces
TC3 Card
Side One
Side Two
Live
Name:
Joe,G I
ID:
122-45-6789
DTG:
24.Jul.2012 13:30
Allergy:
None
Friendly
Unknown
NBC
TQ time:
Elapsed time:
TQ
GSW
MVA
Blast
Burn
Other
Time
AVPU
Pulse (bpm)
Resp (resps/min)
BP Sys/Dia (mmHg)
SpO2 (%)
Start
C:\WINDOWS\system32...
i2i Response Centre v02...
i2i - Patient Incident - ...
10:26

CHAPTER twenty-four

Telehealth in the Central Command Region

DANIEL KRAL, MSMOT, and RON POROPATICH, MD

THE PROBLEM

UNLIKE PRIOR CONFLICTS, MILITARY OPERATIONS in Afghanistan involved small, widely dispersed units fighting on rugged terrain, often with extended lines of communication. After the air and ground campaigns that toppled the Taliban in Afghanistan and Saddam Hussein's regime in Iraq, the wars evolved into widely dispersed insurgencies. It was not feasible to staff every forward operating base and combat support hospital with specialists trained to manage the wide array of conditions encountered in Iraq and Afghanistan (Chapter 6). Rather than bring patients to medical expertise—a hazardous and costly endeavor—it made sense whenever possible to bring medical expertise to the military health system's widely dispersed patients.

THE INNOVATION

The federal Health Resources and Services Administration (HRSA) defines telehealth as "the use of electronic information and telecommunications technologies to support and promote long distance clinical health care, patient and professional health-related education, public health, and health administration."[1] There are two main types of telehealth services:

FIGURE 24.1. [*Opposite*] Medics sent electronic Tactical Casualty Care cards over a tactical network so surgeons can see injuries and what treatment had been performed prior to the patient's arrival. Fort Dix, July 24, 2012. Photo by Edric Thompson, US Army Research, Development and Engineering Command's Communications-Electronics Center. Reproduced from: https://www.dvidshub.net/image/668206/electronic-tc3-card.

1. **"Store and forward" consultations**, in which a provider uses a computer to send a clinical question, digital image, or x-ray to a specialist for an expert opinion. Common in dermatology, radiology, and pathology, this form of telehealth is "asynchronous" because the query can sit on a computer drive for hours before being answered.

2. **"Real-time" interactive services** use video conferencing to enable healthcare providers or patients to converse with a specialist hundreds or even thousands of miles away. Real-time interactions allow the telehealth consultant to directly obtain a medical history, visually assess the patient's condition, and discuss a treatment plan with the patient's on-site provider. Tele-behavioral health is a prime example of this type of telemedicine.

Telemedicine in a deployed military setting was first tried in Somalia in 1993. Based on encouraging results, the US Army Medical Department expanded telemedicine services to locations including Croatia, Macedonia, and Bosnia (1994–1996); Haiti (1995); and Kenya (1998). These operations helped the military recognize telemedicine's value in remote settings, and it was widely deployed in Iraq, Afghanistan, and Kuwait.[2]

IMPACT

2004: "Store and Forward" Telemedicine, the Email Teleconsultation Program

In April 2004, the US Army Medical Department approved use of Army Knowledge Online (AKO), a special email system, to provide teledermatology support to deployed healthcare providers.[3,4] This tele-consult system has since been expanded to serve all overseas locations, including Navy ships at sea. Based on the program's success, the Army adopted an over-arching policy,[5] as follows: To obtain a consult, the deployed healthcare provider submits an email request with a description of the patient's condition and any digital images necessary to illustrate the problem. The appropriate on-duty specialist (for example, a dermatologist) answers a routine request within 24 hours, and more promptly for emergency requests.

The program is designed for use by all Department of Defense (DoD) healthcare providers to support deployed or geographically isolated regions. Because the emails are not encrypted, they cannot contain

VIGNETTE >> On September 12, 2005, Corporal Smith, a Marine stationed in western Iraq, sustained 1st and 2nd degree burns to his right shoulder and armpit when a flare tossed from his vehicle bounced back and lodged in his flak jacket. The healthcare provider at his forward operating base strongly considered evacuating him to the nearest combat support hospital. But first he emailed a telehealth inquiry to a military burn specialist, seeking advice on immediate topical treatments, the role of prophylactic antibiotics, and whether the patient needed advanced burn care and rehabilitation (Figure 24.2).

This information enabled the staff burn surgeon at Brooke Army Medical Center to assess Corporal Smith's burn. The feedback the burn surgeon provided not only allowed the patient to avoid a costly and potentially hazardous MEDEVAC flight, but Corporal Smith also returned to duty several days later, preserving his unit's fighting strength.

FIGURE 24.2. A typical telehealth consult from Afghanistan and the attached clinical image.

Referring Physician's Message >> Pt sustained 1st and 2nd degree burns to the right axilla. He threw a flare; it bounced back and lodged in his flack. Initially treated with silvadene—now on Levoquin for prophylaxis against bacterial infection, with daily wound dressing changes, dry/Telfa. Patient has had gross sensory tenderness throughout post injury course.

1) Any topicals? silvadene, vitamin A, E?
2) Continue Antibiotic Prophylaxis?
3) Daily cleaning? NS or warm water soap?
4) Concerned about Range of Motion in shoulder as ROM limited by pain?
5) Do you have a contact at a Burn Center (Brooks Army Medical Center)?

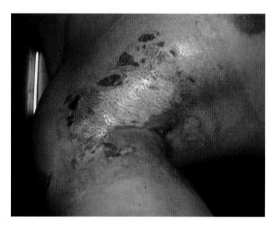

Specialty Physician's Message >> This is a partial thickness burn with budding apparent and should heal in 10 - 21 days. Prophylaxis with antibiotics is not indicated for this or any burns. This can be treated with BID silvidene cream or bacitracin with daily shower and washing the area, no significant scrubbing. If silvidene is used all remaining silvidene from the prior application must be washed off therefore BID washing with soap and water or pseudoeshar will appear (a white to grey appearing film which is a combination of serous discharge and cream). If bacitracin is used only one wash with soap and water is needed and the ointment can be applied BID, no pseudoeshar will appear. Once healed, keep moist with moisturizer BID and PRN and keep ROM of the shoulder during the healing

Referring Physician's Reply >> Thank you for the help. We believe we will be able to take care of this Marine here, as we have supply for the dressing changes and access to showers daily, but will not hesitate to call for help again. Thank you

protected health information. Combat-area providers, including clinicians in Afghanistan, were required to follow policies regarding electronic transfer of patient information and imagery, as well as documenting the consultant's advice in the patient's electronic health record. To facilitate program implementation, the military created an online training program and reference materials for providers.

"Store and Forward" Impact

Corporal Smith's case is a good example of a tele-consult with high-resolution digital images. The pictures helped the consulting burn surgeon make a reliable diagnosis and recommend an effective treatment plan. Between 2004 and 2015, more than 13,000 email tele-consults were completed, linking more than 3,200 remote providers with 20 medical and dental specialties. The average response time for an asynchronous, emailed tele-consult was five hours.[2] During this period, 39 percent of all consults were for dermatologic (skin) problems, followed by orthopedics (9 percent), infectious disease (7 percent), neurology (6 percent), and ophthalmology (5 percent). Army healthcare providers generated slightly more than half of tele-consult requests. The rest were divided among providers in the Marine Corps (10 percent), Navy (10 percent), and Air Force (8 percent).

Accurate decision-making regarding whether or not to evacuate an injured warrior is a key benefit of tele-consultation. Between 2004 and 2015, tele-consultations prevented at least 214 needless MEDEVAC flights, including Corporal Smith's case. At other times, tele-consultants identified a serious or life-threatening problem, leading to a medically appropriate evacuation. During the 11 years of this review, telehealth consultants prompted 645 MEDEVAC flights.

2010: Introduction of Tele-Behavioral Health

Providing behavioral healthcare in forward operating bases is complicated by challenging or contested terrain, travel constraints, and operational considerations. Under such circumstances, tele-behavioral health (TBH) offers the potential to provide behavioral health services without the costs, delays, and hazards of air or ground travel.

Unlike "store and forward" transmission of digital messages and medical images, TBH requires synchronous, real-time interaction between patients, their local healthcare providers, and the telehealth consultant. This requires secure, bi-directional video technology. TBH:

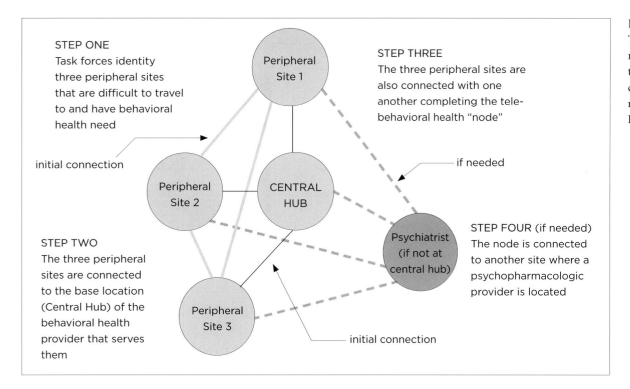

STEP ONE
Task forces identity three peripheral sites that are difficult to travel to and have behavioral health need

initial connection

STEP TWO
The three peripheral sites are connected to the base location (Central Hub) of the behavioral health provider that serves them

STEP THREE
The three peripheral sites are also connected with one another completing the tele-behavioral health "node"

if needed

STEP FOUR (if needed)
The node is connected to another site where a psychopharmacologic provider is located

Peripheral Site 1

Peripheral Site 2

CENTRAL HUB

Peripheral Site 3

Psychiatrist (if not at central hub)

initial connection

FIGURE 24.3.
Tele-behavioral health node design. Courtesy of the US Army Telemedicine and Advanced Technology Research Center, Frederick, Maryland.

- improves access to behavioral health providers for service members who need emergency evaluations;

- extends the providers' reach to far-forward locations without risky travel;

- allows behavioral health providers at remote outposts to continue seeing patients elsewhere when unable to travel due to weather or hostile action; and

- assists with command-directed evaluations of military personnel.

REQUIREMENT: To improve patient access to care at remote FOBs in an active combat theater. Also to reduce travel risk and extended virtual outreach by behavioral health providers.

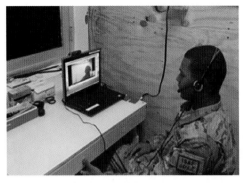

Patient to Provider
TBH Session

→

Dual laptop and
dual network
Technical solutions
MC4/TBH CENTRIXS

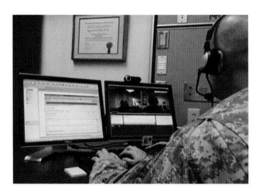

MEDICAL IMPACT: The TBH pilot documented over 1,300 clinical care episodes during the last nine months of FY12. Over 73 percent of these patients would not have been seen without access to "tele," as reported by Public Health Command assessments.

Providers documented encounters in AHLTA-Theater, the MHS electronic record.

The first TBH program was launched in Afghanistan in August 2010. Providers created four task forces in the Joint Force's area of operations. Each consisted of a central "hub" at a larger facility and three peripheral "spokes" in small forward operating bases (Figure 24.3).

To hold down costs, the TBH program used repurposed DoD-issued laptops ($355/unit) equipped with a commercial web-cam, a secure internet network, and commercial software. Healthcare providers in Afghanistan could stream confidential video and audio to TBH consultants elsewhere over a secure network (Figure 24.4).

Tele-Behavioral Health Impact

Troops in Afghanistan reported a reasonable level of satisfaction with TBH, giving it an overall rating of 3.8 on a scale of 1 to 5. Most responding behavioral health providers reported that the email encounters saved them considerable travel time (43 percent reported 1 to 3 days saved per encounter). The most common uses of TBH in Afghanistan included providing psychodynamic therapy (69 percent) and medication management (23 percent).

Based on this success, TBH was extended to Iraq in October 2011. By the end of that year, TBH providers were handling 20 percent of all combat-area mental health encounters. Over the next three years, TBH encounters accounted for more than 2,000 visits per year.

In 2011, the US Army Public Health Command conducted a formal evaluation of the TBH program. Metrics included Soldier perceptions, command acceptance, technical success and failures, number of sessions provided, and travel days saved. The evaluation documented high levels of satisfaction among providers, patients, and commanders. Importantly, it noted that "nearly 72 percent of theater tele-behavior health patients reported they would not have sought BH [behavioral health] care if the telecare option had not been available."[6]

From fiscal year 2012 to fiscal year 2014, a total of 5,313 TBH patients were seen. The program peaked in 2013 with 87 operational sites in Afghanistan. In 2014, the average number of consults per month (102) declined from the preceding year (168).[2]

2011: Tele-Radiology Introduced

Providers need highly specialized training to accurately read computerized tomography (CT) and magnetic resonance imaging (MRI) scans. When the Central Command area of operations expanded access to CT and MRI scanning in war zones, the equipment it deployed used a commercial picture archiving and communication system to capture and store images on computer drives rather than on photographic film. The easy transfer of high-resolution digital images allowed expert radiologists in different locations around the world to read scans.

In 2005, an operational needs statement authorized the Central Command region to acquire the Deployable Tele-Radiology System (DTRS) and a theater image repository to transmit CT, MRI, and digital x-ray images to Landstuhl Regional Medical Center in Germany. This technology was used to send digital images from Iraq, Kuwait, and Afghanistan to Germany and, when necessary, to expert

FIGURE 24.4. [*Opposite*] Theater (a defined area of military operations) tele-behavioral health allows patients in forward operating bases and other remote locations to reach behavioral health providers by streaming confidential video and audio over a secure network. Courtesy of the US Army Telemedicine and Advanced Technology Research Center, Frederick, Maryland.

FOB: forward operating base
TBH: tele-behavioral health
MC4: Medical Communications for Combat Casualty Care
AHLTA: Armed Forces Health Longitudinal Technology Application
CENTRIXS: Combined Enterprise Regional Information Exchange System
FY: fiscal year
MHS: Military Health System

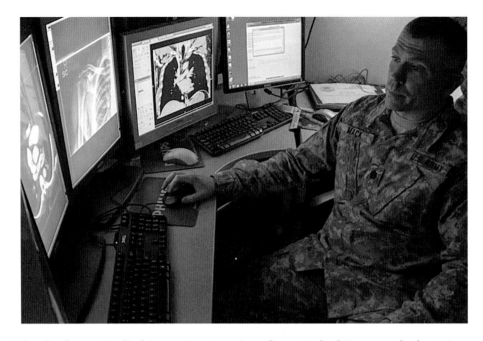

FIGURE 24.5. Lieutenant Colonel Joseph Mack, a radiologist at the 325th Combat Support Hospital in Camp Arifjan, Kuwait, reviews an x-ray showing a blood clot in the heart. "Store and forward" transmission of digital images to and from combat zones allows military radiologists to interpret images from anywhere in the world. Photo by Hendrick Simoes. Reproduced with permission from Stars and Stripes (http://www.stripes.com/army-doctors-warn-that-long-flights-pose-blood-clot-risk-1.207211).

radiologists at Walter Reed Army Medical Center, San Antonio Military Medical Center, and other US facilities. In the later years of the conflicts, declining clinical workloads in the combat theaters allowed deployed radiologists to read digitized images taken at their home station medical treatment facilities (the facility from which they had deployed and at which they were credentialed). This "reverse telemedicine" let them support their home departments and maintain their clinical skills (Figure 24.5).

Tele-radiology also enabled CT and MRI technicians in the United States to remotely monitor the performance of forward-deployed scanning equipment and address impending problems with digital patches or guidance to stationed technical staff.

Tele-Radiology Impact

By December 2011, 13 tele-radiology systems were established in Afghanistan, and 22 sites were established in Iraq. Between 2011 and March 2016, a total of 263,372 digital studies were transmitted from Iraq and Afghanistan to the Landstuhl Regional Medical Center. Of these, 4,441 were MRI scans; 40,674

A PEDIATRICIAN GOES TO WAR

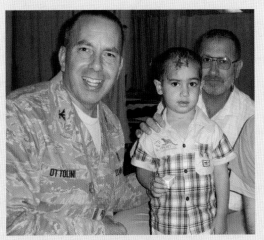
The author with an Iraqi father and child.

In 2008, near the end of my 28-year career as a military pediatrician and infectious disease specialist, I deployed to Iraq to serve as the chief of staff of the 332nd Air Force Theater Hospital in Balad, Iraq, which then was the world's busiest trauma hospital. I was fairly late to the game, not only by age (I was 50 years old), but also because most of my fellow military pediatricians had already deployed multiple times downrange in a variety of settings, from large combat support hospitals like Balad to small forward operating bases.

At Balad, I was part of a leadership team that worked tirelessly with the surgeons, nurses, and others to treat an endless stream of major trauma and lesser problems. I made rounds twice daily with our chief surgeon, chief nurse, and aeromedical transport expert. Besides being a resource on infectious disease, I had several other responsibilities I didn't relish. I was the "gatekeeper" who accepted or rejected the admission of civilians, often children, sometimes literally at the gate. I led the ethics team, which frequently had to make immediate, life-and-death decisions, knowing our resources were finite. We always did everything possible for our own forces, but we had to be more cautious with host nationals and civilians. Otherwise, we could quickly exhaust our supplies and staff and be unable to respond to the next mass casualty event.

I like to think that being a pediatrician helped me make these difficult decisions. Military pediatricians have to be great communicators, a skill that transfers well to battlefield medicine. Also, people tend to forget that children make up a large portion of war's innocent victims. I know that every child I admitted weighed heavily on the minds of our staff. A pregnant mother who delivered a stillborn in our intensive care unit after sustaining shrapnel injuries devastated us for days. Conversely, we were elated when we discharged a two-year-old whose face had been reconstructed by our oral surgeon. These memories and others like them remain fresh in my mind. My time in Iraq was the most intense, focused, and rewarding service I have ever provided.

Martin Ottolini, MD, Colonel (Retired), Medical Corps, US Air Force

were CT scans, and 139,651 were digital x-ray studies. The capability allowed deployed providers to discuss diagnosis and management of complex trauma cases with specialist healthcare providers at Landstuhl, Walter Reed, and other locations.

CONCLUSION

Medical care on the battlefield improves when providers have ready access to specialists' expertise back home. Fifteen years of sustained military operations have demonstrated telehealth's value as a force multiplier. Concept documents, such as the Army's "Force 2025" and the Air Force's "Collaborative Operations in a Denied Environment,"[7,8] detail its potential to support future missions, which will be increasingly characterized by small-unit operations, long distances, and substantial autonomy at the unit level.

While the Army's Telemedicine and Advanced Technology Research Center works on new concepts and technologies, telehealth should be fully integrated into the military health system's day-to-day operations. Widespread adoption of telehealth in military treatment facilities in the continental United States will not only connect military healthcare professionals in the States with their deployed colleagues, but it will also make the military health system more accessible, safe, and efficient (Figure 24.1).

Notes

1. US Health Resources and Services Administration. What is telehealth? http://www.hrsa.gov/healthit/toolbox/RuralHealthITtoolbox/Telehealth/whatistelehealth.html Accessed January 1, 2016.
2. Poropatich R, Lai E, McVeigh F, Bashshur R. The US Army telemedicine and m-health program: making a difference at home and abroad. *Telemed J E Health*. 2013;19:1–7.
3. Office of The Surgeon General, US Army Medical Command. *Use of Tele-Dermatology Consults Prior to Patient Evacuation from Operation Iraqi Freedom (OIF) and Operation Enduring Freedom (OEF) Locations.* May 2004. OTSG/MEDCOM Policy Memo 04-003.

4. Poropatich RK, DeTreville R, Lappan C, Barrigan C. The US Army telemedicine program: general overview and current status in southwest Asia. *Telemed J E Health.* 2006;12:396–408.

5. Office of the Surgeon General, US Army Medical Command. *Use of Army Knowledge Online (AKO) Email in Support of Electronic Telehealth Medical Consultation by Deployed Providers.* March 2005. OTSG/MEDCOM Policy Memo 05-004.

6. Nextgov.com. Army telebehavioral project broadens access to mental health care. http://www.nextgov.com/health/2011/04/army-telebehavioral-project-broadens-access-to-mental-health-care/48937/. Accessed January 24, 2017.

7. US Army Training and Doctrine Command. *Force 2025 and Beyond: Unified Land Operations Win in a Complex World.* Fort Eustis, VA: TRADOC: 2014 http://www.arcic.army.mil/app_Documents/tradoc_ausa_force2025andbeyond-unifiedlandoperations-wininacomplexworld_07oct2014.pdf. Accessed January 24, 2017.

8. Lede JC. Collaborative operations in denied environment. Defense Advanced Research Projects Agency website. http://www.darpa.mil/program/collaborative-operations-in-denied-environment. Accessed January 24, 2017.

Recommended Reading

Lappan CM. The US Army Medical Department email teleconsultation program. *US Army Med Dep J.* 2016;Apr-Sep:140–147.

Acknowledgement

In appreciation to Lieutenant Colonel (Retired) Chuck Lappan, Health Systems Specialist, for his many years of service to the Army Medical Department in managing the US Army Office of The Surgeon General Teleconsultation Program, and for providing telemedicine data for this book chapter.

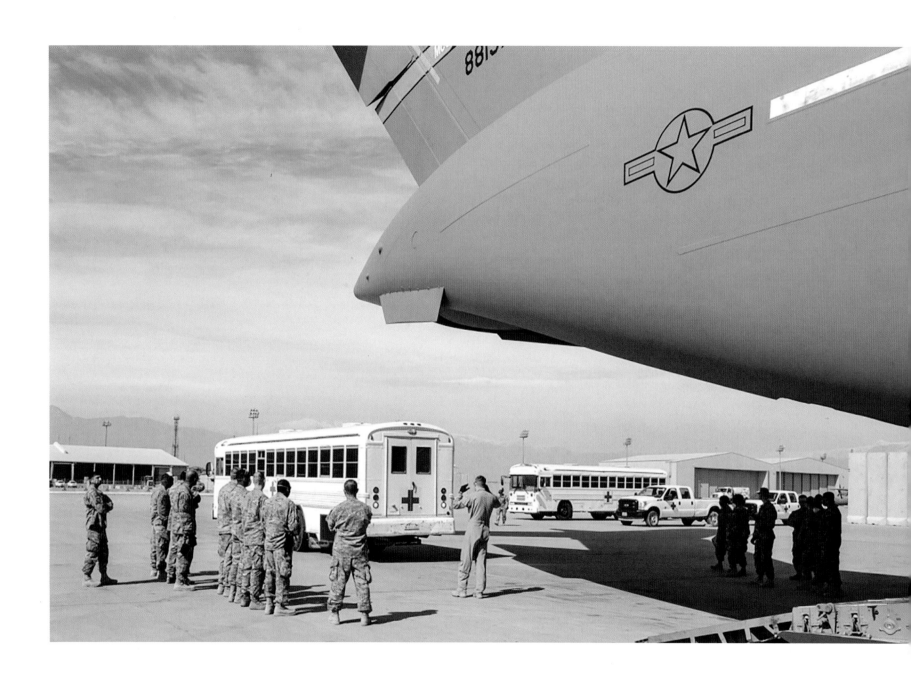

CHAPTER twenty-five

Critical Care Air Transport Teams

JAY JOHANNIGMAN, MD, and PAUL K. CARLTON JR, MD

OVERVIEW

THE FIRST CRITICAL CARE AIR TRANSPORT TEAMS (CCATTs) were developed shortly after the first Gulf War. A CCATT team consists of a critical care physician, a critical care nurse, and a respiratory therapist. They are responsible for providing seamless critical care for up to six patients during evacuation (three of whom may be supported on a breathing machine or ventilator). The last decade of conflict proved the value of these teams in providing rapid and sophisticated en route care to severely injured service members. This Air Force innovation enabled the military health system to swiftly transport wounded, ill, and injured warfighters from far-forward areas in Iraq and Afghanistan to major military hospitals in Germany and the United States.

THE CHALLENGE

In previous conflicts, wounded troops were often held for a prolonged period of time in hospitals near the combat zone. Casualties remained at these facilities until deemed stable enough for the lengthy evacuation flights. This process often required months in World War II and Korea, and still took weeks in Vietnam. The goal of these facilities was to provide definitive treatment of wounded and ill personnel so that they would be strong enough to withstand the rigors of transport back to the United States. The

FIGURE 25.1. [*Opposite*] Loading a Critical Care Air Transport Team patient from the AMBUS (ambulance bus) onto an awaiting C-17 Globemaster. Photograph: Reproduced from Defense Video Imagery Distribution System. US Air Force photo by Technical Sergeant Nicholas Rau.

VIGNETTE >> While on patrol in southern Afghanistan, Sergeant Jones stepped on an improvised explosive device (IED). The blast severed his right leg below the knee and his left leg above the knee. He also lost parts of his right hand and forearm and sustained multiple wounds to his abdomen and pelvis. His fellow soldiers immediately applied tourniquets to his mangled legs and arms and called a MEDEVAC (medical evacuation) helicopter. Forty-five minutes later, he reached a Forward Surgical Team (FST) (see Chapter 14), where he received blood transfusions and medicine to help his blood clot (see Chapters 16 and 17). In the single-table operating room tent, the surgical team stopped the bleeding and placed a small tube (shunt) across a damaged artery in his right leg to restore blood flow to what remained of his leg. Using the principles of damage control surgery (see Chapter 15), the surgical team explored his abdomen to stop internal bleeding and address any immediately life-threatening injuries. Then, they applied a temporary abdominal dressing and moved Sergeant Jones to the nearby intensive care unit (ICU) tent to await transfer.

As Sergeant Jones entered surgery, other FST personnel issued a radio request for a Critical Care Air Transport Team (CCATT) team to board a military transport plane. About two hours after Sergeant Jones emerged from surgery, CCATT members entered his tent, met with the surgical team, then hooked him up to their equipment in preparation for the one-hour flight to a large combat support hospital in northern Afghanistan. In flight, the CCATT team supported Sergeant Jones on a ventilator and closely monitored his condition with a handheld blood analysis unit. He continued to receive balanced infusions of blood and plasma as the team checked his abdominal and leg dressings.

At the larger hospital, surgeons returned Sergeant Jones to the operating room to inspect and revise his wounds. Once in the ICU, the hospital team prepared him for transport via a C-17 cargo plane to Germany's Landstuhl Regional Medical Center. A second CCATT team, tasked with caring for Sergeant Jones and two other critically injured patients throughout the flight, loaded them on the plane last so they would be the first offloaded when the flight touched down in Germany. Throughout the flight, Sergeant Jones was sedated and supported by a ventilator.

Landing at Ramstein Air Base in Germany, the CCATT team accompanied Sergeant Jones and his fellow patients onto the base ambulance bus for the 20-minute trip to the hospital. Only 28 hours after being critically injured in Afghanistan, Sergeant Jones was in the ICU of Landstuhl Regional Medical Center.

Over the next three days, he was twice taken back to surgery for further treatment of his wounds. His family arrived from the United States and stayed by his bedside. On the third day, yet another CCATT team accompanied him on the flight from Ramstein to Andrews Air Force Base in Maryland, followed by a short ground trip to Walter Reed National Military Medical Center (Bethesda, MD). Only 90 hours had elapsed between his wounding in Afghanistan and his return to the United States. During that time, Sergeant Jones had four operations, traveled more than 7,000 miles, and spent 22 hours in the air accompanied first by a MEDEVAC crew and subsequently by three different CCATT teams. Over the next two weeks, Sergeant Jones moved from Walter Reed's ICU to a regular hospital room where he began a long, but ultimately successful, process of recovery and rehabilitation (see Chapters 28 and 31).

large size, scale, and complexity of these facilities made them costly to support and difficult to protect, particularly in unconventional conflicts where there is no "frontline."

To stay close to the troops they serve, modern Forward Surgical Teams (see Chapter 14) maintain a lean footprint. This limits their capacity to hold postoperative patients. CCATT teams are designed to safely move critically injured combat casualties most hospitals would consider too ill to transport from one ward to the next, let alone thousands of miles. The challenge involves ensuring that these teams, their equipment, and their training consistently meet their patients' needs.

THE INNOVATION

CCATT teams were developed around the principle that local conditions and the logistical challenges of long-distance aeromedical evacuation must not compromise a patient's care. They are designed to match the level of treatment that occurs in the intensive care unit (ICU) of a combat support hospital in the cargo bay of an intercontinental transport jet, over thousands of miles of flight (Figure 25.1). To maintain the necessary level of care, each CCATT team is expected to treat up to six critically injured patients—three of which may require support on a breathing machine—for up to 24 hours. A few teams provide even more specialized care, such as extracorporeal membrane oxygenation (ECMO) (Figure 25.2).

Typically, CCATT teams work at night, in dark, noisy, and vibrating cargo holds, at altitudes that provide limited oxygen. The temperature can rise and fall sharply. Equipment must be hardy and capable of working with limited resupply of electricity. For all these reasons, as well as the complexity of the patients they treat, CCATT teams are trained to compensate for all sorts of challenges while providing an unwavering level of "critical care in the air" (Figure 25.3).

Training
Providing critical care to severely wounded patients can challenge the most experienced and savvy physicians and nurses. This makes training, preparation, and sustainment of CCATT skills a paramount concern. Introductory training occurs at the US Air Force School of Aerospace Medicine at Wright Patterson Air Force Base. This training emphasizes flight physiology and the rigors imposed by aeromedical transport. Before deployment, each CCATT team member must complete a two-week advanced course that includes clinical experience within a busy academic Level I urban trauma center.

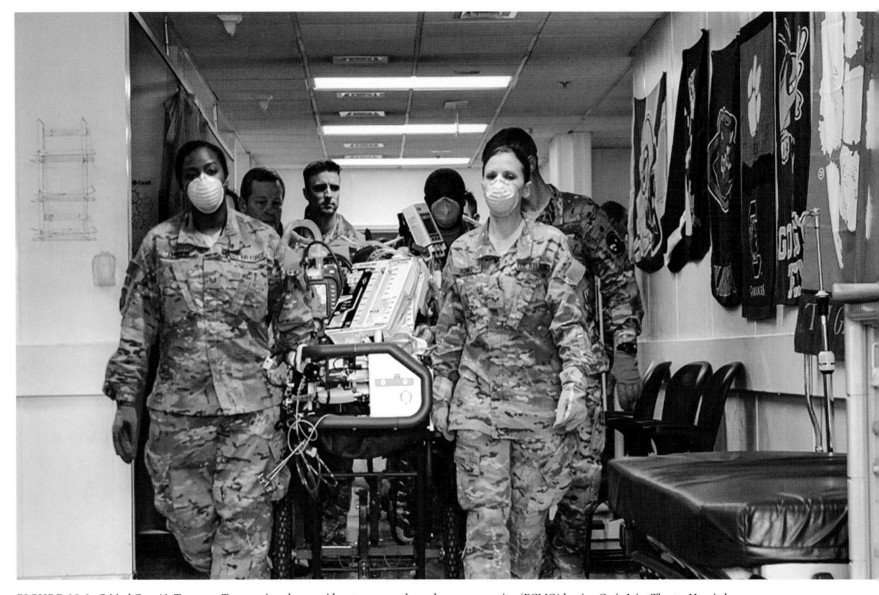

FIGURE 25.2. Critical Care Air Transport Team equipped to provide extracorporeal membrane oxygenation (ECMO) leaving Craig Joint Theater Hospital, Bagram Airfield, Afghanistan. Photograph: Reproduced from Defense Video Imagery Distribution System. US Air Force photo by Technical Sergeant Nicholas Rau.

Course material and lectures emphasize protocols and clinical guidelines of care. Training venues include the Emergency Department, the surgical ICU, and the operating room. Finally, before deploying, each CCATT team spends hours practicing inside a high-fidelity simulation environment (Figure 25.4) that hones skills, team dynamics, and resource management. In the second week, students complete a simulated CCATT mission, including an actual flight in a C-130.

Equipment

Providing critical care at high altitude requires equipment that is durable, lightweight, portable, and battery-capable (Figure 25.5). Every CCATT team must maintain *situational awareness* (continuous monitoring) of patients' medical conditions in an environment that limits sight, sound, and physical examination. CCATT teams have devised a variety of techniques to overcome the difficulties caused by low light (displays that cannot be seen or read), vibration (equipment failure and/or error), noise (alarms that cannot be heard), and altitude (ventilators and equipment failing due to low cabin pressures). Research and innovation underscore the need for new equipment that enables delivery of safe and effective ICU care during lengthy medical evacuations. Additionally, CCATT equipment is evolving to provide reliable information and offset the provider distractions that commonly occur during missions.

IMPACT

Since the 2001 terror attacks, more than 5,600 CCATT patient transports have occurred, with an astounding transport mortality rate of less than 0.25 percent. During peak periods of conflict in Iraq or Afghanistan, it was commonplace for casualties to undergo two or three operations during the initial phases of care and still arrive in Germany within the 36 hours of injury. (See "A Different Paradigm.") A recent review demonstrated that 93 percent of all CCATT patients reached Landstuhl within 72 hours of wounding.[1] Even more remarkably, nearly all (98.5 percent) critically injured service members reached Ramstein Air Base by the 96-hour mark.

CCATT teams have amply demonstrated that it is feasible to transport critical patients within hours of injury and/or major surgery without jeopardizing their medical condition. On the strength of these results, the US military has incorporated the techniques

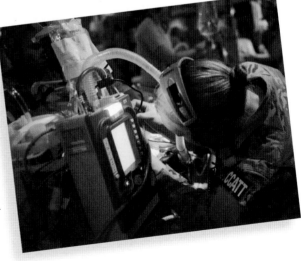

FIGURE 25.3. US Air Force Captain Deann Hoelscher, 455th Expeditionary Aeromedical Evacuation Squadron Critical Care Air Transport Team physician deployed from the 60th Medical Group at Travis Air Force Base, California, checks on a patient's status during an aeromedical evacuation mission aboard a C-17 Globemaster III aircraft from Bagram Airfield, Afghanistan, to Ramstein Air Base, Germany, August 9, 2015. Photograph: Reproduced from Defense Video Imagery Distribution System. US Air Force photo by Major Tony Wickman.

FIGURE 25.4. [*Opposite*] A US Air Force Critical Care Air Transport Team practices securing a tube in preparation for simulated transport missions at the Gulfport Combat Readiness Training Center, Mississippi, during Exercise Southern Strike 16, October 27, 2015. Photograph: Reproduced from Defense Video Imagery Distribution System. US Air Force photo by Staff Sergeant Marianique Santos.

A DIFFERENT PARADIGM

In Vietnam, we had hundreds of hospital beds in country, or nearby, and patients would be in the hospital for weeks before being brought home. The average was 45 days. Now, we keep as few beds as possible in theater, and the average transport time is just a few days. It is not unusual for a critically wounded patient to be back in the United States at a military medical center with family at the bedside within 48 to 72 hours. They get the right care in theater, but then get loaded onto a C-17 staffed by highly trained Critical Care Air Transport Teams (CCATTs), an Air Force innovation and game changer.

The C-17s that make these flights do double duty. After bringing military equipment, supplies, and personnel into the war zone, they quickly convert into flying ICUs (intensive care units) that carry special litters equipped with ventilators, monitoring equipment, and vital medications. The three-member CCATT teams that staff these flights are composed of a critical care physician, a critical care nurse, and a respiratory technician. This combination of skilled personnel and special equipment allows critically injured or ill patients to begin healing as they are flown thousands of miles to major medical centers in Germany and, ultimately, the United States.

This innovation transformed combat casualty care far forward and revolutionized how quickly we bring patients back. Now, it isn't how many beds we have available in theater, it's the flow rate of patients being brought back by the best-trained and best-equipped flying teams in the world. Between 9/11/2001 and April 2014, the Air Force logged an astounding 194,300 patient movements, including 7,900 critical care patients.

Thomas W. Travis, MD, MPH
Lieutenant General (Retired), US Air Force
21st US Air Force Surgeon General

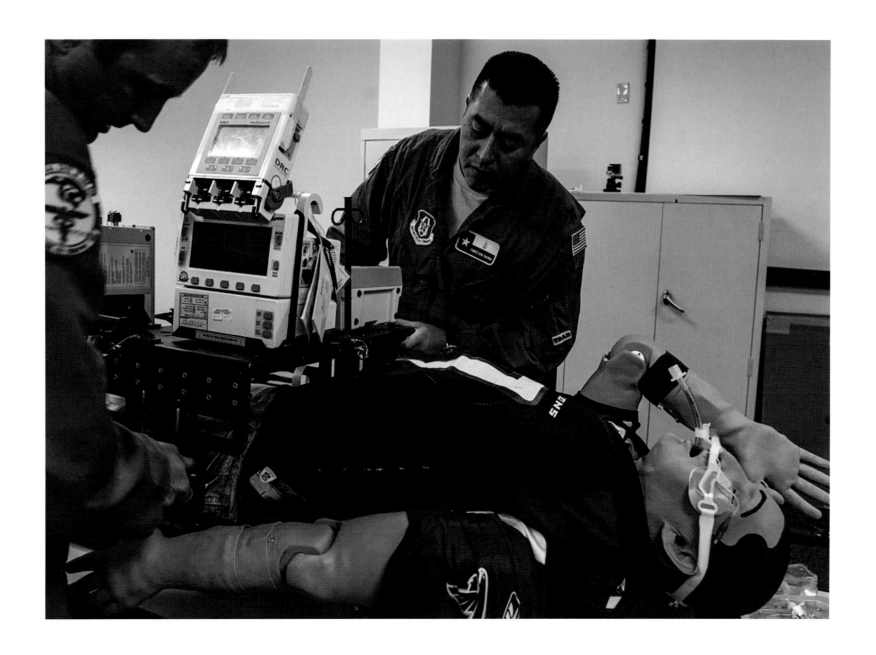

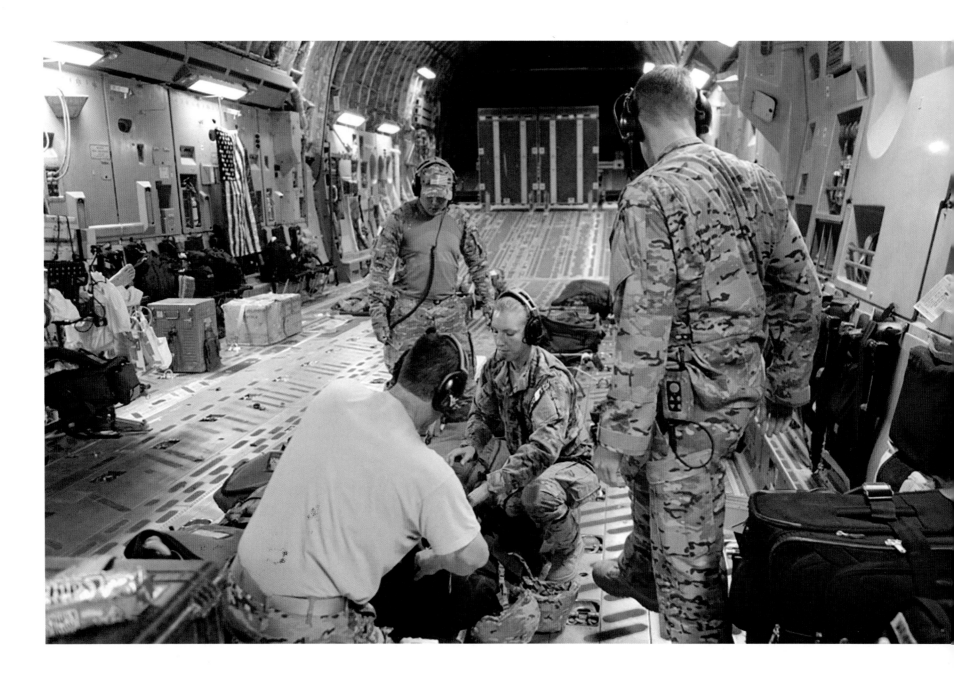

it so swiftly developed and refined during Operation Enduring Freedom and Operation Iraqi Freedom into the principles and practices that drive CCATT operations.

CONCLUSION

This success is a tribute to the dedication of the Air Force CCATT teams, the coordinated use of transport aircraft, and the robust chain of survival established by the US military and the medical departments of the Army, Navy, and Air Force. This chain begins with a medic providing care under fire, progresses through MEDEVAC (medical evacuation) and forward surgery, and continues until the injured service member returns home. The promise of the CCATT community is to provide unparalleled critical care in the air to wounded Soldiers, Sailors, Airmen and Marines. Our challenge now is to ensure that the skills and techniques perfected at great cost are retained and strengthened so that CCATT teams are always ready to provide every casualty, anywhere in the world, the greatest opportunity to survive.

FIGURE 25.5. [*Opposite*] US Airmen assigned to the 455th Expeditionary Aeromedical Evacuation Squadron repack aeromedical evacuation equipment and supplies after an aeromedical evauction mission aboard a C-17 Globemaster III aircraft at Ramstein Air Base, Germany, August 9, 2015. Photograph: Reproduced from Defense Video Imagery Distribution System. US Air Force photo by Major Tony Wickman.

Note

1. Ingalls N, Zonies D, Bailey JA, et al. A review of the first 10 years of critical care aeromedical transport during Operation Iraqi Freedom and Operation Enduring Freedom: the importance of evacuation timing. *JAMA Surg*. 2014;148:807–813.

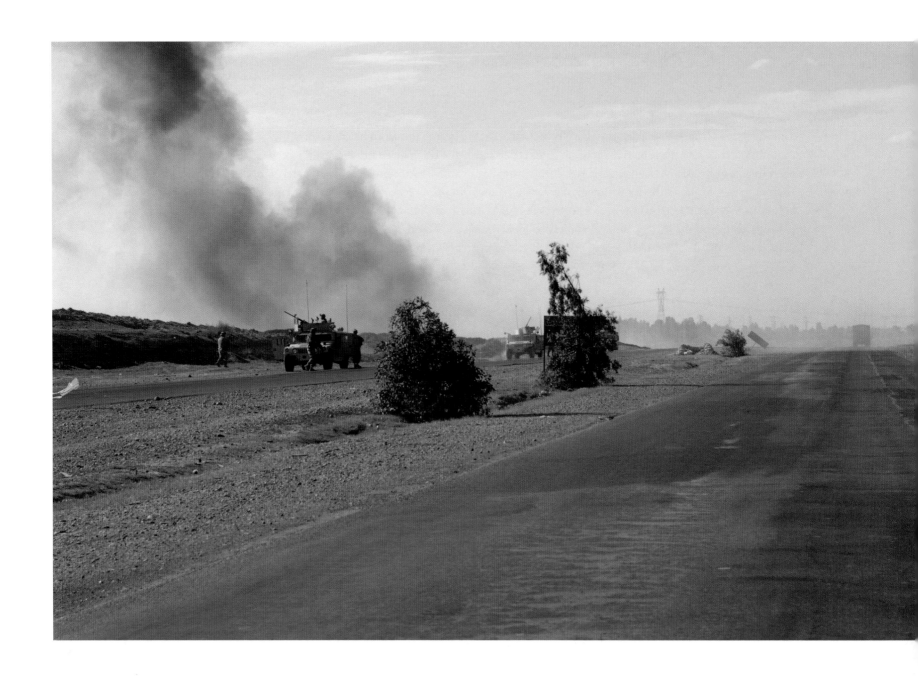

CHAPTER twenty-six

Limb Salvage and Reconstruction

BENJAMIN K. POTTER, MD, and ROMNEY C. ANDERSEN, MD

THE CHALLENGE

MODERN BODY ARMOR, RAPID PLACEMENT OF TOURNIQUETS, aeromedical evacuation, far-forward "damage control" surgery, and other advances have dramatically increased rates of survival from severe combat injuries. One consequence of these advances, however, is a massive increase in the number of wounded warriors with damaged, mangled, and "threatened" limbs, which remain exposed to blasts. Indeed, extremity injuries accounted for most combat-related injuries in Iraq and Afghanistan.[1] In addition, blasts from improvised explosive devices and conventional ordnance such as mortars and rocket-propelled grenades caused nearly three-fourths of the wars' serious battlefield injuries. As a result, most arm and leg fractures were open, and the average wounded warrior sustained three extremity wounds. Most were complex injuries often contaminated with dirt, bomb fragments, fragments of clothing, and large quantities of bacteria.

THE INNOVATION

Techniques for limb salvage surgery advanced dramatically during Operations Enduring Freedom (OEF) and Iraqi Freedom (OIF). In most cases, management passes through three distinct but overlapping phases:

FIGURE 26.1. [*Opposite*] Smoke and dust waft through the air after an improvised explosive device detonated and damaged a Humvee belonging to 3rd Platoon, Delta Company, 1st Battalion, 187th Infantry Regiment, 101st Airborne Division on patrol in Bayji, Iraq, March 27, 2006. US Army photo by Specialist Charles W. Gill, 55th Combat Camera/Released. Reproduced from: https://www.dvidshub.net/image/1438116/patrol-bayji-iraq.

VIGNETTE >> Iraq, 2006. A 32-year-old Marine sergeant was driving a Humvee when it was struck by a massive improvised explosive device (Figure 26.1). The blast penetrated the vehicle floor's armor plate, shattering the main bones in both of the Marine's legs, shredding his leg muscles, and destroying both knee caps and the ligaments that support standing. To prevent him from bleeding to death on the scene, his fellow Marines applied tourniquets on both legs (Chapter 10) and summoned a MEDEVAC helicopter (Chapter 13) to fly him to the nearest combat support hospital. There, he received balanced resuscitation with a 1:1:1 mix of blood products (Chapter 16). After his blood pressure stabilized, a combat surgeon repaired tears in the major blood vessels in both legs, and made incisions in the leg muscles to allow badly damaged tissue to swell without shutting off the blood supply (Chapter 15). Rather than amputating both legs, as might have been done in prior conflicts, an orthopedic surgeon drilled

temporary pins through the broken bones and connected them to external braces. Within 72 hours, a Critical Care Air Transport Team (CCATT, Chapter 25) flew the Marine to the United States. He received four rounds of surgical debridement en route.

After the sergeant arrived at Walter Reed Army Medical Center, doctors debrided his wounds again. They also started powerful antibiotics to treat an early wound infection caused by methicillin-resistant Staphylococcus aureus (the dreaded MRSA, Chapter 27). Once this problem was cleared up, the doctors took the sergeant back to surgery for definitive repairs. First, surgeons fixed the bones around his shattered knee joints with plates and screws. Next, they placed special antibiotic-cement spacers to fill the defects where he was missing parts of his knee joint (on the right leg) and both knee caps (Figure 26.2).

To replace tissue lost in the blast, doctors rotated the calf muscles of both legs to the front of his knees, and covered them with synthetic skin—a cow-derived matrix of cells that provided a framework for his body to regrow its skin. Once this synthetic skin was in place, doctors covered the wound with skin grafts. Walter Reed doctors also used human donor (cadaver) bone and tendons to rebuild his shattered knees and replace the missing part of his right knee joint (Figure 26.3).

In total, the sergeant underwent more than 60 operations to salvage and ultimately rebuild his legs. After extensive rehabilitation, he was able to walk without assistance and had good strength in both legs (Figure 26.4).

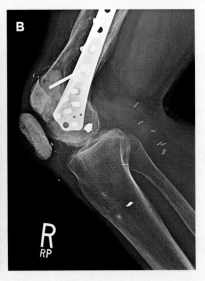

FIGURE 26.2. Anterior-posterior (A) and lateral (B) radiographs of the right knee after plate and screw fixation and healing of fractures, with antibiotic cement spacers placed at the site of the missing knee cap and medial femoral condyle.

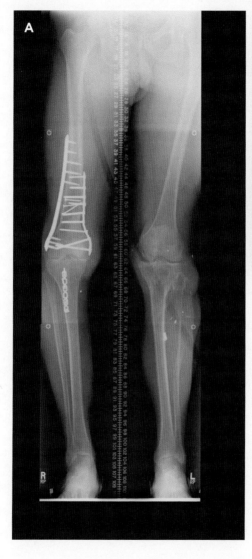

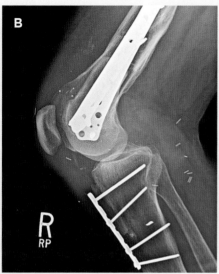

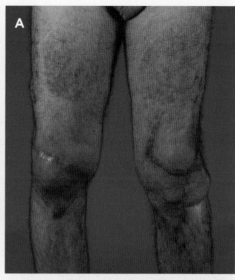

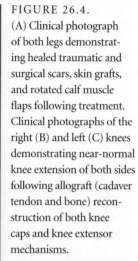

FIGURE 26.4.
(A) Clinical photograph of both legs demonstrating healed traumatic and surgical scars, skin grafts, and rotated calf muscle flaps following treatment. Clinical photographs of the right (B) and left (C) knees demonstrating near-normal knee extension of both sides following allograft (cadaver tendon and bone) reconstruction of both knee caps and knee extensor mechanisms.

FIGURE 26.3. (A) Standing full-length anterior-posterior radiograph of both legs demonstrating healed fractures and allografts. The surgical fixation implants were removed from the left leg after fracture healing due to infection. (B) Lateral radiograph of the right knee demonstrating replacement of the missing bone and antibiotic cement spacers with cadaver bone and tendon, which has healed and resulted in near-normal knee extension and function.

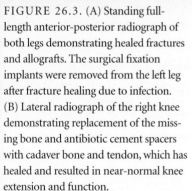

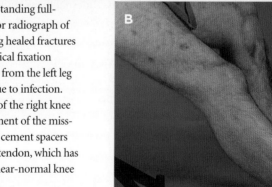

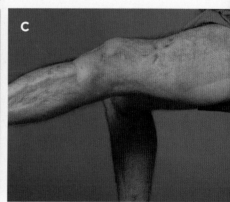

1. The first phase is **stabilization.** It coincides with resuscitating the patient and, often, performance of damage-control surgery (Chapter 15). During this phase, surgeons control major bleeding, clean and clear wounds of debris, and stabilize fractures. If the limb looks potentially salvageable and immediate amputation is not absolutely necessary to save the service member's life, surgeons will treat major vascular injuries by placing temporary plastic tubes to restore blood flow. This keeps the limb alive until more definitive vascular and limb reconstruction can take place.[2] If post-traumatic swelling of an injured leg or arm becomes severe, it may shut off blood flow to key muscle groups and nerves, a phenomenon called compartment syndrome. To prevent this from happening, surgeons sometimes make a series of incisions that relieve the buildup of pressure. To hold badly damaged long bones in place, surgeons drill pins through broken bones and apply external fixators (basically a type of "erector set") to hold the parts together. This reduces pain and helps prevent secondary injury.[3] Finally, the recent wars demonstrated that open combat-related wounds almost inevitably become infected and will fail to heal if they are closed too soon. As a result, military surgeons learned to leave the wounds open early on, but covered with either moist gauze, a negative pressure (suction) dressing, and/or bone cement with antibiotic "pouches." Typically, patients with these injuries need several rounds of wound debridement before their wounds are sufficiently clear of germs to be safely closed or covered.

2. In the second phase, **definitive treatment**, surgeons use a combination of internal and/or external fixation to heal fractures and close wounds. Some patients require local or remote tissue flaps (complete with their blood vessel supply), or application of standard skin grafts. Internal fixation using plates, rods, and screws is typically used only for less complex and less contaminated injuries, because putting permanent implants in a contaminated wound can lead to severe infection. Depending on the patient and his or her spectrum of injuries, the definitive treatment phase may stretch over weeks and numerous surgical procedures. This requires a close partnership between various surgeons and teams, including orthopedic, plastic, urological, microsurgical, and general surgery/trauma teams. In many cases, doctors won't attempt definitive external fixation until the wound or flap is showing promising initial healing, because these devices provide greater fracture stability and enable earlier weight-bearing. Using this staged approach, circular external fixation has allowed us to salvage grievously wounded limbs.[4] This complex sequence of surgeries has been made possible by multimodal anesthesia and analgesia, including aggressive use of peripheral nerve blocks and regional anesthetics (Chapter 22). These have allowed surgeons to substantially reduce the use of painful bedside dressing changes during the first two phases of limb salvage without compromising pain control.

3. The third and final phase of limb salvage is **rehabilitation and regeneration.** Although patients typically begin rehabilitation therapy long before this phase commences, the third phase is typically marked by more aggressive and focused

mobilization to restore function. Surgical treatments continue, and sometimes require halting the progress of physical therapy. Sometimes, additional operations are inevitable as a result of complications such as infection or the development of heterotopic ossification (the growth of abnormal bone within soft tissues, which can cause severe pain or ulcers and limit motion). Heterotopic ossification occurs in nearly two-thirds of severely blast-injured patients.[5] When this happens, the abnormal bone growth must often be cut away. Early and successful management of these complications is crucial to maintain a sense of progress and prevent despair, since delayed amputations account for about 15 percent of all amputations.[6] Other common operative procedures during the rehabilitative/regenerative phase include release of contractures to improve joint range of motion; bone grafting to accelerate the fusion of slow-healing fractures; nerve repairs and tendon transfers to compensate for de-innervated or lost muscle groups; reconstruction of missing tendons, ligaments, and bone; and excision of failed skin grafts.

The goal of limb salvage is a satisfied patient with a viable and functional extremity. It is rarely possible to restore normal function completely after devastating injuries, but we can achieve remarkable outcomes using the modern techniques summarized above.

For those left with some impairment, dynamic braces and orthoses can often compensate for problems such as limited strength or motion, and permit wounded warriors to pursue high-end athletic and military activities that would not have been possible before 9/11. One of the most innovative of these devices is the Intrepid Dynamic Exoskeletal Orthosis (IDEO brace)–a novel dynamic brace that was entirely developed and refined at the Center For the Intrepid in San Antonio. Its ingenious design stores energy with each step and returns it when the foot lifts, mimicking normal walking and thereby compensating for structural deficits. It has enabled many wounded warriors with salvaged limbs to achieve a level of recovery no one thought possible (Figure 26.5).

Ultimately, successful limb salvage requires a dedicated, multidisciplinary team of providers and therapists, as well as a motivated and persistent wounded warrior.

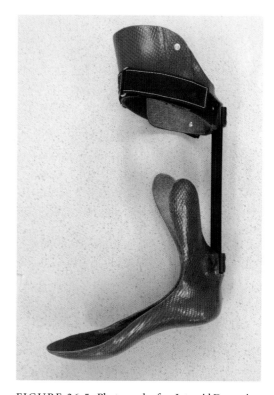

FIGURE 26.5. Photograph of an Intrepid Dynamic Extraskeletal Orthosis (IDEO brace), developed at the Center for the Intrepid at San Antonio Military Medical Center during recent conflicts to compensate for deficits, relieve pain via offloading, and improve function for many limb salvage patients. The brace is now in both clinical and research use at Walter Reed National Military Medical Center and Naval Medical Center San Diego, as well as San Antonio Military Medical Center, the three US military medical centers performing definitive treatment for the vast majority of combat casualties from Operations Enduring Freedom, Iraqi Freedom, and New Dawn. Photograph courtesy of Walter Reed National Military Medical Center.

IMPACT

During OEF and OIF, more than 1,600 wounded warriors endured over 2,200 major extremity amputations. However, more than *five times* that number suffered severe extremity injuries that were successfully managed with limb salvage techniques. As a result of the advances in surgical technique, a far higher percentage of mangled extremities were salvaged during these conflicts than during any prior wars.

Many medical advances made this possible. These include tourniquet use, damage control surgery and orthopedics, vascular shunts, negative pressure wound therapy, regenerative medicine techniques, and coordinated multidisciplinary care. All were developed or refined within the Military Health System. In fact, many wounded warriors with salvaged limbs, as well as dozens of amputees, recovered so well that they were able to return to action, often in combatant roles, following successful treatment and rehabilitation.

Many of the techniques developed or refined by military surgeons during this period of intense conflict are being adopted by civilian orthopedic surgeons and other surgical specialists (Chapter 43). This progress underscores the benefits of encouraging active and ongoing collaboration between military and civilian surgeons, product developers and innovators.

Notes

1. Owens BD, Kragh JF, Wenke JC, Macaitis J, Wade CE, Holcomb JB. Combat wounds in Operation Iraqi Freedom and Operation Enduring Freedom. *J Trauma.* 2008;264:295–299.
2. Borut J, Acosta JA, Tadlock M, Dye JL, Galarneau M, Elshire D. The use of temporary vascular shunts in military extremity wounds: a preliminary analysis with 2-year follow-up. *J Trauma.* 2010;69:174–178.
3. Possley DR, Burns TC, Stinner DJ, Murray CK, Wenke JC, Hsu J. Temporary external fixation is safe in a combat environment. *J Trauma.* 2010;69:S135-S139.
4. Keeling JJ, Gwinn DE, Tintle SM, Andersen RC, McGuigan FX. Short-term outcomes of severe open wartime tibial fractures treated with ring external fixation. *J Bone Joint Surg Am.* 2008;90-A;2643–2651.
5. Potter BK, Forsberg JA, Davis TA, et al. Heterotopic ossification following combat-related trauma. *J Bone Joint Surg Am.* 2010;92 Suppl 2;74–89.
6. Stinner DJ, Burns TC, Kirk KL, Scoville CR, Ficke JR, Hsu J. Prevalence of late amputations during the current conflicts in Afghanistan and Iraq. *Mil Med.* 2010;175:102–1029.

CHAPTER twenty-seven

Preventing and Treating Infectious Complications in Wounded Warriors

CLINTON K. MURRAY, MD; DANIEL R. ROBLES; and DAVID R. TRIBBLE, MD, DRPH

BACKGROUND

WOUND INFECTIONS ARE A COMMON COMPLICATION of battlefield injuries.[1,2] Although wounded warriors are similar in certain respects to civilian trauma patients, the complex nature of battlefield injuries and the unusual microorganisms encountered in combat zones add an extra level of complexity. The wars in Iraq (Operation Iraqi Freedom) and Afghanistan (Operation Enduring Freedom) illustrate this point. US troops not only sustained complicated wounds, but they also encountered challenging disease processes such as invasive fungal wound infections and multidrug-resistant organisms (MDROs).[3] The Military Health System responded by rapidly developing and disseminating new approaches, guidelines, and techniques to prevent, detect, and treat these infections—hallmarks of a "learning healthcare system."

Infectious complications have been a challenge in every war.[2] Gas gangrene was associated with a 28 percent mortality rate in World War I and a 15 percent mortality rate in World War II. Septic shock was the third-leading cause of death among wounded service members in Vietnam. Initial wound infection rates in Vietnam averaged 4 percent during the early phase of care, but reached as high as 30 percent among high-risk wounded after their evacuation to Japan.

VIGNETTE >> Iraq, April 8, 2006. Army Master Sergeant Robles was patrolling outside Baghdad in an up-armored Humvee when a road-side bomb hit his vehicle. He survived thanks to the vehicle's armor and his protective vest, but the explosion penetrated the floorboard and sprayed his legs with ballistic fragments. His injuries included mangled lower legs, fragment injuries and burns to his right buttock and posterior thigh, left wrist fragment injuries, and corneal abrasions in both eyes. But for the prompt application of tourniquets, he would have bled to death on the scene (see Chapter 10) (Figure 27.1). He was immediately evacuated by helicopter.

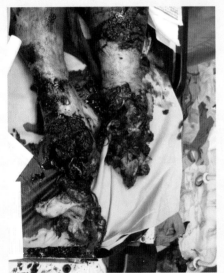

Arriving at the combat support hospital in Baghdad 40 minutes after his injury, Robles was met by fellowship-trained trauma and orthopedic surgeons. His initial care included balanced infusion of 16 units of fresh whole blood, fresh frozen plasma and packed red blood cells (Chapter 16), bilateral below-the-knee amputations, and administration of antibiotics to prevent infection. Shortly thereafter, a Critical Care

FIGURE 27.1. Master Sergeant Robles' lower leg injuries.

Air Transport Team (CCATT) flew him to Landstuhl Regional Medical Center in Germany (Chapter 25). After six days of wound management there, he was transferred on a second CCATT flight to Brooke Army Medical Center in San Antonio.

Unfortunately, Master Sergeant Robles' already complex situation was further complicated by severe wound infections that did not respond to standard antibiotics. Operative wound cultures provided the answer: three weeks into his hospitalization, he had become infected with multiple strains of antibiotic-resistant bacteria. His cultures grew several dangerous organisms: multidrug-resistant *Acinetobacter baumannii*, multidrug-resistant *Pseudomonas aeruginosa*, multidrug-resistant *Klebsiella pneumoniae*, and methicillin-sensitive *Staphylococcus aureus* (MSSA). To treat these infections, Robles required powerful antibiotics with potentially harmful side effects. During this phase of care, he developed antibiotic-induced kidney failure. Fortunately, once his wounds responded and the antibiotics were stopped, his kidney function improved. At that point, he was fitted for prosthetic legs (Chapter 28).

One year later, Master Sergeant Robles returned to the hospital because one of his stumps was infected with *P aeruginosa*. Doctors started powerful antibiotics to clear the infection, but they caused bone marrow toxicity. Fortunately, after switching to a different antibiotic, his bone marrow responded, and that stump never showed infection again. Unfortunately, his other stump later developed an infection with methicillin-resistant *S aureus* (MRSA). Instead of further surgery, Robles opted for chronic antimicrobial suppressive therapy to keep it under control.

Thanks to advances in combat casualty care, case-fatality rates for US battlefield casualties have dropped from 19 percent in World War II to less than 9 percent in Iraq and Afghanistan, despite greater injury severity. However, as more wounded warriors survive devastating injuries, the risk of subsequent wound infections is probably higher than in prior conflicts (although lack of information from earlier wars makes direct comparisons difficult).

THE CHALLENGE

In Iraq and Afghanistan, trauma-related infections occurred in roughly one-third of injured personnel during their initial hospitalization. The rate approached 50 percent if the service member was injured severely enough to require intensive care unit admission at Landstuhl or a major military hospital in the United States.

One reason for this high rate of trauma-related infections was the complexity of the underlying injuries, which posed an added challenge. As the conflict in Afghanistan evolved, a new injury pattern called "dismounted complex blast injuries" emerged. These injuries happened when a service member on foot patrol triggered an improvised explosive device. The injuries were characterized by traumatic amputation of one or both legs, often the associated loss of part or all of an arm, and severe pelvic and/or urogenital injuries. Because many of these injuries were contaminated by ballistic fragments, soil, and other contaminants, they often become infected (25 to 50 percent).

Moreover, even when the initial infections were controlled, these patients often developed recurrent or new infections long after leaving the hospital. A concerning number of patients developed invasive fungal wound infections (6.8 percent of trauma admissions from 2009 to 2011), which are particularly hard to treat.[4] These cases tended to have higher rates of mortality (up to 8 percent) and greater disability because doctors often had to take the patient back to the operating room to debride infected tissue. Some required higher-level amputations, up to the hip or even the pelvis. Given the severity of these infections, surgeons start aggressive surgical debridement and early systemic antifungal treatment if there is any suspicion of fungal involvement.

Another challenge in the Iraq and Afghanistan wars was a sharp rise in infections involving MDROs, particularly gram-negative bacteria.[5] One such outbreak, which involved a multidrug-resistant strain of *Acinetobacter* among injured military personnel in Iraq, was probably due to inadvertent hospital transmission. Other outbreaks of MDROs included extended-spectrum β-lactamase–producing *Escherichia coli* and *K pneumoniae*. To combat the emergence and transmission of MDROs, military doctors in war zones and at US hospitals have implemented strict infection-control protocols, including standardized approaches to screening at-risk patients as they are admitted to the hospital. Those found to be colonized or infected with MDROs are placed in medical isolation and cared for in very precise ways that reduce the risk of inadvertently transmitting drug-resistant organisms to other patients. Unfortunately, the challenge of combatting MDROs is not limited to military healthcare settings. It is a serious health problem worldwide.

THE INNOVATIONS

The driving force in countering infectious complications in trauma patients was the establishment, in November 2004, of the Department of Defense (DoD) Joint Theater Trauma System (now referred to as the Joint Trauma System or JTS; see Chapter 8).[6] By systematically collecting and sharing data, the JTS enabled military surgeons and infectious disease experts to identify concerns and implement numerous initiatives to improve care. Over the subsequent decade, JTS-led clinical practice guidelines were disseminated worldwide.

 The first evidence-based clinical practice guidelines specific to preventing infections following combat-related injuries were published by the JTS in 2008, and subsequently revised in 2011.[7] Developed by JTS-convened military and civilian experts, the guidelines focused on the immediate care of patients in the combat zone during the first few days after evacuation to Landstuhl Regional Medical Center or US hospitals. The guidelines emphasized the importance of prompt surgical treatment, early use of appropriate antibiotics to prevent infection, and stringent practice of infection control. To prevent or delay the emergence of resistance, the guidelines strongly discouraged the indiscriminant use of broad-spectrum antibiotics.

Another important JTS innovation was the creation of the DoD Trauma Registry (DoDTR). As noted in Chapter 8, the DoDTR collects detailed clinical data from wounded military personnel across levels of care. When rates of infection began to rise, military health leaders realized that this registry could help them collect comprehensive data on these infections. To capitalize on this capability, the military launched the Trauma Infectious Disease Outcomes Study (TIDOS). Devised and run by the Infectious Disease Clinical Research Program at the Uniformed Services University of the Health Sciences (Chapter 4), this ongoing, multicenter DoD/Veterans Administration cohort study is funded by the Navy Bureau of Medicine and Surgery Wounded, Ill, and Injured Program and the National Institute of Allergy and Infectious Diseases. TIDOS is designed to study the short- and long-term consequences of trauma-related infections in wounded military personnel. Wounded warriors enrolled in the study are followed for years to determine their long-term outcomes and the risk of developing recurrent infections. The supplemental data required to support this study, including infection diagnoses, antimicrobial treatment, and wound microbiology, are captured through a special infectious disease module created to supplement the DoDTR.

IMPACT

TIDOS found that the complications of trauma-related wound infections can affect patients long after their initial hospitalization. Problems include new or recurrent wound infections as well as the need for additional hospitalizations or surgeries—much like Master Sergeant Robles' experience. The TIDOS project, in collaboration with the JTS, led outbreak investigations to inform practice guidance for diagnosis and management of invasive fungal wound infections. This evidence has supported early risk characterization leading to earlier diagnosis, which is critical in reducing morbidity and mortality. Further research will be needed to identify modifiable factors to prevent wound infections as well as to devise effective countermeasures to achieve better outcomes.

A LOOK AT THE FUTURE

The complex injuries encountered in modern warfare and the expanding capabilities of global terrorist organizations pose substantial challenges for military health professionals (Chapter 34). The extent and complexity of combat wounds, many of which are grossly contaminated with fragments, soil, or debris, and the added risk of acquiring healthcare-associated infections make it imperative for military surgeons and other healthcare providers to focus on preventing and aggressively managing wound infections. Once trauma-associated infections occur, as illustrated in Master Sergeant Robles' case, they can have serious short- and long-term consequences. The US military and the National Institute of Allergy and Infectious Diseases are actively engaged in joint research to develop improvements in patient care. This is the best way to assure that our military health system will be ready to identify, manage, and overcome a wide array of infectious disease threats.

EPILOGUE

Fortunately, Master Sergeant Robles eventually recovered from his lengthy fight with infections, and thanks to his remarkable resilience and ongoing care, is doing well. He has continued to see the same military infectious disease doctor (CKM) for ongoing chronic antimicrobial therapy for 10-plus years.

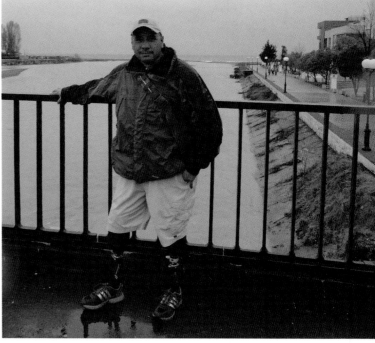

FIGURE 27.2. Master Sergeant (Retired) Robles today.

He recently retired from active duty after 20 years of service (Figure 27.2). During this time, the surgeon progressed in rank from major to colonel, and continued to care for patients with chronic combat-related wound infections at Brooke Army Medical Center. Together, this wounded warrior and military doctor saw each other's daughters grow from preteens to college students. Lessons learned from this courageous Soldier have helped prepare a generation of military orthopedic surgeons and infectious disease physicians to handle infectious complications of combat-related injuries.

Notes

1. Blyth DM, Yun HC, Tribble DR, Murray CK. Lessons of war: combat-related injury infections during the Vietnam War and Operation Iraqi and Enduring Freedom. *J Trauma Acute Care Surg.* 2015;794:S227–S235.

2. Murray CK, Hinkle MK, Yun HC. History of infections associated with combat-related injuries. *J Trauma.* 2008;64:S221–S231.

3. Tribble DR, Li P, Warkentien TE, et al. Impact of operational theater on combat and noncombat trauma-related infections. *Mil Med.* 2016;181:1258–1268.

4. Tribble DR, Rodriguez CJ. Combat-related invasive fungal wound infections. *Curr Fungal Infect Rep.* 2014;8:277–286.

5. Hospenthal DR, Crouch HK, English JF, et al. Multidrug-resistant bacterial colonization of combat-injured personnel at admission to medical centers after evacuation from Afghanistan and Iraq. *J Trauma.* 2011;71:S52–S57.

6. Eastridge BJ, Jenkins D, Flaherty S, Schiller H, Holcomb JB. Trauma system development in a theater of war: experiences from Operation Iraqi Freedom and Operation Enduring Freedom. *J Trauma.* 2006;61:1366–1372.

7. Hospenthal DR, Murray CK, Andersen RC, et al. Guidelines for the prevention of infections associated with combat-related injuries: 2011 update: endorsed by the Infectious Diseases Society of America and the Surgical Infection Society. *J Trauma.* 2011;71:S210–S234.

Recommended Reading

Murray CK, Gross K, Russell RJ, Haslett RA. Dismounted complex blast injuries including invasive fungal infections. *US Army Med Dep J.* 2016;Apr-Sep:24–28.

Yun JC, Murray Ck. Infection prevention in the deployed environment. *US Army Med Dep J.* 2016; Apr-Sep:114–118.

CHAPTER twenty-eight

Advances in Combat Amputee Care

PAUL F. PASQUINA, MD, and BENJAMIN K. POTTER, MD

THE CHALLENGE

SINCE MILITARY OPERATIONS BEGAN IN IRAQ AND AFGHANISTAN, numerous medical advances implemented over the course of the wars produced historically high battlefield survival rates.[1] As a result, service members now survive complex injuries that in prior conflicts would have been fatal. Many of these wounded warriors face enormous short- and long-term challenges with recovery and rehabilitation.

Limb amputation due to combat trauma or subsequent infection has been a common consequence of war through most of human history (Figure 28.1). To date, nearly 1,700 US service members have lost close to 2,300 limbs from combat injuries in Iraq and Afghanistan. Particularly challenged are those who sustain "dismounted complex blast injuries" (DCBIs). DCBIs are caused when an IED explodes below or next to a service member on foot patrol. The unique injury pattern of DCBIs includes the traumatic amputation of one or both legs above the knee; concurrent pelvic and genitourinary injuries; and upper extremity dysfunction or amputations.[2]

Military amputees differ in many ways from their civilian counterparts. More than half of civilian amputations involve older individuals and result from peripheral vascular disease, frequently due to diabetes.[3] War trauma hits a far younger, physically fit population, and is frequently complicated by

VIGNETTE >> Lance Corporal "T" was a 20-year-old active duty Marine who stepped on an improvised explosive device (IED) while on foot patrol in Afghanistan. The blast amputated both of his legs above the knee and mangled his hands and arms, resulting in the loss of his left middle finger and right index and middle fingers. He also sustained an open fracture to his right arm with damage to the ulnar nerve, plus extensive soft tissue wounds to his pelvis, abdomen, and all four extremities. Thanks to expert treatment at the point of injury and throughout his subsequent evacuation from Afghanistan to Germany and then the United States, he survived to reach Walter Reed National Military Medical Center.

His rehabilitation was complicated by large blood clots in both legs, a pulmonary embolus, complex pain, insomnia, and heterotopic ossification (bone formation in the soft tissue where bone does not normally exist) in the stump of his right leg, which had to be surgically removed about 10 months after his original injury. Despite the severity of his multiple injuries, he exhibited remarkable courage and resilience. Still, he will always be affected by the loss of many comrades, including his best friend.

Since his injury, he has received extensive rehabilitation, becoming independent in all daily activities. After initially operating both power and manual wheelchairs, he mastered walking with advanced, microprocessor-controlled prosthetic legs. Playing adaptive sports helped his recovery. Today, he lives with his wife in a specially adapted home provided by public donations and one of the many nonprofits that support wounded warriors.

other injuries, including traumatic brain injury, vision or hearing loss, and other orthopedic injuries. Furthermore, the trauma of the attack and the stressful period that follows often lead to posttraumatic stress disorder and other long-term psychological problems, which are reported in nearly six of ten warriors who lose a limb.[4] In addition, women service members, previously underrepresented in war casualty statistics, are sustaining injuries that lead to extensive impairment, including amputation.[5]

THE INNOVATION

Early, Comprehensive Rehabilitation

Faced with a large and sustained influx of service members with missing limbs, the Military Health System had to quickly develop **Advanced Rehabilitation Centers** (ARCs) and strategically position them across the continental United States. Current ARCs include Walter Reed National Military Medical Center in Bethesda, Maryland; the Center for the Intrepid in San Antonio, Texas; and the Comprehensive Combat and Complex Casualty Care program in San Diego, California. Together with the Department of Veterans Affairs (VA) PolyTrauma Rehabilitation Centers, the ARCs provide comprehensive rehabilitative care to service members with amputations and other complex injuries. Distinguishing ARCs from other regional medical facilities is their ability to combine acute medical and surgical care with comprehensive rehabilitation and behavioral health support. They have highly specialized interdisciplinary teams composed of rehabilitation physicians, therapists, surgical and medical specialists, prosthetists, orthotists, nurses, social workers, and pain and behavioral health specialists. A team approach is vital to treating service members with multiple complex physical, neurological, and behavioral health problems (see Chapters 29–31).

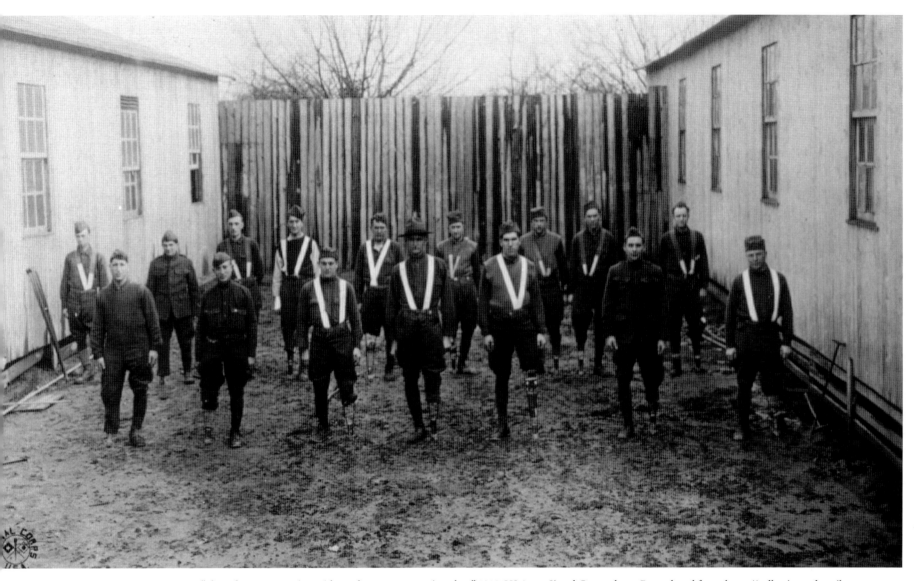

FIGURE 28.1. "Above knee amputation with peg legs: reconstruction class," 1919. US Army Signal Corps photo. Reproduced from: https://collections.nlm.nih.gov/catalog/nlm:nlmuid-101397824-img.

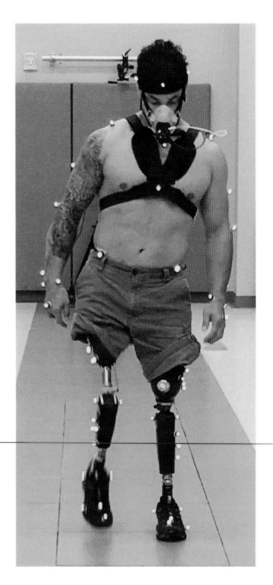

Family members also play critical roles in promoting maximal physical, emotional, and psychological recovery (Chapter 33). Over the past decade the military has provided unprecedented support to family members, who are officially designated "non-medical attendants," so they can join their loved ones during the frequently lengthy inpatient and outpatient stays at military treatment facilities. This support includes monthly monetary stipends, access to healthcare, and free on-base lodging, often at "Fisher Houses" (provided by public donations; see Americans Helping Wounded Warriors, by Arnold Fisher, in Chapter 29).

Each patient's individualized **rehabilitation goals** are based on multiple factors, including the level of amputation, the number and nature of any associated injuries, and the patient's personal aspirations. For all patients, particularly those with upper limb loss, the rehabilitation goals (with or without an artificial limb or "prosthesis") initially involve promoting independence with "activities of daily living," such as bathing, dressing, eating, and using the toilet. Later, more advanced "instrumental activities of daily living" are taught. These include housekeeping skills, shopping, managing finances, driving, and returning to a vocation. For those with lower limb amputations, initial goals include restoring independent mobility with a wheelchair, prosthesis, or both. Patients later engage in rehabilitative programs to promote higher-level activities, such as running and participating in sports and other recreational activities using specialized prosthetics or other adaptive equipment. These activities are often guided by sophisticated gait and motion-analysis systems (Figure 28-2).

Modern rehabilitation for military amputees starts as soon as possible, because waiting until all medical and surgical issues are resolved can worsen outcomes.[6] Caregivers typically start rehabilitative interventions early in the intensive care environment, long before the patient is ready to be fitted with a prosthesis. We've learned that aggressive rehabilitation, started

FIGURE 28.2. A DCBI casualty undergoing state-of-the-art biomechanical and metabolic analysis. Photograph: Courtesy of Ben Harrow (pictured).

early, helps prevent deconditioning and joint stiffness (contractures), improves pain management, and minimizes secondary complications such as pressure ulcers and loss of bone density. It also promotes general health, wound healing, and psychological recovery. Further, rather than communicate to the warfighter that he or she is permanently "disabled," early rehab signals the military's commitment to help them recover to their maximum potential.[7]

Early rehabilitative intervention should continue through the prosthetic phase of treatment as well. After the wounds from amputation surgery have adequately healed, patients are more likely to accept and use prosthetics if they are fitted promptly. This is particularly true for upper extremity amputations.[8] Newer prosthetic technologies allow patients to return to activities that were unlikely a few years ago. Advanced technologies can also be incorporated into customized "smart" homes to improve independence despite severe disabilities.[9]

Fitting patients with prosthetics, and training them to use them, are crucial steps. Good care also includes strategies to minimize or prevent secondary health complications that commonly occur in patients with major limb losses. These include the increased long-term risk of obesity, cardiovascular disease, arthritis, low back pain, chronic pain, and psychological problems.[10]

Advanced Technology

The options for prosthetic limbs today are vastly better than they were at the start of the wars in Afghanistan and Iraq. This is because over the past 10 years, rehabilitation specialists, prosthetists, and biomechanical engineers have achieved remarkable advances in prosthetic technology. Much of this progress is a direct result of substantial investments by the Department of Defense (DoD) and VA.

Examples include:

- *Microprocessor variable dampening prosthetic knees*. These knees are equipped with sensors that detect how fast a patient is walking or running. They send the information to an internal computer (microprocessor) that controls the knee's resistance to flexion and extension. This allows the prosthesis to accommodate variable walking speeds, which creates a more normal and efficient gait, and reduces the risk of stumbles and falls, especially when negotiating stairs and ramps.[11]

- *Powered prosthetics.* Advanced motor actuators have been incorporated into powered prosthetic knees and ankles. These devices can replace the function of thigh and calf muscles lost to amputation. What was once considered science fiction is now commercially available.

- *Enhanced prosthetic sockets.* Newer, lighter-weight composite materials—including carbon fiber, silicon imbedded fabrics, and novel suction devices—allow better customized fit of various residual limb sizes and shapes as well as improved prosthetic suspension. Additional advances are being achieved through computer-assisted design, computer-assisted manufacturing, and 3-dimensional printing. The result is better-fitting, more comfortable, and more wearable prostheses.

- *Coming soon: direct skeletal attachment.* Despite advances in socket technology, some patients with very proximal amputations or poor soft tissue coverage of their residual limb encounter significant challenges with use of conventional prosthetics. *Osseointegration* involves the direct skeletal implantation of a prosthesis, with a metal post permanently protruding through the skin. The technique has proven effective in certain subgroups with limb loss, particularly in Europe and Australia.[12] In 2015, military and VA clinicians and researchers, working in collaboration with academic and industry partners, received initial Food and Drug Administration approval to begin clinical trials of this technology in the United States.[13]

- *Robotic hands and arms.* The frequency of upper limb loss among Operation Enduring Freedom (OEF) and Operation Iraqi Freedom (OIF) combat casualties prompted the Defense Advanced Research Projects Agency to sponsor research to revolutionize the design and functionality of prosthetics. This ignited research in upper limb prosthetics, leading to the development of two advanced robotic arms: the DEKA arm[14] and the modular prosthetic limb (MPL).[15] The MPL contains 17 independent actuators (motors) that drive 27 joints (Figure 28.3). While both devices are currently used primarily for research, they provide a road map for future advances in the field.

- *Advanced human-machine interfaces.* Early feasibility studies have shown that more advanced control may be possible between humans and their prosthetic/robotic limbs. Enhanced "human-machine" interface systems allow a person to think about moving their prosthetic limb and have the limb perform the activity. Future prostheses may even allow tactile feedback from the prosthetic hand to the user. This approach involves implanting sensors within the nervous system (brain, spinal cord, peripheral nerve, or peripheral muscle) that transmit signals to and from the human and machine. Future applications may help not only those with limb loss, but those with paralysis as well.[16]

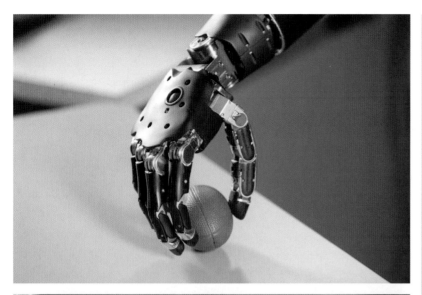

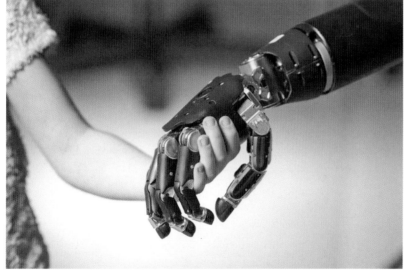

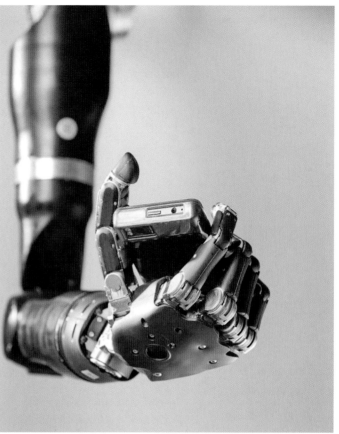

FIGURE 28.3. The modular prosthetic limb, designed to support below and above elbow (up to shoulder) level amputation. Reproduced with permission from Johns Hopkins Applied Physics Laboratory. Copyright 2014 Johns Hopkins University/Applied Physics Laboratory LLC. All rights reserved. For permission to use, modify, or reproduce, contact the Office of Technology Transfer at JHU/APL

A MESSAGE FROM BOSTON

"Our prayers are with the injured; so many wounded, some gravely. From their beds, some are surely watching us gather here today. And if you are, know this: As you begin this long journey of recovery, your city is with you. Your commonwealth is with you. Your country is with you. We will all be with you as you learn to stand and walk and, yes, run again . . . Your resolve is the greatest rebuke to whoever committed this heinous act."

President Barack Obama
Boston, Massachusetts, April 18, 2013

On April 15, 2013, three people were killed and more than 230 injured when two bombs exploded near the finish line of the Boston Marathon. Although the death rate was mercifully low, many who survived suffered grievous injuries rarely seen by doctors who have not served in a war zone.

Despite the skills and dedication of the Boston-area medical professionals who cared for us, many had never treated patients with complex blast-related injuries. And even Boston's world-renowned healthcare system lacked the infrastructure needed to provide integrated, comprehensive care that links specialists across various disciplines, including surgery, rehabilitation, therapy, nursing, pain management, prosthetics, and behavioral health. This made the process of navigating from doctor to doctor, and clinic to therapist, extremely difficult.

The two of us sustained, among other injuries, traumatic amputations, ruptured eardrums, shrapnel wounds, depression, anxiety, mild traumatic brain injury, and posttraumatic stress. Many other Boston survivors shared similar experiences. We two were fortunate. Thanks to the persistent efforts of many, we were eventually granted Secretary of Defense Designee Status. This allowed us, despite being civilians, to receive care from the military healthcare system.

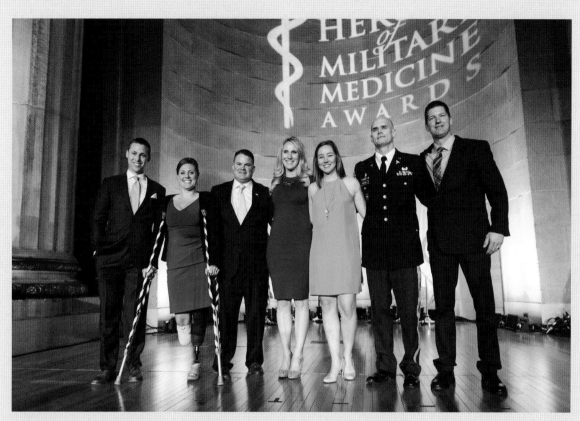

2016 Henry M. Jackson Foundation Heroes of Military Medicine Awards Dinner, Washington, DC. Left to right: Patrick Downes; Jessica Kensky, RN; Captain (Retired) Ferris Butler; Annemarie Orr, OTD; Kelly McGaughey, DPT; Lieutenant Colonel Benjamin Kyle Potter, MD; Art Molnar, CPO. Photograph: Courtesy of the Henry M. Jackson Foundation for the Advancement of Military Medicine.

We benefited in four important ways:

1. Military trauma surgeons consulted with our civilian trauma surgeons at home. Their advice on orthopedic and soft tissue care helped improve our long-term functionality and prosthetic use.

2. We were granted access to inpatient and outpatient surgical and rehabilitative treatment at Walter Reed National Military Medical Center for a year on a space-available and fully reimbursable basis, with the possibility for yearly renewal.

3. Our care was highly integrated and interdisciplinary. Walter Reed's staff not only assessed all of our ongoing medical, surgical, rehabilitation, and mental health needs; they also formulated a comprehensive plan to treat them in a coordinated and efficient manner.

4. We were welcomed into a deeply supportive community. At Walter Reed, we found ourselves surrounded by health professionals, therapists, and wounded warriors focused on our recovery.

We are grateful for all we've received. But we cannot help but think of our fellow survivors who did not have this opportunity. Recently, the Health and Medicine Division of the National Academies of Sciences, Engineering, and Medicine issued a major report on fostering a national trauma system. One of the report's recommendations is that "... the Secretary of Defense should direct the Military Health System to pursue the development of integrated, permanent joint civilian and military trauma system training platforms to create and sustain an expert trauma workforce."[1] We strongly agree with this recommendation, but urge that it not be limited to emergency trauma care. To give victims of terrorism the best chance for recovery, military and civilian health systems should partner to provide expert rehabilitation as well. Here are three ways that could happen:

- First, establish formal protocols to allow military experts in surgery and rehabilitation medicine to offer consultative assistance to civilian hospitals caring for victims of terrorist attacks.
- Second, create an expedited process, on a space-available basis, to allow US survivors of terrorist attacks to access the military's medical, surgical, and rehabilitation resources. This will not only assure that victims of terrorism receive world-class care, it will also help military healthcare providers keep their skills sharp for future deployments.
- Third, offer these services free of charge. As a group, the Boston Marathon bombing survivors received no federal funds to assist in our recovery. What financial assistance we received came from caring and generous individuals and organizations. This begs the question: when terrorists strike, should victims rely on private charity, or will our nation, through the federal government, care for its own?

Tragically, more terrorist attacks may be inevitable. We believe there is no bigger rebuke to terrorism than when Americans respond as one to assure that survivors thrive. Terrorists strive to divide us. We will defeat them by standing together.

Sincerely,
Jessica Kensky and Patrick Downes
Boston Marathon bombing survivors

Note

1. National Academies of Sciences, Engineering, and Medicine. *A National Trauma Care System: Integrating Military and Civilian Trauma Systems to Achieve Zero Preventable Deaths After Injury*. Washington, DC: National Academies Press; 2016: S21. http://www.nationalacademies.org/hmd/Reports/2016/A-National-Trauma-Care-System-Integrating-Military-and-Civilian-Trauma-Systems.aspx. Accessed August 17, 2016.

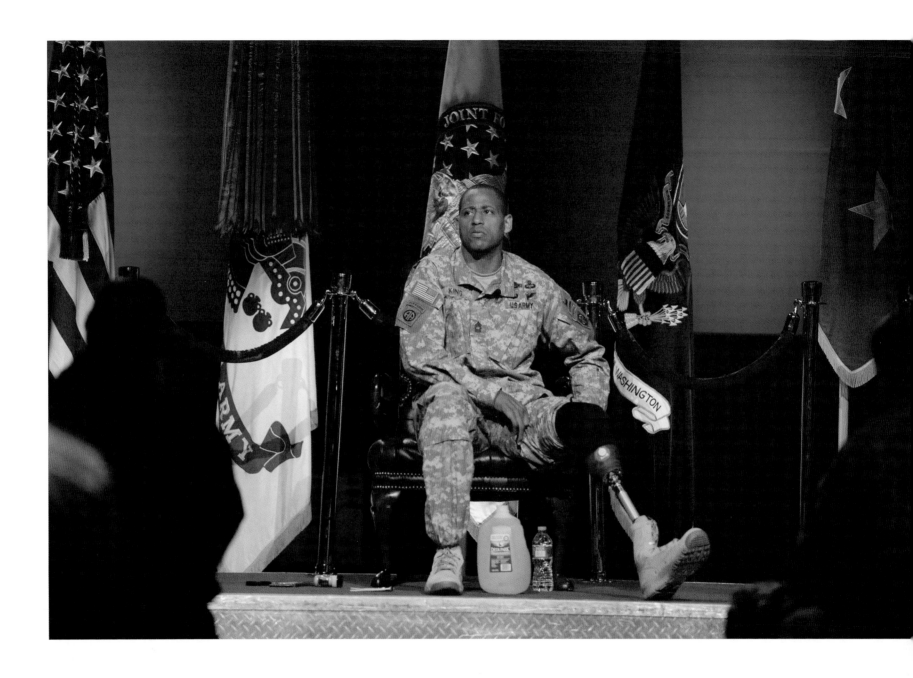

IMPACT

Historically, advances in military medicine have ultimately benefitted civilian healthcare. Nowhere is this more evident than with amputations. Whether influencing the surgical management of residual limbs, the timing of rehabilitation, or the development of advanced technology, the DoD, in partnership with the VA and other public and private organizations, has dramatically improved the quality of care, and resulting quality of life, for those who have lost one or more limbs. Lessons learned during OIF and OEF demonstrate that technological advances are only one component of a comprehensive and holistic approach to caring for service members with limb loss. The coordination of interdisciplinary teams in military treatment centers, especially the DoD's ARCs, is critical to success. These programs are committed to helping each injured service member achieve his or her maximal functional recovery, independence, and participation in society, whether this involves returning to active duty or transitioning to a rewarding civilian career (Figure 28.4 and Chapter 31).[17]

Much remains to be done. Many individuals with amputation still face lifelong challenges to their overall health, independence, and quality of life. Sustained commitment to these dedicated heroes, and ongoing research to advance rehabilitation science, will ensure continued progress to advance their recovery and benefit current and future generations.

FIGURE 28.4. [*Opposite*] US Army Master Sergeant Cedric King, Warrior Transition Brigade, Bravo Company, Walter Reed National Military Medical Center, speaks during a Ready and Resilient Training event at Conmy Hall, Joint Base Myer Henderson Hall, Arlington, Virginia, January 13, 2015. Just 21 months after losing both legs, King completed the Boston Marathon, running on prosthetic blades. He has gone on to compete in a 70.3-mile Half Ironman Triathlon, the 2014 New York City Marathon, and the 48.6-mile Disney Marathon series. US Army photo by Specialist Michael Mulderick/Released. Reproduced from: https://www.dvidshub.net/image/1722696/ready-and-resilient-training.

Notes

1. Holcomb JB, Stansbury LG, Champion HR, Bellamy RF. Understanding combat casualty care statistics. *J Trauma.* 2006;60:397–401.
2. Dismounted Complex Blast Injury Task Force. *Dismounted Complex Blast Injury: Report of the Army Dismounted Complex Blast Injury Task Force.* Fort Sam Houston, TX: Office of the Army Surgeon General; June 18, 2011. http://armymedicine.mil/Documents/DCBI-Task-Force-Report-Redacted-Final.pdf. Accessed January 1, 2016.
3. Ziegler-Graham K, MacKenzie EJ, Ephraim PL, Travison TG, Brookmeyer R. Estimating the prevalence of limb loss in the United States: 2005 to 2050. *Arch Phys Med Rehabil.* 2008;89(3):422–429.
4. Stevelink SA, Malcolm EM, Mason C, Jenkins S, Sundin J, Fear NT. The prevalence of mental health disorders in (ex-)military personnel with a physical impairment: a systematic review. *Occup Environ Med.* 2015;72:243–251.

5. Katon JG, Reiber GE. Major traumatic limb loss among women veterans and service members. *J Rehabil Res Dev.* 2013;50:173–182.

6. Pasquina PF, McAuliffe C, Fitzpatrick K, Isaacson B. Chapter 51: Rehabilitation. In: Moore EE, Feliciano DV, Mattox KL, eds. *Trauma.* 8th ed. New York, NY: McGraw-Hill Education; 2016.

7. Doukas WC, Hayda RA, Frisch HM, et al. The Military Extremity Trauma Amputation/Limb Salvage (METALS) study: outcomes of amputation versus limb salvage following major lower-extremity trauma. *J Bone Joint Surg Am.* 2013;95A:138–145.

8. Solarz MK, Thoder JJ, Rehman S. Management of major traumatic upper extremity amputations. *Orthop Clin North Am.* 2016;47:127–136.

9. Ding D, Cooper RA, Pasquina PF, Fici-Pasquina L. Sensor technology for smart homes. *Maturitas.* 2011;69:131–136.

10. Pasquina PF, Hendershot BD, Isaacson BM. Secondary health effects of amputation. In: *Atlas of Amputations and Limb Deficiencies.* 4th ed. Rosemont, IL: American Academy of Orthopedic Surgeons. In press.

11. Sawers AB, Hafner BJ. Outcomes associated with the use of microprocessor-controlled prosthetic knees among individuals with unilateral transfemoral limb loss: A systematic review. *J Rehabil Res Dev.* 2013;50:273–314.

12. Hagberg K, Hansson E, Brånemark R. Outcome of percutaneous osseointegrated prostheses for patients with unilateral transfemoral amputation at two-year follow-up. *Arch Phys Med Rehabil.* 2014;95:2120–2127.

13. FDA authorizes use of prosthesis for rehabilitation of above-the-knee amputations [news release]. Washington, DC: Food and Drug Administration; July 16, 2015. http://www.fda.gov/NewsEvents/Newsroom/PressAnnouncements/UCM455103. Accessed January 1, 2016.

14. Bionic DEKA Arm, mind-controlled prosthetic, approved by FDA. CBS News website. http://www.cbsnews.com/news/bionic-deka-arm-mind-controlled-prosthetic-approved-by-fda. Published May 12, 2014. Accessed January 1, 2016.

15. Prosthetics: Modular prosthetic limb. Johns Hopkins Applied Physics Laboratory website. http://www.jhuapl.edu/prosthetics/scientists/mpl.asp. Accessed January 1, 2016.

16. Collinger JL, Kryger MA, Barbara R, Betler T, et al. Collaborative approach in the development of high-performance brain-computer interfaces for a neuroprosthetic arm: translation from animal models to human control. *Clin Transl Sci.* 2014;7:52–59.

17. Pasquina PF, Cooper RA, eds. *Care of the Combat Amputee.* Washington, DC: Borden Institute, 2009.

Recommended Reading

Pasquina PF, Shero JC. Rehabilitation of the combat casualty: lessons learned from past and current conflicts. *US Army Med Dep J.* 2016;Apr-Sep:77–86.

CHAPTER twenty-nine

Rehabilitation of Blast Casualties with Traumatic Brain Injury

PAUL F. PASQUINA, MD; LOUIS M. FRENCH, PSYD; and RORY A. COOPER, PHD

THE PROBLEM

ALONG WITH IMPROVEMENTS IN TRAUMA CARE, modern protective gear dramatically reduced combat-related fatalities in Iraq and Afghanistan. Studies show that a casualty wearing a Kevlar combat helmet is 2.7 times less likely to sustain a fragmentation wound to the head than those who are unprotected. Casualties wearing a body armor vest are more than four times less likely to sustain a fragmentation wound to the chest or abdomen.[1] However, body armor does not provide complete protection, particularly from the effects of blasts.

"Polytrauma" refers to casualties with injuries to multiple body systems. The term "polytrauma triad" encompasses three long-term consequences of severe blast injuries: chronic pain, posttraumatic stress disorder (PTSD), and persistent symptoms from traumatic brain injury (TBI).[2] This constellation of symptoms generally exceeds the capabilities of a single rehabilitation provider, no matter how skilled.

TBI has been termed one of the "signature injuries" of Operations Enduring Freedom, Iraqi Freedom, and New Dawn (OEF/OIF/OND). It has been detected in more than 20 percent of combat-deployed soldiers and over 60 percent of polytrauma patients returning from Afghanistan and Iraq.[3] Although TBI has long been associated with war, mild TBI, also known as a "concussion," is a common complica-

FIGURE 29.1. [*Opposite*]
The Veterans Health Administration (VHA) Polytrauma/Traumatic Brain Injury (TBI) System of Care (PSC) is an integrated network of specialized rehabilitation programs dedicated to serving veterans and service members with both combat- and non-combat-related TBI and polytrauma. Specialized TBI and polytrauma care is provided at the facility closest to the veteran's home with the expertise necessary to manage his or her rehabilitation, medical, surgical, and mental health needs. The PSC provides a continuum of care from acute rehabilitation to community reintegration through five regional Polytrauma Rehabilitation Centers as well as polytrauma network sites, support clinic teams, and points of contact located at Veterans Affairs medical centers across the country.

tion of blast injuries. Surveillance data from the Defense and Veterans Brain Injury Center indicates that more than 300,000 TBIs were noted in military medical records between September 2001 and the second quarter of 2014. In contrast to the more serious moderate and severe TBIs, mild brain injuries are often subtle and difficult to detect, especially since the symptoms they produce overlap with those of posttraumatic stress (Chapter 30).[4]

THE INNOVATIONS

Polytrauma Rehabilitative Teams

In addition to meeting the acute medical and surgical care needs of the large number of complex casualties returning home at the height of OEF and OIF, the US military organized *polytrauma rehabilitative teams* consisting of specialists in physiatry, psychiatry, neuropsychology, physical and occupational therapy, nursing, nutrition, speech/language pathology, audiology, orthotics/prosthetics, rehabilitation engineering, assistive technology, peer support, sports and recreation therapy, case management, and social work. This coordinated team approach became essential to delivering high-quality effective care for complex war casualties, with early rehabilitative interventions demonstrating improved outcomes.[5] Research has found that early and aggressive interdisciplinary involvement is safe, does not increase net costs, results in shorter intensive care unit and hospital stays, and achieves better long-term outcomes.[6]

The Department of Defense/Veterans Affairs Rehab Partnership

To best meet the needs of the growing influx of injured veterans of OEF and OIF, especially those with TBI and polytrauma, the Department of Veterans Affairs (VA) developed specialized *polytrauma rehabilitation centers*. The most intensive of these VA polytrauma rehabilitation centers are located in Richmond, Virginia; Tampa, Florida; San Antonio, Texas; Minneapolis, Minnesota; and Palo Alto, California. Each offers intensive interdisciplinary inpatient rehabilitation services as well as residential outpatient rehab programs to help individuals with complex injuries transition from inpatient to outpatient status. The VA also supports comprehensive inpatient and outpatient rehabilitation centers that specialize in spinal cord injury and vision and hearing loss. Formal agreements between the Department of Defense (DoD) and the VA allow service members with polytrauma, amputation, or spinal cord injury to transfer freely between DoD and VA facilities, even while still on active duty (Figure 29.1).

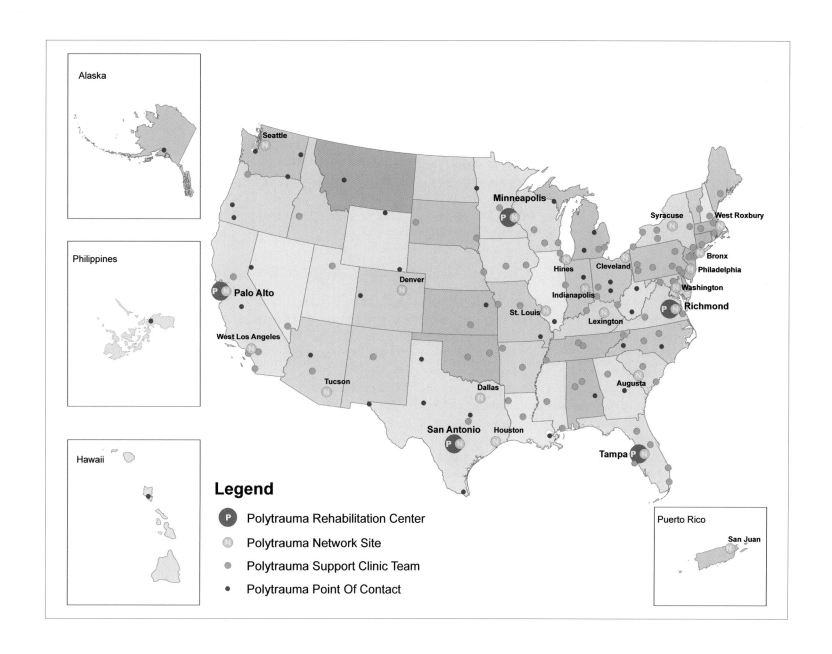

Alaska

Philippines

Hawaii

Seattle

Minneapolis

Syracuse West Roxbury

Palo Alto

Hines Cleveland Bronx

Denver Philadelphia

Indianapolis Washington

West Los Angeles St. Louis Richmond

Lexington

Tucson

Dallas Augusta

San Antonio Houston

Tampa

Puerto Rico

San Juan

Legend

P Polytrauma Rehabilitation Center

N Polytrauma Network Site

● Polytrauma Support Clinic Team

• Polytrauma Point Of Contact

AMERICANS HELPING WOUNDED WARRIORS

It has long been my conviction that no matter what your political beliefs may be, as Americans, we need to support the Soldiers, Sailors, Airmen, and Marines who have stepped forward to defend our nation. That is why I am incredibly proud that my family has been able to partner with the American people in forming the Intrepid Fallen Heroes Foundation.[1] Together, we've raised close to $200 million to build state-of-the-art facilities across the United States to not only support exceptional care for our wounded warriors, but also to serve as testament of our gratitude for their service and sacrifice.

We don't take any money from the government, because then the government would tell us what to do. The first thing I say when I get a signed agreement from a secretary of defense is to tell him, "Stay out of my way, because I can build these things in half the time at half the cost and twice the quality as the government."

These facilities include:
* The Center for the Intrepid in San Antonio, Texas, built in 2007, is a monumental, world-class facility that provides comprehensive interdisciplinary outpatient care to wounded warriors with amputations, limb trauma, and burns.
* The National Intrepid Center of Excellence in Bethesda, Maryland, built in 2010, is a 72,000 square foot, two-story facility on the campus of Walter Reed National Military Medical Center. This facility specializes in the diagnosis and treatment of wounded warriors with traumatic brain injury and psychological health conditions.
* A network of nine Intrepid Spirit centers extend state-of-the-art care to service members with traumatic brain injury and psychological health conditions across the nation. The first Intrepid Spirit center opened at Fort Belvoir, Virginia, in August 2013. Camp Lejeune, North Carolina, followed in August 2013. Fort Campbell, Kentucky, opened in August 2014; Fort Hood, Texas, opened March 2016; and Fort Bragg, North Carolina, opened in March 2016. Additional centers are under construction at Joint Base Lewis-McChord, in Washington state, and Camp Pendleton, in California, and two more are planned. Once complete, these Intrepid Spirit centers will treat thousands of patients annually, providing wounded warriors and their families the most advanced care possible.

Throughout my travels across the globe, including in war zones, it has been truly a privilege to meet and talk with countless service members and their families. Whenever I meet those who suffer from visible or invisible wounds, I am reminded that

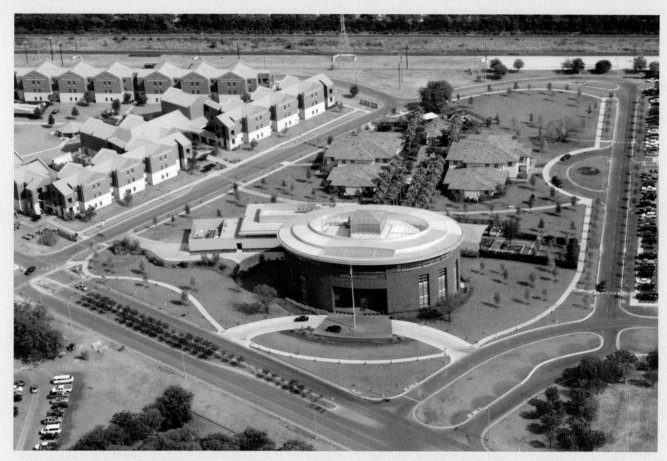

Aerial view, Center for the Intrepid. The facility is located next to the San Antonio Military Medical Center at Fort Sam Houston in San Antonio, Texas. Photo courtesy of the Intrepid Fallen Heroes Foundation.

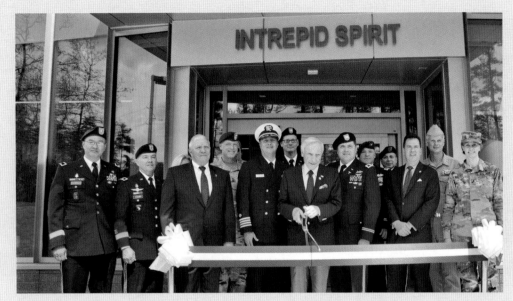

Arnold Fisher cutting the ribbon at the opening ceremony for the new Intrepid Spirit center at Fort Bragg, North Carolina, March 31, 2016. Photo courtesy of the Intrepid Fallen Heroes Foundation.

more must be done. Caring for our wounded warriors is not just the responsibility of the military health care system, it is an obligation our entire country shares. I am proud that we are still contributing to this effort. While many Americans may be tired of war, our commitment to help our wounded warriors and their families must continue.

Arnold Fisher, Honorary Chairman
Intrepid Fallen Heroes Foundation

Note
1.   Intrepid Fallen Heroes Fund website. https://www.fallenheroesfund.org/. Accessed November 28, 2016.

Comprehensive Screening Programs

To improve TBI treatment and rehabilitation, the military established several joint, inter-service initiatives, including the *Defense and Veterans Brain Injury Center* (Chapter 39), the *Armed Forces Health Surveillance Center,* and the *Joint Trauma Analysis and Prevention of Injury in Combat Directorate* (Chapter 9). Together, these programs and other teams expanded the military's knowledge of the frequency and impact of TBI, whether related to blasts, motor vehicle collisions, training accidents, sports, falls, or recreational activities. As a consequence of this surveillance data, DoD policy now requires mandatory screening of service members exposed to a significant blast or other concussive events.[7]

To improve the objectivity of assessments, formal tools, such as the *Military Acute Concussion Evaluation (MACE)* were devised for use in combat zones. These tools allow military health personnel to consistently screen service members for concussions, protect their health, and assess their readiness to return to duty. The military also put *postdeployment health surveillance* in place to detect previously undocumented concussive events and initiate early and effective treatment of returning service members. Collectively, staff of these programs discovered that upon returning from deployment, a soldier is eight times more likely to be diagnosed with having sustained a TBI that was either unreported during deployment or occurred as a result of risky behavior within the first four weeks of returning to the United States.[8] This finding underscores the need for careful monitoring of TBI among military forces because many injuries are likely underreported.

Research and Development

DoD and VA scientists and clinicians have led efforts to *standardize diagnostic criteria for TBI* (Table 29.1) and validate clinical outcome measures.[9] This work has been a catalyst in forming partnerships between the DoD, VA, National Institutes of Health, and other public and private organizations such as the NCAA and NFL. Over the past decade, the DoD has been heavily invested in efforts to improve TBI prevention and assessment, including advanced diagnostic imaging, discovery of biomarkers of injury, and development of more effective treatments (Chapter 39).

Nonpharmaceutical Treatments

Although medical science has not yet developed an effective medication to improve recovery from TBI, a variety of nonpharmacologic measures help. *Assistive technology* has been found to help rehabilitation and achievement of functional autonomy. During OEF and OIF, two major forms of assistive technology were found to be useful in polytrauma: *cognitive assistive technology* (CAT) and *recreational/fitness technology* (RFT). Using the computing power of smart phones, researchers have built CAT software and wearable sensors into handheld devices that help sense the user's mood, organize daily activities, and assist with care. RFT has also become a core part of rehabilitation for service

TABLE 29.1. Traumatic Brain Injury Classification and Veterans Health Administration/Department of Defense Clinical Practice Guideline for Management.

Injury Severity	Glasgow Coma Scale	Posttraumatic Amnesia	Structural Imaging	Loss of Consciousness	Alteration of Consciousness/ Mental State
Mild	13–15	< 24 h	Normal	0–30 min	A moment to 24 h
Moderate	9–12	1–7 days	Normal or abnormal	>30 min and < 24 h	> 24 h
Severe	3–8	>7 days	Normal or abnormal	> 24 h	> 24 h

members and veterans who come from a culture that honors "tactical athletes." Adaptive technologies now help service members with polytrauma return to a variety of sports and recreational activities that greatly enhance their health, confidence, and well-being (Figure 29.2). In addition, new technologies such as virtual reality (VR) are also being applied to rehabilitation. The computer-assisted rehabilitation environment (CAREN) is an example of full-immersion VR that is able to engage patients with a variety of physical and cognitive rehabilitation tasks (Figure 29.3).

Policy Coordination

The ultimate goal of rehabilitation is to successfully reintegrate service members into their military units, or alternatively, to facilitate their transition back to civilian life (Chapter 31).[10] This requires extensive communication and planning between specialized, interdisciplinary healthcare teams and community support programs, including the patient's support network (eg, family, friends, and military unit; Chapter 33). To support these efforts, the DoD created the Office of Warrior Care Policy, where each military branch has a dedicated command that works with the VA to help service members successfully transition back to their civilian community. Additional programs, such as the VA Vocational Rehabilitation and Education Program, promote education and job training after injury. In all such programs, it is important to set realistic and attainable goals, with milestones along the way.

VIGNETTE >> Sergeant "R," a 24-year-old, single, active duty Soldier in Iraq, was wearing full body armor and a Kevlar (DuPont, Wilmington, DE) helmet when a rocket-propelled grenade struck the Humvee he was driving. Although severely injured, he was able to exit the vehicle, which was on fire. The flames ignited ammunition in the vehicle, preventing him from rescuing his severely injured gunner and a rear passenger. As a result, he watched them die in the fire. As a second Humvee approached to provide assistance, it detonated an improvised explosive device about 25 meters from Sergeant R. He recalled nothing after that until he awoke at Landstuhl Regional Medical Center. His injuries required lower amputations of both legs, and he also sustained a moderate traumatic brain injury (TBI) complicated by a subdural hematoma (blood clot on his brain) and severe soft tissue injuries to his face.

After flying under the care of a Critical Care Air Transport Team (CCATT; Chapter 25) to Walter Reed Army Medical Center (WRAMC), he required six weeks of additional surgery and inpatient care to treat his facial and dental injuries and manage multiple bacterial infections (Chapter 27). While his surgical care continued, he began rehabilitation, which included physical and occupational therapy as well as neuropsychological testing, preventative psychiatric assessments, and behavioral interventions to ward off depression and help foster the resiliency he would need to facilitate his recovery. Despite this, he had frequent nightmares compounded by feelings of guilt that he could not help the occupants of his vehicle and a recurring fear that he would never be "whole again."

Because of his lower extremity injuries and concern about occult genital injuries, the hospital's sexual health team provided a thorough evaluation. Bedside cognitive testing and a consulting neuropsychologist identified attention and memory issues. The patient also suffered reduced hearing.

When his acute care was completed, the treatment team decided Sergeant R needed continued care at the Department of Veterans Affairs (VA) Polytrauma Rehabilitation Center in Tampa, Florida. After two months there, he returned to WRAMC to continue his rehabilitation, including prosthetic fitting, pain management, advanced activity training, and cognitive rehabilitation.

One year after his combat injuries, he had good use of his prostheses and was mobile and active. He participated in therapeutic recreation activities and responded well to a peer support network. Although his cognitive problems largely resolved and his sleep improved, he continued to see a mental health counselor for help with posttraumatic stress symptoms.

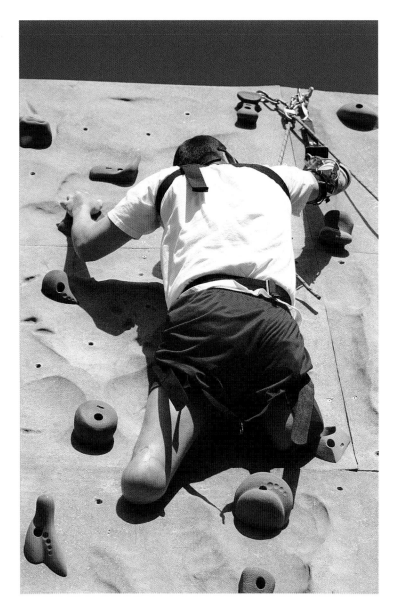

IMPACT

Lessons learned over the past decade underscore the importance of screening active duty service members and veterans for TBI and psychological health disorders.[11] The development of *common definitions and validated TBI outcome measures* improved the accuracy of diagnosis, allowed for the detection of far more cases than were previously recognized, and enhanced our ability to assess treatments and identify predictors of a good outcome.

Starting rehabilitation early and improving the coordination of care between the DoD and VA significantly enhanced recovery from complex polytrauma with TBI. Besides improving our understanding and management of polytrauma, these interdisciplinary programs demonstrated that early, intensive rehabilitation shortens hospital stays and improves long-term outcomes.[8] Following release from the hospital, programs that support and enhance cognitive and behavioral recovery by providing animal assistive therapy (Figure 29.4), other assistive technology, peer visitation, vocational rehabilitation, and sports and recreation programs improve injured veterans' quality of life, help prevent social isolation, and facilitate their successful reintegration into the community.[12,13]

CONCLUSION

As the story of Sergeant R illustrates, the consequences of TBI and PTSD can complicate recovery from polytrauma and cause ongoing symptoms long after the more visible wounds of war have healed. Fortunately, our capacity to help wounded warriors recover is substantially better than when the United States entered Iraq and Afghanistan more than a decade ago. Those of us who are privileged to work with these patients and their families remain determined to

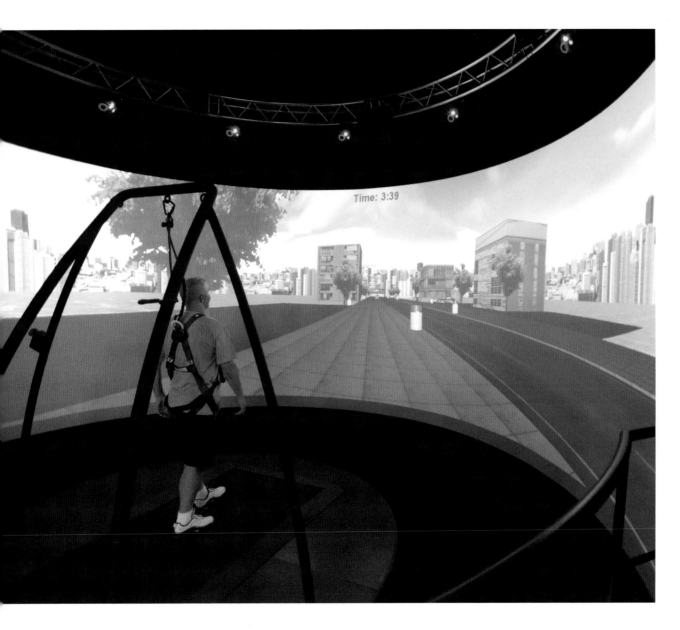

Time: 3:39

FIGURE 29.2. [*Opposite*] After release from the hospital, a veteran climbs a wall as part of a program that supports recovery. Photo courtesy of Nick Lancaster, Department of Veterans Affairs.

FIGURE 29.3. A "computer-assisted rehabilitation environment" (CAREN) uses a sophisticated multidimensional treadmill platform and wrap-around visual screen, as well as a multi-speaker array behind the screen, to recreate common scenes in the community, but in a controlled and harnessed environment. It allows for clinical evaluation and multimodal rehabilitation in cases of physical, neurosensory, and/ or cognitive-behavioral injuries. There are only about a dozen such devices in the world, including four within the military healthcare system. Photo courtesy of the National Intrepid Center of Excellence at Walter Reed National Military Medical Center.

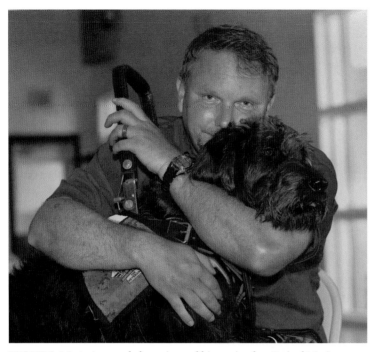

FIGURE 29.4. A wounded warrior and his service dog. Retired Marine Staff Sergeant Dean Suthard's 2-year old Labradoodle, Esther, spent almost a year training for her new mission as part of the Carolina Canines for Service program. Photo by Senior Airman Ashlee Galloway, May 17, 2012. Reproduced from: https://www.dvidshub.net/news/88553/wounded-warrior-receives-helping-paw.

help them advance in their recovery and achieve the highest quality of life while we develop even better approaches to rehabilitation in the years to come.

Notes

1. Breeze J, Allanson-Bailey LS, Hepper AE, Midwinter MJ. Demonstrating the effectiveness of body armour: a pilot prospective computerised surface wound mapping trial performed at the Role 3 hospital in Afghanistan. *J R Army Med Corps.* 2015;161:36–41.

2. Cifu DX, Taylor BC, Carne WF, et al. Traumatic brain injury, posttraumatic stress disorder, and pain diagnoses in OIF/OEF/OND Veterans. *J Rehabil Res Dev.* 2013;50:1169–1176.

3. Terrio H, Brenner LA, Ivins BJ, et al. Traumatic brain injury screening: preliminary findings in a US Army Brigade Combat Team. *J Head Trauma Rehabil.* 2009;24:14–23.

4. Stein MB, McAllister TW. Exploring the convergence of posttraumatic stress disorder and mild traumatic brain injury. *Am J Psychiatry.* 2009;166:768–776.

5. Sayer NA, Chiros CE, Sigford B, et al. Characteristics and rehabilitation outcomes among patients with blast and other injuries sustained during the Global War on Terror. *Arch Phys Med Rehabil.* 2008;89:163–170.

6. Parker A, Sricharoenchai T, Needham DM. Early rehabilitation in the intensive care unit: preventing physical and mental health impairments. *Curr Phys Med Rehabil Rep.* 2013;1:307–314.

7. Helmick KM, Spells CA, Malik SZ, Davies CA, Marion DW, Hinds SR. Traumatic brain injury in the US military: epidemiology and key clinical and research programs. *Brain Imaging Behav.* 2015;9:358–366.

8. Regasa LE, Thomas DM, Gill RS, Marion DW, Ivins BJ. Military deployment may increase the risk for traumatic brain injury following deployment. *J Head Trauma Rehabil.* 2016;31:E28–35.

9. National Institute of Neurological Disorders and Stroke. NINDS common data elements: traumatic brain injury. https://commondataelements.ninds.nih.gov/tbi.aspx#tab=Data_Standards. Accessed January 1, 2016.

10. Cooper RA, Pasquina PF, Drach R, eds. *Warrior Transition Leader Medical Rehabilitation Handbook.* Washington, DC: Borden Institute; 2011.

11. Scholten J, Cernich A, Hurley RA, Helmick K. Department of Veterans Affairs' traumatic brain injury screening and evaluation program: promoting individualized interdisciplinary care for symptomatic veterans. *J Head Trauma Rehabil.* 2013;28:219–222.

12. Pasquina PF, Tsao JW, Collins DM, et al. Quality of medical care provided to service members with combat-related limb amputations: report of patient satisfaction, *J Rehabil Res Dev.* 2008:47:953–960.

13. Laferrier JZ, Teodorski E, Cooper RA. Investigation of the impact of sports, exercise and recreation participation on psychosocial outcomes in a population of veterans with disabilities: a cross-sectional study. *Am J Phys Med Rehabil.* 2015;94:1026–1034.

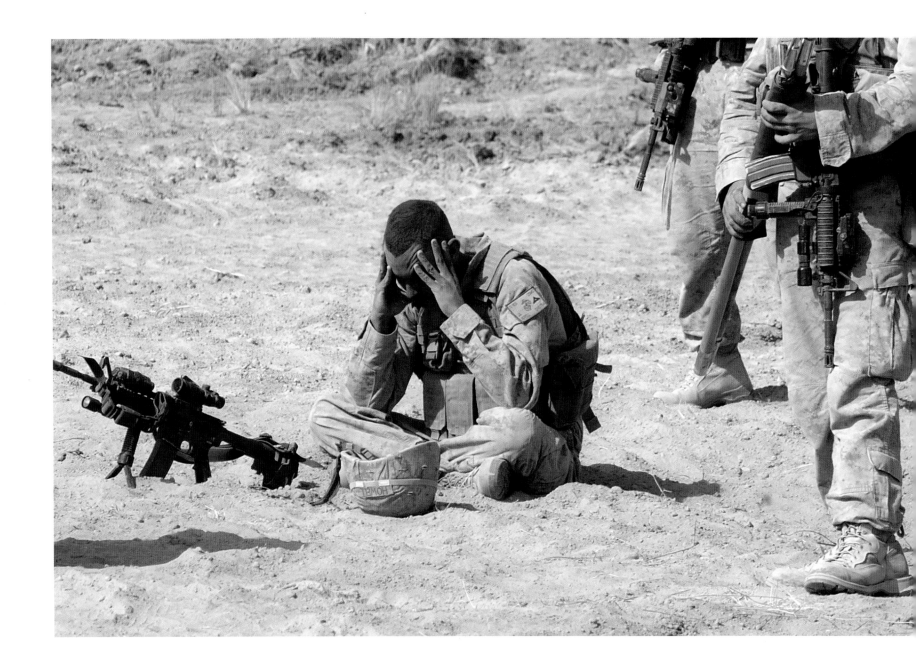

CHAPTER thirty

Recognition and Management of Posttraumatic Stress Disorder and Combat-Related Stress Reactions

JAMES C. WEST, MD; GARY H. WYNN, MD; and DAVID M. BENEDEK, MD

THE CHALLENGE

PSYCHOLOGICAL CONSEQUENCES OF COMBAT have been observed for millennia. At various points in human history, cognitive, emotional, and behavioral changes after battle have been attributed to gods, the concussive force of artillery shells, contagion, and most recently, changes to brain circuitry that process sensations of threat, fear, and memory.[1] The progression of diagnostic terms from "shell shock" to "posttraumatic stress disorder" (PTSD) and "combat-stress disorder"—terms that appeared before the wars in Iraq and Afghanistan—mirror our evolving understanding of these phenomena. Since the onset of Operations Enduring Freedom (OEF) and Iraqi Freedom (OIF), 14 years of war have produced a new generation of casualties, and expanded our understanding of these conditions and their neurological and psychological consequences (Figure 30.1).

THE INNOVATIONS

Today, we know far more about the origins and treatment of PTSD and combat stress disorder than we did only a decade ago. This progress is due, in large part, to government investments in research to improve the diagnosis and treatment of PTSD. The Walter Reed Army Institute of Research Land

FIGURE 30.1. [*Opposite*] Khan Neshin Rig District, Helmand Province, south Afghanistan. A US Marine buries his head in his hands following a memorial service for two US Marines with Delta Company 2nd Light Armored Reconnaissance Battalion, Master Sergeant Jerome D. Hatfield and Lance Corporal Pedro A. Barbozaflores, who were killed in action in Helmand Province, Afghanistan, Monday, July 13, 2009, when an improvised explosive device exploded. Photo by Nikki Kahn/The Washington Post/Getty Images. Reproduced with permission from Getty Images.

VIGNETTE >> Toward the end of a difficult combat tour, Sergeant "B," an experienced Marine Corps small unit leader, experienced two improvised explosive device blasts. Less than 12 hours later, his immediate supervisor radioed the battalion's combat stress control psychiatrist to report that Sergeant B was "behaving erratically" at their forward operating base. Concerned, the doctor helicoptered out to evaluate him. Sergeant B reported headaches and confusion, but denied psychotic or suicidal thoughts. His exam was notable for confusion and difficulty concentrating and remembering things. The psychiatrist determined that Sergeant B needed to return to the United States under the supervision of unit medical personnel for further evaluation.

Eight months later, when the same psychiatrist visited the battalion back in the United States, Sergeant B approached him and asked to speak privately. He said he was concerned about continued cognitive impairment and anxiety. He said he'd been "putting up a front" of being a capable Marine leader, but felt he "couldn't hold it together anymore." He was concerned that he might put his fellow Marines in danger due to impaired decision-making. Sergeant B added that the only reason he approached the psychiatrist was because he recalled their interaction in Iraq and sensed he could trust him.

Together, Sergeant B and the psychiatrist approached the battalion commander. Sergeant B underwent another full evaluation that confirmed ongoing moderate impairment. After six months of limited duty and comprehensive treatment, Sergeant B returned to duty and served effectively without further difficulty.

Combat Study[2] and the subsequent series of Mental Health Advisory Team (MHAT) reports it spawned between 2005 and 2013 compiled anonymous combat zone surveys and focus group interviews with deployed service members, healthcare providers, and unit leaders to identify and track health trends on the battlefield.[3] These studies, and others like them, focused media and government attention on the prevalence and significance of posttraumatic stress. For example, these studies estimated 5.5 percent of troops from various nations returning from deployment had PTSD, but the comparable figure in infantry units was over 13 percent.[4] The studies also noted inadequacies in the distribution and availability of mental health resources to deployed units. They described how stigma and other barriers impede access to care, and they noted that PTSD symptoms often overlap with those caused by blast-related traumatic brain injury (TBI).

Spurred by these findings, military and government leaders boosted efforts to screen returning troops for PSTD symptoms by implementing the Post Deployment Health Assessment and Post Deployment Health Reassessment programs.[5] They also implemented multiple outreach programs to encourage those in need to seek care, improve access when such care is desired, and improve the diagnosis and management of PTSD symptoms in combat zones and upon return home (Figure 30.2).

CHANGING THE PARADIGM FOR DIAGNOSIS AND TREATMENT

Reports produced by the MHATs supported previous anecdotal observations that traditional mental health treatment delivered in hospital-based clinics is hard to access, lacks credibility among service members, and tends to stigmatize those who seek care. To overcome these barriers, the Marine Corps and Army initiated pilot programs to assess the feasibility of embedding behavioral healthcare providers in settings more accessible to units. This approach represents a dramatic departure from the traditional "specialty clinic" approach that relies on primary care referrals and requires service members to travel to specialty treatment facilities in the combat zone.

The Army's effort began in the 1990s, when it developed combat stress control (CSC) detachments. These units consisted of personnel specifically trained to identify and manage combat-related stress reactions and augment standard division-level medical assets. Initially, CSCs struggled to win trust and credibility, but they slowly gained ground.

During OIF and OEF, the Army began deploying smaller, more mobile brigade combat teams rather than full divisions. To keep pace, CSCs created similarly nimble behavioral health teams. During the wars in Iraq and Afghanistan, the Army took the concept one step further by embedding behavioral health teams in units before they deployed to the battlefield. Preliminary data from this innovation demonstrated a net reduction in inpatient hospitalizations and improved rates of fitness for duty.[6] Encouraged by these findings, the Army embedded behavioral health teams in units throughout Iraq and Afghanistan (Figure 30.3). Because the number of units on forward operating bases exceeded the number of CSCs, the Army expanded the reach of CSCs with tele-behavioral health (Chapter 24).

The Marine Corps followed a similar path. In the decade before the wars, it piloted the Operational Stress Control and Readiness (OSCAR) program, which embedded behavioral health providers in combat units to bridge the divide between providers and line personnel. This reduced the stigma of talking to a mental health professional and greatly improved access to care. The Marines' program embraced many of the principles of combat stress control articulated by Army doctrine. With the onset of the OIF, the OSCAR program was expanded to all three Marine divisions, placing additional psychiatrists and psychologists within infantry units. These mental health providers worked, trained, and deployed alongside Marines, developing credibility as sources of help and simultaneously gaining a deeper appreciation for the challeng-

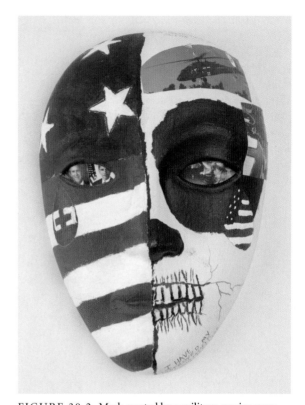

FIGURE 30.2. Mask created by a military service member during art therapy sessions at the National Intrepid Center of Excellence, Walter Reed National Military Medical Center. It was displayed in a temporary exhibit of art therapy masks at the National Museum of Health and Medicine, Silver Spring, Maryland, August to September, 2016. Its caption read, "An Army flight medic. The mask represents our country shedding tears for our military on one side, and our military shedding tears for our country on the other side. Reproduced from: https://www.dvidshub.net/image/2808093/art-therapy-masks-nicoe-walter-reed-display-nmhm-aug-sept-2016.

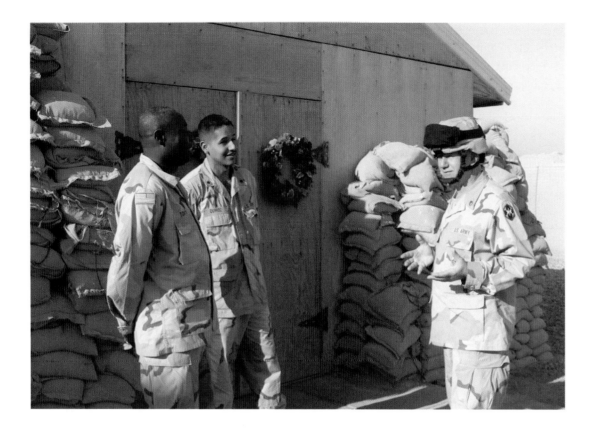

FIGURE 30.3. [*Right to left*] Staff Sergeant Philip Burke speaks with Specialist Juan Quiroz and Staff Sergeant Festus Doki, all of the 883rd Medical Company (Combat Stress Control), about classes they are conducting at their base on mental health fitness. Forward Operating Base McKenzie, Northern Iraq, December 14, 2005. Reproduced from: https://www.dvidshub.net/image/13850/883.

ing environments in which Marines operate. In 2011, the OSCAR program was expanded to include commissioned and noncommissioned officers with special training in combat and operational stress control. Preliminary data indicate that the OSCAR programs increased Marines' willingness to seek help.[7]

DRUG TREATMENTS

When the US military first deployed to Afghanistan in 2002 and Iraq the following year, clinicians had little guidance for treating acute combat stress and PTSD. At the time, the only medications approved by the Food and Drug Administration (FDA) for these conditions were paroxetine and sertraline. It was not clear what forms of psychotherapy, if any, could help. Although some published studies had included Vietnam War veterans with complicated medical and psychiatric conditions, the primary focus of PTSD research at the time was on civilian victims of sexual assault, motor vehicle crashes, or natural disasters. Likewise, concussion guidelines were based on studies from the worlds of sports medicine and civilian trauma (mainly blunt trauma from falls or motor vehicle crashes). Few reports were derived from combat experience.

As a growing number of service members returned with symptoms of PTSD and/or TBI, the Departments of Defense (DoD) and Veterans Affairs (VA) recognized that they needed to collaborate to study the overlap between these injuries and develop new practice guidelines.[8] This led to the development and implementation of the first protocols for the battlefield treatment of concussions. Congressional appropriations dedicated to improving veterans' treatment supported many studies that subsequently advanced treatment of TBI and PTSD—conditions often called the "signature injuries" of the wars in Iraq and Afghanistan.

Although there are still only two FDA-approved medications for the treatment of PTSD, researchers have made substantial progress in identifying effective pharmacologic treatments. Much of this research involves off-label use of therapeutic agents. In the American Psychiatric Association's 2004 Guideline for the Treatment of Acute Stress Disorder and Posttraumatic Stress Disorder, the only class of medications that received the strongest level of endorsement for efficacy was selective serotonin reuptake inhibitors (SSRIs). These medications include antidepressants such as Prozac (Eli Lilly and Company, Indianapolis, IN) and Zoloft (Pfizer, New York, NY). In the most recently published (2010) edition of the *VA/DoD Clinical Practice Guideline for Post Traumatic Stress*, SSRIs and serotonin-norepinephrine reuptake inhibitors received the strongest recommendation, while older classes of medications previously recommended were downgraded to "fair" (mostly due to frequent side effects).[9] Also receiving modest endorsement (ie, "fair evidence") were mirtazapine, prazosin (for sleep/nightmares), and nefazodone. Equally important, the list of medications identified as "ineffective" or even harmful for these conditions—initially limited only to benzodiazepines like lorazepam and typical antipsychotics such as chlorpromazine and haloperidol—was expanded to include tiagabine, guanfacine, valproate, topiramate, and risperidone.[9] Determining which psychiatric medications work for PTSD and which do not was not a simple task; it required countless hours of painstaking research. More work is needed to build on these gains.

PSYCHOTHERAPY

Psychotherapy for PTSD was intensively studied as well. Over the course of the wars, several major clinical trials assessed the effectiveness of commonly used treatments for PTSD as well as promising new interventions. As with pharmaco-therapy, the evolution of practice attests to the pace and scale of progress. In 2004, the American Psychiatric Association's guideline gave its strongest endorsement (significant benefit) to cognitive therapy, exposure therapy, stress inoculation training, and eye movement desensitization and reprocessing. By 2013, the strongest level of support went to "any trauma-focused psychotherapy that includes components of exposure and/or cognitive restructuring as well as stress inoculation."[10] Because psychotherapy is not as easily quantified as is the use of medications, the Association's endorsement represents a clearer understanding of the beneficial components of effective psychotherapies. Beyond these treatments, other interventions identified as potentially having benefit without evidence of harm include: patient education, imagery rehearsal therapy, psychodynamic therapy, hypnosis, relaxation techniques, and group therapy. There was no discussion of harmful or ineffective psychotherapeutic interventions, although critical incident stress debriefing, long believed to be a valuable intervention after trauma, has not been found to prevent PTSD.[10]

COMPLEMENTARY AND ALTERNATIVE MEDICINE

Before the recent wars, there was little evidence—or interest—in using complementary and alternative medicine (CAM) modalities to treat combat-related PTSD. However, given the stigma surrounding traditional mental health treatment and increasing evidence of the value of "meeting the patient where he or she is at," interest in CAM grew. Today, interventions such as yoga, acupuncture, meditation, animal therapy, and recreational therapy have moved from the fringes of clinical thinking to being relatively commonplace. They are increasingly available at military and VA treatment facilities.

Rigorous evidence on the efficacy of these interventions for combat-related PTSD is sparse, but several modalities show promise in military populations. For example, acupuncture was evaluated in a recent well-designed randomized controlled study and found to provide clear benefit for PTSD. Yoga and meditation are potentially beneficial, although methodological challenges make measuring their effects difficult.[11] Nonetheless, the safety of most CAM approaches gives clinicians a level of comfort for recommending them, particularly when they are integrated into a broader treatment plan. There is some evidence that incorporating CAM into treatment increases participation in traditional care. Thus, focusing on the desires and needs of war veterans has expanded the range of treatment options, and rigorous synthesis of evidence helps clinicians and patients assess the effectiveness of various options[12] (Figure 30.4).

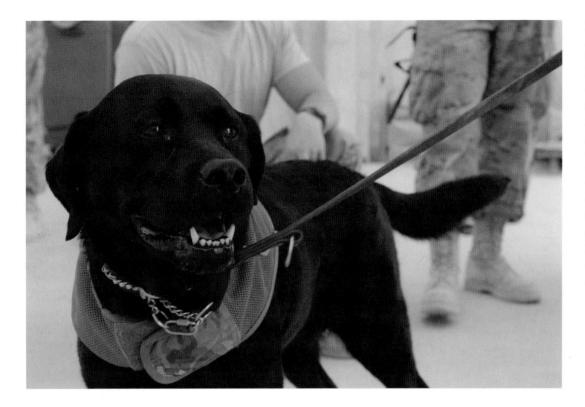

FIGURE 30.4. Sergeant 1st Class Zeke, a therapy dog with the 113th Combat Stress Control team, visited Forward Operating Base Spin Boldak on September 23, 2011, to greet Soldiers and help alleviate some of the stress they incur while deployed. In addition to getting to pet Zeke and play with him, the Soldiers learned about his role as a therapy dog and about the programs the combat stress control teams offer when it comes to dealing with tough times. Photo by Specialist Darryl Montgomery, 504th Battlefield Surveillance Brigade. Reproduced from: https://www.dvidshub.net/image/470366/therapy-dog-visits-spin-boldak.

IMPACT

A decade-plus of intensive PTSD research, combined with clinical experience treating combat veterans in war zones and after their return home, has substantially increased our understanding of this challenging condition. We have identified effective treatments, developed a broader array of options, reduced stigma, and increased access to care (Figure 30.5). This has increased patient engagement, produced better control of symptoms, and achieved higher rates of recovery. The result is a more effective fighting force, lower rates of disability, more rapid recovery, and a higher percentage of service members who are able to return to duty after experiencing symptoms of PTSD.

FIGURE 30.5. A weathered sign indicates members of the Combat Stress Control Detachment at Forward Operating Base Fenty, Afghanistan, are assisting someone in need of their expertise, December 28, 2007. Photo by Captain Monika Comeaux, Combined Joint Task Force–82 Public Affairs Office. Reproduced from: https://www.dvidshub.net/image/70823/if-you-cant-come-them-they-will-come-you.

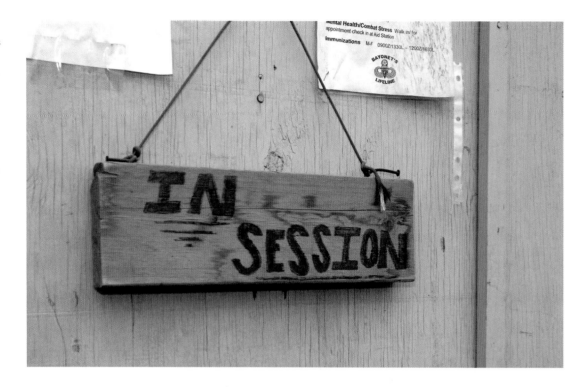

CONCLUSION

America's involvement in Iraq and Afghanistan dramatically accelerated efforts to identify and reduce the immediate and long-term effects of traumatic combat experiences on service members. The innovations this produced include better ways to recognize symptoms and screen for illness in combat zones and upon return, placement of behavioral health providers within units to improve access to care, improved communication between health providers and line commanders, and greater appreciation of the overlap between PTSD and symptoms of TBI. A steady stream of research more clearly defined pharmacologic, psychosocial, and CAM treatments and interventions that are effective in PSTD and combat stress reactions, and those that are not. As a result, the odds that a wounded warrior will receive timely and effective behavioral healthcare and fully recover are much better today than a decade ago. With continued investments in research and treatment, they will be even better in the years to come.

Notes

1. Benedek DM, Wynn GH. *Clinical Manual for the Management of PTSD*. Washington, DC: American Psychiatric Publishing; 2010.
2. Hoge CW, Castro CA, Messer SC, McGurk D, Cotting DI, Koffman RL. Combat duty in Iraq and Afghanistan, mental health problems and barriers to care. *N Engl J Med*. 2004;351:13–22.
3. Operation Iraqi Freedom Mental Health Advisory Team. *MHAT-II Report*. Washington, DC: Office of The Surgeon General; January 2005. http://armymedicine.mil/Pages/Mental-Health-Advisory-Team-II-Information.aspx. Accessed November 29, 2016.
4. Kok BC, Herrell RK, Thomas JL, Hoge CW. Posttraumatic stress disorder associated with combat service in Iraq or Afghanistan: reconciling prevalence differences between studies. *J Nerv Ment Dis*. 2012;200:444–450.
5. Milliken CS, Achterloine JL, Hoge CW. Longitudinal assessment of mental health problems among active duty and reserve component soldiers returning from the Iraq war. *JAMA*. 2007;298:2141–2148.
6. Russell DW, Whalen RJ, Riviere LA, et al. Embedded behavioral health providers: an assessment with the Army National Guard. *Psychol Serv*, 2014;11(3):265–272. doi: 10.1037/a0037005.
7. Vaughan C, Farmer C, Breslau J, Burnette C. *Evaluation of the Operational Stress Control and Readiness (OSCAR) Program*. Santa Monica, CA: RAND Corporation; 2015.
8. Stein MB, McAllister TW, Exploring the Convergence of posttraumatic stress disorder and mild traumatic brain injury. *Am J Psychiatry*. 2009;166:768–776.
9. Department of Veterans Affairs, Department of Defense. *VA/DoD Clinical Practice Guideline for Management of Post Traumatic Stress*. Version 2.0. Washington, DC: VHA, DoD; 2010.
10. Department of Veterans Affairs, Department of Defense. *Posttraumatic Stress Disorder Pocket Guide: To Accompany the 2010 VA/DoD Clinical Practice Guideline for Management of Post Traumatic Stress*. Washington, DC: DC: VHA, DoD; 2013.
11. Wynn GH. Complementary and alternative medicine approaches in the treatment of PTSD. *Curr Psychiatry Rep*. 2015;17:600.
12. Benedek DM, Wynn GH, eds. *Complementary and Alternative Medicine for PTSD*. New York, NY: Oxford University Press; 2016.

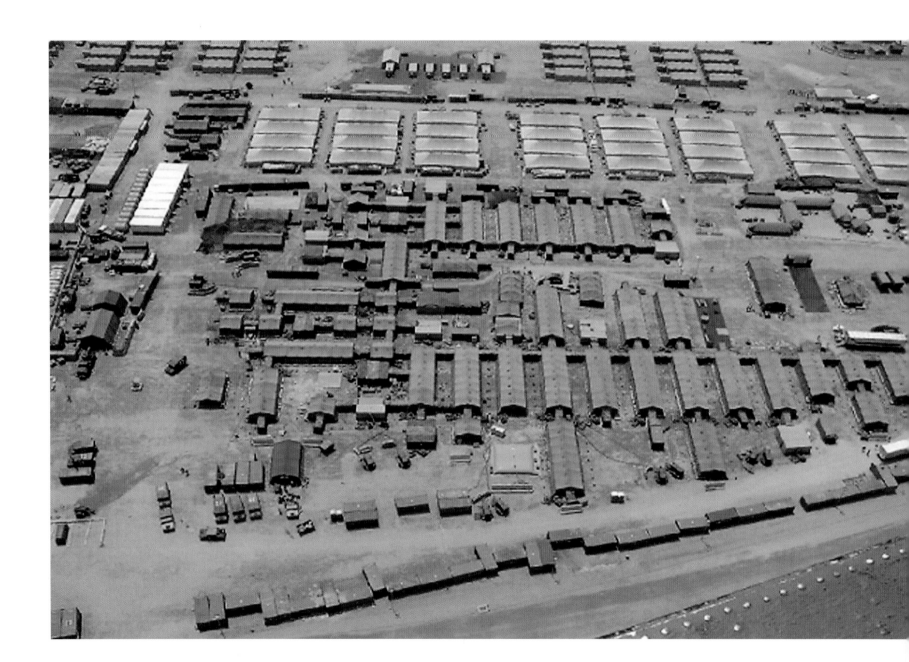

CHAPTER thirty-one

Warrior Care and Transition: Patient-Centered Care for Wounded, Ill, and Injured Warriors

ERIC B. SCHOOMAKER, MD, PHD

THE PROBLEM

THE PERSIAN GULF WAR (1991–1992) AND THE BALKANS contingency operations (1993–2004) demonstrated the feasibility of quickly evacuating casualties from the point of injury on a distant battlefield to definitive care at a European or stateside military hospital. These innovations foreshadowed the dramatic improvements implemented during Operations Enduring Freedom (OEF), Iraqi Freedom (OIF), and New Dawn (OND) that are described elsewhere in this book. These changes allowed the military health system to reduce its "medical footprint" in the combat zone, doing more with less—fewer doctors, nurses, allied health professionals, hospitals, beds, and medical equipment (Figure 31.1).

Not fully appreciated at the time was the impact these advances would have on the number, severity, and complexity of war-associated casualties returning to the United States within days of being injured. In past wars, severely injured service members either died on the battlefield or spent weeks recuperating in large field hospitals before being deemed "stable enough" to make the long flight home. Now, they were returning stateside within days.

FIGURE 31.1. [*Opposite*] Khan View from a MEDEVAC helicopter of the 47th Combat Support Hospital (CSH), Camp Wolfe, Kuwait, 2003–2004. The hospital had 300-bed capability, which was typical for major field hospitals at the time. The subsequent maturation of critical care air transport allowed the US military to quickly evacuate severely wounded, ill, and injured troops to Landstuhl Regional Medical Center in Germany and to the United States, reducing the need for large CSHs in combat zones. Photograph courtesy of Major General (Retired) Richard Thomas, MD.

GRIDLOCK IN STATESIDE MILITARY HOSPITALS

As the transit point for home-bound patients, Landstuhl Regional Medical Center in Germany devoted substantial effort to ensuring the safety and stability of inbound patients, while moving them swiftly back to major military medical centers in the continental United States, notably, Walter Reed Army Medical Center in the District of Columbia; the National Naval Medical Center in Bethesda, Maryland; Brooke Army Medical Center in San Antonio, Texas; and Naval Medical Center-San Diego, California.[1]

Often, family members quickly arrived to serve as non-medical attendants for their loved ones. It was not uncommon for spouses and children, fathers and mothers, and close friends to converge on a patient undergoing repeated surgical procedures, lengthy medical care, and specialized nursing and rehabilitation services. The disruption of families' lives was often profound, with suspension or loss of employment, interruptions in schooling, and multiple financial, social, physical, and psychological challenges (Chapter 33). While their extra hands were always welcome, the clinical staff of these hospitals were ill-equipped to manage the complex psychosocial dimensions of care introduced by severely wounded warriors and their families.

In the early years of OEF and OIF, Soldiers facing long-term care for problems that rendered them temporarily or permanently unable to return to active duty were transferred out of their units and administratively attached to MEDHOLD. This was intended to ensure continuity in the myriad personnel actions required of active duty and mobilized Reserve and National Guard Soldiers. Although some of these Soldier-patients were seriously ill or injured, most were ambulatory with varying degrees of self-sufficiency (Figure 31.2). The sparse staff of enlisted medical personnel assigned to this duty—sometimes supplemented by the more physically capable patients—tried to shepherd MEDHOLD patients through the complex process of coordinating outpatient care and, if need be, transitioning to civilian life and subsequent care in the Department of Veterans Affairs.

Although the MEDHOLD approach made sense during the first months of the war, the few untrained staff assigned to this duty were no match for the growing flow of casualties as the conflicts intensified. Complicating the challenge was the fact that the military health system, patterned after its civilian health system counterparts, compartmentalized care into "inpatient" and "outpatient" domains, and its various specialty services managed each patient as they saw fit, with little effort to coordinate treatment with other specialty services. When a patient improved enough to leave the hospital, this fragmented approach forced wounded, ill, and injured warfighters to pick their way through a labyrinth of specialty and subspecialty clinics, disjointed schedules, and confusing messages about treatment.

VIGNETTE >> October 2005: On patrol in Iraq, an Army National Guard member was severely injured by an exploding improvised explosive device. He sustained an open fracture to his right femur (leg bone) and an arterial injury to his right arm at the elbow. Immediate care on the battlefield, followed by a prompt MEDEVAC flight to a nearby combat support hospital, saved his life. Soon thereafter, he was flown by a Critical Care Air Transport Team (CCATT) to the historic Walter Reed Army Medical Center (WRAMC) in Washington, DC. There a multi-specialty team of surgeons repaired his arterial injury and placed a leg rod to unite the two ends of his broken leg bone. Following a satisfactory postoperative course, the Soldier was told he would be discharged from the hospital the following morning and move to on-campus housing while he received outpatient rehabilitative treatment. During this final phase of his care, he would be part of a medical holding company (MEDHOLD) before separating from the Army.

Unfortunately, he was discharged later that night because the hospital needed beds to accommodate an inbound CCATT flight. Not yet able to walk on his badly broken leg, he was placed in a manual wheelchair without an attendant and given a map to the Army hotel two blocks away. Because the aging hospital's campus lacked many curb wheelchair ramps, the trip to his hotel required an hour of hard labor.[1] The door to his room had a narrow entrance, making it difficult to navigate in his wheelchair. His mother could not come to Washington to help him because she was caring for her father, who was dying of Alzheimer's disease.

A few days following this transfer, while trying to get through the doorway, he over-extended his right arm and tore open the arterial repair, nearly bleeding to death in the hotel hallway. He was readmitted to WRAMC for a second operation on his damaged artery. After recovery, he was discharged again—in another hand-driven wheelchair. After the Soldier was readmitted a second time due to another preventable postoperative problem, his surgeon kept him in the hospital until he could be discharged in ambulatory condition. In the interim, the surgeon personally found him a motorized wheelchair.

THE TURNING POINT

Matters came to a head in early 2007, when a series of investigative reports in the *Washington Post*[2] about care at WRAMC drew national and international attention to the problems faced by returning casualties, particularly once they were discharged from the hospital and moved to temporary base housing. The revelations prompted the Army to relieve several senior Army uniformed and civilian leaders of their duties, and the military health system suffered serious damage to the trust and respect it had

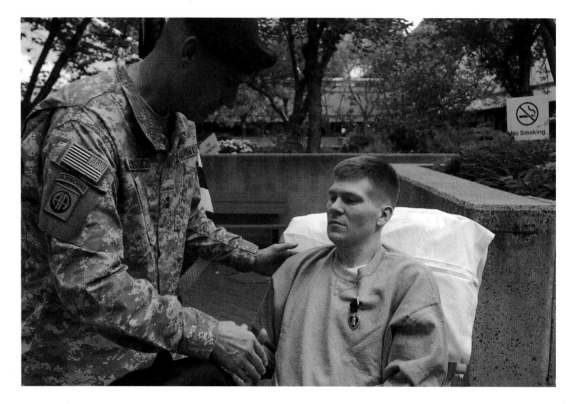

FIGURE 31.2. The 82nd Airborne Division commander, Major General David Rodriguez, shakes hands with Staff Sergeant Bryan McNees, Headquarters and Headquarters Company, 1st Battalion, 325th Airborne Infantry Regiment, at Walter Reed Army Medical Center after pinning on his Purple Heart, October 17, 2006. Photo by Sergeant 1st Class Randy Randolph, 2nd Brigade Combat Team, 82nd Airborne Division. Reproduced from: https://www.dvidshub.net/image/31807/wounds-bring-life-lessons.

earned in the current and prior conflicts. Several congressional oversight committees held hearings, and national-level task forces sought the root causes of the problem and recommended steps to correct apparent deficiencies.

THE INNOVATION: "WARRIOR TRANSITION UNITS"

In response, the Army created a medical action plan aimed at mobilizing medical and non-medical support for a more effective, efficient, and patient- and family-centered multidisciplinary approach to caring for wounded, ill, and injured Soldiers. The warrior-patient was placed in the center of a process that combined clinical care, emotional support, family support, and close administrative oversight to ensure a continuum of treatment, recovery, rehabilitation, and reintegration[3] (Figure 31.3).

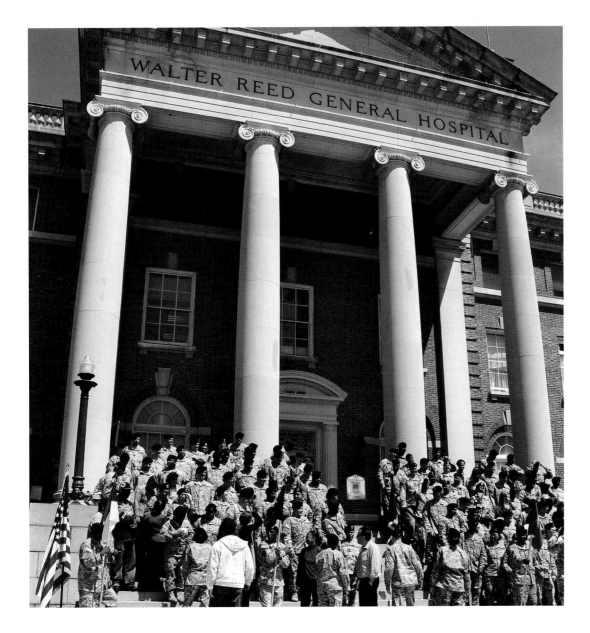

FIGURE 31.3. Civilians and troops attached to Walter Reed Army Medical Center's warrior transition brigade gather for a group photo in front of the post's original hospital in Washington, DC, in recognition of the hospital's 100th anniversary, April 21, 2009. Photo by Samantha Quigley, Office of the Secretary of Defense Public Affairs. Reproduced from: https://www.dvidshub.net/image/169118/home-warrior-care-hits-century-mark.

The MEDHOLD companies were abolished. In their place, a new major Army medical command, the "Warrior Transition Command," was established under the initial command of a non-medical general officer. Hand-picked officers and enlisted personnel were brought in to staff specialized "warrior transition units" of various sizes and tasked with providing administrative attention to the full spectrum of needs of wounded, ill, and injured warriors and their families (Figure 31.4). In addition to medical care and rehabilitation, these issues included pay, employment, housing, and transportation, as well as non-medical attendants, family counseling, and family engagement in care planning.

PATIENT-CENTEREDNESS AND THE TRIAD OF CARE

To promote individualized attention for each patient in a warrior transition unit, the military created a "triad of care" consisting of a primary care manager (physician, nurse practitioner or physician assistant); nurse case manager; and a non-medical noncommissioned officer. To correct deficiencies in post-discharge housing, the Army and other armed services built or designated new barracks that enabled universal access in compliance with the Americans with Disabilities Act. Administrators closely monitored key performance measures such as clinical access, coordination of care, duration of recovery, rehabilitation, and disability adjudication. These measures greatly improved wounded, ill, and injured warriors' post-hospital care, and helped more of them move forward to successful post-injury careers[3] (see "A Former Wounded Warrior's Personal Journey").

DEPARTMENT OF DEFENSE-VETERANS BENEFITS ADMINISTRATION DISABILITY ADJUDICATION

One of the most challenging administrative hurdles was the need to reconcile the military health system's approach to disability adjudication and awarding of compensation with the very different approach used by the Veterans Benefits Administration (VBA). Although these organizations employ identical schemes for assessing loss of

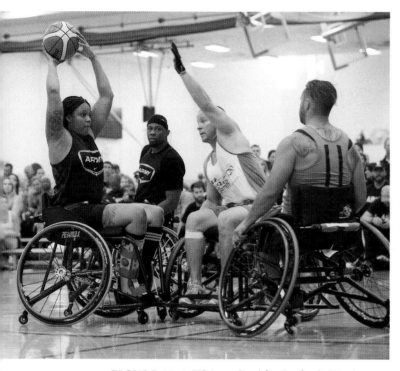

FIGURE 31.4. US Army Specialist Stephanie Morris, assigned to a warrior transition battalion at Walter Reed National Military Medical Center, Bethesda, Maryland, holds up a basketball during a Department of Defense Warrior Games wheelchair basketball competition, in Arvin Gym, at the US Military Academy, West Point, New York, June 18, 2016. US Army photo by Private First Class Tianna S. Wilson/ Released. Reproduced from: https://www.dvidshub.net/image/2674862/dod-warrior-games-2016.

IDES Timeline

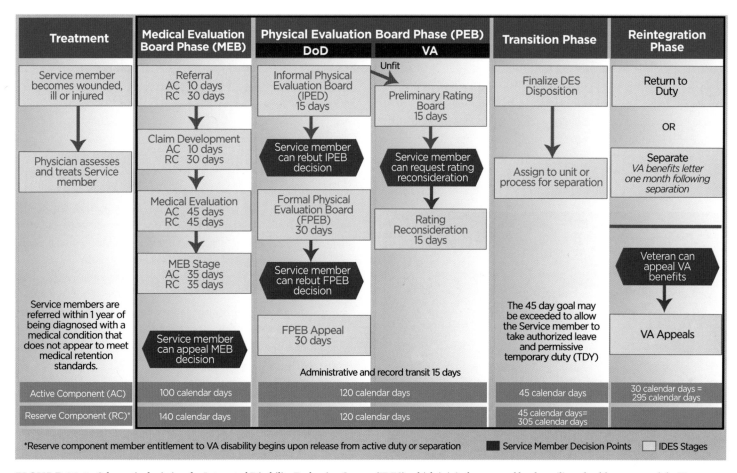

FIGURE 31.5. Schematic depicting the Integrated Disability Evaluation System (IDES), which is jointly managed by the military health system and the Veterans Benefits Administration.

A FORMER WOUNDED WARRIOR'S PERSONAL JOURNEY

My journey of recovery, rehabilitation, and transition has been long and arduous, but so full of hope and renewed strength that I no longer consider myself a "wounded warrior." I don't like to see people use the "victim card"; I bristle at the reference. I think of myself as a retired career Soldier and artilleryman, a motivational speaker, a photographer, a businessman, and an actor.

My "alive day" was May 7, 2007, in Baghdad. Returning from a memorial service for two in a sister battalion in my brigade, I was

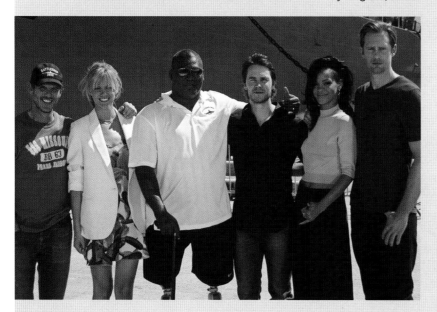

struck by a roadside bomb or improvised explosive device that severely mangled my legs and injured my arm. My well-trained medics ensured that I did not bleed to death, saving my life and getting me quickly to forward surgical care.

I recall little of the ensuing days that took me by Air Force medical evacuation through Landstuhl Regional Medical Center in Germany to Walter Reed Army Medical Center (WRAMC) in Washington, DC, on May 11. I awakened very confused and combative with my wife Kim, son Jaelen, and daughter Gabriella at my bedside. On May 18, my left leg further worsened and the doctors amputated it above the knee to save my life. I decided my quality of life would be better without my severely damaged right leg as well, so on May 24 the doctors amputated my remaining leg above the knee. My three pillars of strength—faith, family and friends—allowed me to accept and make sense of what had happened to me. My family has been there to support me 100 percent. That unconditional love and friendship has allowed me to continue to serve. They helped me get through each day—one at a time.

From left, Peter Berg, director of the 2012 science fiction naval war film Battleship, along with cast members Brooklyn Decker, Greg Gadson, Taylor Kitsch, Rihanna, and Alexander Skarsgard, stand in front of the USS Missouri Memorial at Joint Base Pearl Harbor-Hickam in Hawaii, April 28, 2012. The cast and crew attended events in Hawaii to promote the film's opening in the United States. US Navy photo by Mass Communication Specialist 3rd Class Dustin W. Sisco. Reproduced from: https://www.dvidshub.net/image/574105/battleship-cast-and-crew-promotes-film.

Nothing at West Point, my career on the Army football team, nor my previous deployments to Operations Desert Shield/Desert Storm (Kuwait), Operation Joint Forge (Bosnia-Herzegovina), and Operation Enduring Freedom (Afghanistan) prepared me completely for the challenges of this journey. I arrived at WRAMC as the Army and Department of Defense were transforming care of their wounded, ill, and injured. I was resolved to recover from my wounds, rehabilitate to walk again, and remain on active duty. I knew I had far more to contribute as an Army officer and an experienced leader. But I also knew I had to complete my transition to a new life. I could not go back.

Within a year of being wounded, I joined the Joint Chiefs of Staff internship program at Georgetown University in 2008, earning a Master's degree in policy management in May 2009. A West Point football classmate and New York Giants coach asked me to address the Giants the night before they played the Washington Redskins. We bonded, and they were inspired to win that game—and ten games to follow, including Super Bowl XLII. After 22 surgeries and the benefit of the newest generation of computer-assisted prostheses, I fought to remain in uniform. The Army understood the lessons in resilience and transition I could teach, and assigned me to lead the Army's Wounded Warrior Program.

I finished my Army career as a brigade commander—the commander of the Fort Belvoir (Virginia) garrison. In the interim, I was privileged to act in the movie Battleship (defeating the alien invasion!) and to refine my skills as a speaker and photographer, ultimately

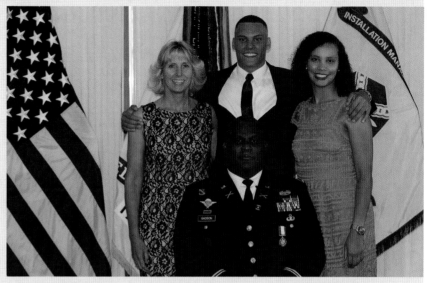

Colonel Greg Gadson and family at the time of his retirement. Used with permission of Colonel (Retired) Gadson.

leading to my retirement from uniform. I turned my full-time attention to being a husband, father, businessman, and motivational speaker committed to helping others. Faith, family, and friends remain my inspiration. Army and military medicine enabled me to survive potentially life-ending (and certainly career-ending) combat wounds and return as a public servant and advocate for those seeking to overcome adversity and achieve their full human potential.

Greg Gadson, Colonel, US Army (Retired)

function and diminished earning power due to injuries or illnesses sustained during military service, they differ on how to take various elements of disability into account. The military is primarily concerned with the way injuries or illness compromise a warrior's ability to continue serving in uniform, while the VBA is primarily concerned with aggregating the cumulative impact of *all* physical and psychological impairments. The level of disability each organization awards has a major impact on a warfighter's compensation, taxable income, and benefits, including healthcare for a medically disabled warrior and his or her family. Disability ratings can be appealed in both organizations.

Persistent differences in approach fueled a widespread perception of unfairness across the two federal agencies. Inevitable delays in administrative processes and the inability to secure speedy adjudication were seen by some as deliberate administrative tactics to deny warriors their just compensation. Because these concerns contributed to the implosion of warrior care centered at WRAMC in 2007, substantial effort was given to devising an Integrated Disability Evaluation System (IDES) jointly conducted by the military and the VBA (Figure 31.5). The system is better today.

IMPACT

The breakdowns that occurred at WRAMC in 2007 prompted the military health system to develop a highly coordinated approach that promotes warrior recovery, rehabilitation, and reintegration. Key elements of this transformation included explicit medical command and accountability; close coordination of inpatient, outpatient and rehabilitation services; and a stronger partnership with the Department of Veterans Affairs. As a result of these efforts, the continuum of care that saved warriors' lives in Iraq and Afghanistan and swiftly brought them home to the United States does not end when these heroes are discharged from the hospital. Between its formation in 2007 and February 2016, more than 70,000 Soldiers have been supported by the Army's Warrior Care and Transition Program (the Navy and Air Force programs are commanded separately). Of these, 43 percent returned to duty (Figure 31.6).[4]

CONCLUSION

Not every advance in combat casualty care during OEF, OIF, and OND involved new technology or biomedical research. The organizational changes made in post-discharge care, most notably the creation of warrior transition units, ensure that America's wounded, ill, and injured warriors and veterans receive care that is closely aligned with their needs and the sacrifices they've made for our nation's defense.

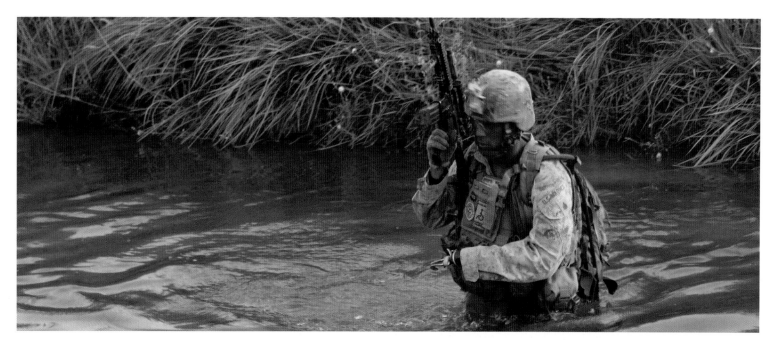

FIGURE 31.6. Sergeant Ricardo Ramirez, a combat replacement for 1st Battalion, 5th Marine Regiment, wades through an irrigation canal to move into a night observation post in Sangin, Helmand Province, Afghanistan, August 5, 2001. In February 2006, Ramirez was wounded in action while serving in Iraq with 3rd Battalion, 5th Marines, and 2 years later became the first hand-amputee to reenlist in the Marines Corps. Reproduced from: https://www.dvidshub.net/image/453012/back-work-hand-amputee-deploys-set-example-wounded-warriors.

Notes

1. Under the Base Realignment and Closure Act (BRAC) of 2005, the Department of Defense was required to combine four National Capital Region inpatient hospitals—WRAMC, National Naval Medical Center, Malcolm Grow Air Force Medical Center at Joint Base Andrews, Maryland, and DeWitt Army Community Hospital at Fort Belvoir, Virginia—into two institutions while maintaining the same patient care capacity. The resulting inpatient facilities, Walter Reed National Military Medical Center in Bethesda and the Fort Belvoir Community Hospital now serve the Washington, DC, metropolitan area. After its passage, the 2005 BRAC law prohibited any substantive improvements in the physical plant of the former WRAMC campus before its closure.

2. Priest D, Hull A. Soldiers face neglect, frustration at Army's top medical facility. *The Washington Post*. February 18, 2007. http://www.washingtonpost.com/wp-dyn/content/article/2007/02/17/AR2007021701172_4.html. Accessed January 12, 2017.

3. Callahan C. To stay a soldier. *Parameters*. 2009:39(3):95–104.

4. US Army Warrior Care and Transition program. Warrior transition units fact sheet.

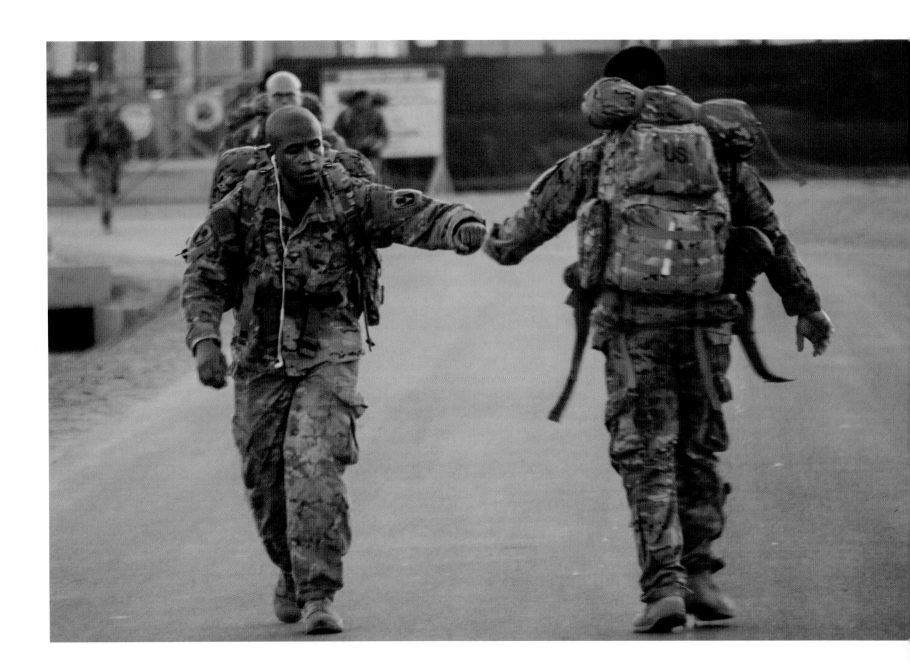

CHAPTER thirty-two

Assessing Suicide Risk and Resilience in Service Members: The Army STARRS Program

ROBERT J. URSANO, MD; PAUL E. HURWITZ, MPH; ROBERT K. GIFFORD, PHD; and MURRAY B. STEIN, MD, MPH

THE PROBLEM

HISTORICALLY, THE RATE OF SUICIDE among US service members has been substantially lower than in the civilian community. However, with the onset of the wars in Iraq and Afghanistan, Army suicide rates started to climb (Figure 32.2). From 2003 to 2009, suicide was the third-leading cause of death in the Army. In 2008, for the first time in recent history, the Army's rate of suicides exceeded that of the demographically matched general population.[1] Despite substantial efforts to publicize the problem, engage command support, and encourage Soldiers to access mental health services, the problem persists (Figure 32.3).

THE INNOVATION

In hopes of finding answers, Army leadership asked the National Institute of Mental Health (NIMH) to identify a group of scientists who could design and conduct a research program comprehensive enough to tackle this complex problem. After a highly competitive process, the NIMH selected a team of experts

FIGURE 32.1. [*Opposite*] US Army Specialist Sherman Dyer, Alpha Company, 1st Battalion, 124th Infantry Regiment, bumps fists with a fellow soldier while performing a ruck march at Camp Lemonnier, Djibouti, Djibouti, October 31, 2016. Photo by Staff Sergeant Christian Jadot, Combined Joint Task Force–Horn of Africa. Reproduced from: https://www.dvidshub.net/image/2960236/cjtf-hoa.

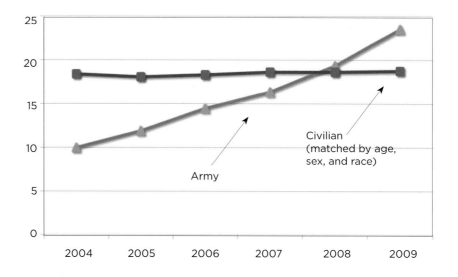

FIGURE 32.2. Rates of suicide in the US Army versus comparable civilian population (suicides per 100,000 person years) between 2004 and 2009. Army figures from Army STARRS calculations; civilian figures from the Centers for Disease Control and Prevention.

from the Uniformed Services University of the Health Sciences; the University of California, San Diego; Harvard University; and the University of Michigan's Institute for Social Research. The project they devised is called the "Army Study to Assess Risk and Resilience in Servicemembers," or Army STARRS. It is the largest research study of suicidality, mental health risk, and resilience ever conducted among military personnel.

From the beginning, Army STARRS set out to produce findings that can be used to prevent suicides. The magnitude, complexity, and comprehensiveness of the project were unprecedented. Suicidal behavior is a function of many interrelated risk factors, including neurobiology, environmental influences, and psychological health, so the Army STARRS research team brought together multiple disciplines to examine outcomes across a wide range of suicide-related behaviors, including suicidal ideation (thoughts), nonfatal suicide attempts, completed suicides, and accidental injuries. The study also conducted a wide variety of assessments, including survey questionnaires, neurocognitive tests, collection of biological specimens, and a review of administrative records (2004–2009). Ultimately, more than 107,000 Soldiers provided data to the team.

Because Army STARRS was created to get answers, it included a process for rapidly communicating interim findings to senior Army leaders and the broader medical community. Throughout the project, researchers briefed senior Army leadership about findings as they became available. These briefings often included the secretary of the Army, the Army chief of staff, and the vice chief of staff.

Since suicidal behaviors develop through complex processes, the research team designed Army STARRS as a multicomponent set of integrated studies.[2] Soldiers' training schedules are busy, so the Army imposed constraints on researchers' time with Soldiers. This forced the team to make difficult decisions about which risk and protection factors to assess, the length of each assessment, and the total length of the data collection effort. To choose items wisely, the team engaged workgroups that ranked potential risk factors in order of expected importance, with particular attention paid to identifying modifiable factors that might be promising targets for intervention.

The design of these sub-studies was, for the most part, conventional. But the close coordination of these projects created unique opportunities to crosscheck and confirm findings. In addition, the vast majority of Army STARRS participants gave researchers permission to link their administrative records to their self-reported (questionnaire) data, and agreed to be re-contacted at later points in time to provide longitudinal follow-up. Consent to access confidential administrative data was particularly important, because this allowed researchers to conduct several sub-studies that would otherwise be impossible. It will also allow them to track outcomes well into the future.

ARMY STARRS COMPONENT STUDIES

- **The Historical Administrative Data Study.** Using 38 Army and Department of Defense administrative data systems for all of the roughly 1.6 million Soldiers on

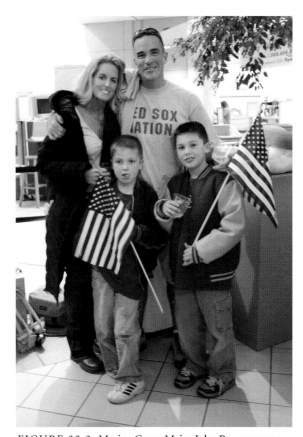

FIGURE 32.3. Marine Corps Major John Ruocco poses for a picture with his wife, Kim, and children, Joey, right, and Billy, in November 2004. The major committed suicide in 2005 after a long battle with depression. His wife has devoted herself to suicide prevention and assisting survivors. Office of the Secretary of Defense Public Affairs photo, June 11, 2010. Reproduced from: https://www.dvidshub.net/image/288786/survivor-shares-story-combat-troop-suicides.

active duty from 2004 to 2009, the Army STARRS team created an integrated individual-level dataset to examine associations between administrative data and a Soldier's subsequent risk of suicide ideation, suicide attempts, and suicide. Researchers examined other adverse outcomes as well, including sexual assault, other violent crimes, and accidental death.

> **VIGNETTE >>** An enlisted Army Soldier, recently returned from combat, bought an expensive new revolver, which he enjoyed shooting at a local target range. Three weeks later, on a Sunday afternoon, his fellow Soldiers found him dead in his barracks with the revolver at his side. Despite the Soldier's widely-recognized skill with firearms, his buddies insisted it must have been an accident. One even said it couldn't be a suicide, because he was wearing his Class A uniform, with all his ribbons, at the time.

- **The New Soldier Study** (NSS). The NSS included assessments of more than 55,000 Soldiers entering basic combat training at each of three basic training installations in 2011 and 2012. Respondents completed a self-administered questionnaire and computer-administered neurocognitive tests. Beginning in late 2011, Soldiers also provided blood samples. The NSS was done while Soldiers were in reception battalions, where new Soldiers go during their first few days of active duty for physical exams, immunizations, fitness tests, and other processing steps before beginning basic combat training.

- **The All Army Study** (AAS). The AAS was a cross-sectional study that used self-administered questionnaires of active duty Army personnel in 2011 and 2012. To increase coverage, the AAS was also administered to a sample of Soldiers deployed in Iraq and Afghanistan by holding group-administered sessions while they were in Kuwait for mid-tour leaves. To ensure coverage of the reserve component, the AAS included a supplemental sample of activated US Army Reserve and Army National Guard units in the continental United States, either just before or just after deployment to Afghanistan. More than 41,000 Soldiers participated in the AAS (Figure 32.1).

- **The Soldier Health Outcomes Studies A and B** (SHOS-A/B) were retrospective case-control studies examining non-fatal suicide attempts (SHOS-A) and death by suicide (SHOS-B). Each sought a targeted sample of 150 cases and 300 matched controls. The studies were designed to quickly identify potentially important risk and resilience factors. SHOS-A cases were psychiatric inpatients at selected military hospitals admitted for one or more suicide attempts. SHOS-

B cases were selected from the administrative records of all Army suicides. Matching controls for both studies were selected from participants in the AAS. For SHOS-B cases and controls, researchers conducted telephone interviews with the next of kin and Army supervisors. Both studies looked at critical junctures in the progression to attempted or completed suicide.

- **The Pre-Post Deployment Study** (PPDS) was a four-wave longitudinal panel survey conducted from 2012 through early 2014. It involved more than 10,000 Soldiers in three combat brigade teams. PPDS collected baseline data and blood samples from the Soldiers shortly before deployment to Afghanistan. Three postdeployment follow-up data collections were scheduled to occur within one month of their return from deployment, two months later, and six months later. Importantly, the PPDS includes many Soldiers who have transitioned back to civilian life, a process that is often stressful and may become more so in the future, since the Army is in the process of downsizing. In contrast to the other sub-studies, this project hopes to follow participants for years.

In addition to these projects, two targeted studies validated key instruments used in Army STARRS research.

IMPACT

Army STARRS has already made a substantial contribution to our understanding of suicide risk and resilience, as reflected by numerous command briefings and peer-reviewed scientific publications. Ultimately, Army STARRS will generate hundreds of scientific reports. Here are some of more than 140 relevant findings reported to the Army:

- Receiving a waiver to enter the Army is not associated with increased risk of suicide.

- Enlisted Soldiers deployed during their first year of service have a significantly higher risk of suicide.

- Almost 14 percent of currently active, non-deployed regular Army Soldiers have considered suicide at some point in their lives; 5.3 percent made a suicide plan, and 2.4 percent attempted suicide.

TABLE 32.1. Examples of Risk Factors for Death by Suicide

- male gender (but females make more suicide attempts)
- lower rank, especially if demoted in rank in previous two years
- less than high school education
- having been deployed at least once
- criminal offenses
- prior suicide attempts
- mental health diagnoses
- substance abuse

TABLE 32.2. Examples of Risk Factors for Making Nonfatal Suicide Attempts

- female gender
- enlisted rank rather than officer
- as with death by suicide, lower rank, younger age, and less education
- risk is highest early in career
- prior mental disorder, especially preenlistment

- A preexisting mental disorder is the strongest predictor of self-reported suicidal behavior among newly-enlisted Soldiers. In a multivariate analysis, preenlistment mental disorders predict postenlistment first suicide attempts. This suggests that preenlistment mental disorders may be important targets for early screening and intervention.

- Other important predictors of nonfatal suicide *attempts* among enlisted Soldiers include female gender, younger current age, older age at Army entry, lower education, and being a non-Hispanic white.[3,4]

- Surprisingly, the team found that Soldiers with a relatively short length of service and those who have never deployed are at higher risk of making nonfatal suicide attempts, despite the fact that having deployed is a risk factor for death by suicide. Suicide attempts are also more likely among those with a recent mental health diagnosis. Risk is highest early in an Army career.[3,4]

- A risk algorithm for predicting who will complete suicide within 12 months of inpatient treatment for a psychiatric disorder determined that 5 percent of hospitalized patients account for more than half (52.9 percent) of all post-hospitalization suicides. This ultra-high risk group also generates a high proportion of other adverse outcomes, including fatal accidents, repeat suicide attempts, and additional psychiatric hospitalizations.

Findings like these provide a wealth of information to the Army and the Department of Defense that can be used to fashion more effective suicide prevention programs. Examples of risk factors for both suicide and nonfatal attempts found in Army STARRS data are in

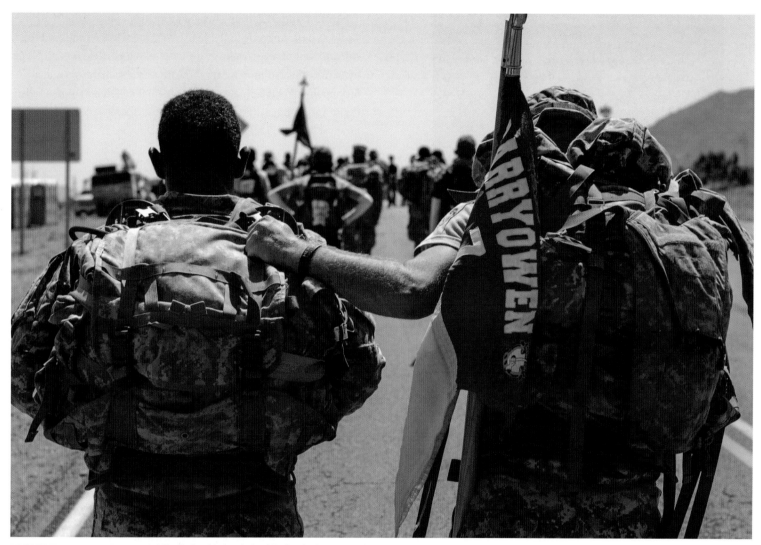

FIGURE 32.5. A US Army Soldier helps his battle buddy finish the 26.2-mile Bataan Memorial Death March, at White Sands Missile Range, New Mexico, on March 20, 2016. Approximately 6,600 people participated in the march. US Air Force photo by Senior Airman Harry Brexel. Reproduced from: https://www.dvidshub.net/image/2489693/bataan-battle-buddy.

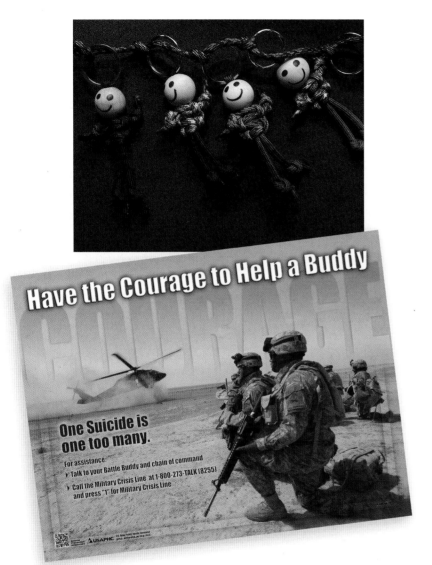

Tables 32.1 and 32.2. Many insights probably apply to the civilian world as well. Apart from the high-value knowledge produced to date, the fact that a sizeable group of research participants is willing to be re-contacted makes Army STARRS an invaluable resource for ongoing, longitudinal studies of mental health and, potentially, the connection between exposure to combat stress and long-term physical health (Figure 32.4).

A LOOK TO THE FUTURE

Recently, the Department of Defense decided to fund a continuation of Army STARRS, called the "STARRS-Longitudinal Study," or STARRS-LS. This will keep the research program going until at least June 2020. The extension makes Army STARRS not only the largest study of military suicides ever conducted, but it will also now provide an ongoing source of findings and insights for mental health providers as our nation strives to better understand and prevent suicides (Figures 32.5 and 32.6).

FIGURE 32.4. [*Top*] Paracord links key chains called "battle buddies" at an exposition featuring the art of wounded warriors in Washington, DC, November 16, 2016. Air Force retiree Victor Rivera created the popular key chains. Department of Defense photo by EJ Hersom. Reproduced from: https://www.dvidshub.net/image/2994902/wounded-warrior-arts-expo.

FIGURE 32.6. [*Bottom*] US Army Public Health Command suicide prevention poster. Reproduced from: https://usaphcapps.amedd.army.mil/HIOShoppingCart/viewItem.aspx?id=247.

Notes

1. Alvarez L. Suicides of soldiers reach high of nearly three decades. *New York Times.* January 30, 2009: A19.
2. Ursano RJ, Colpe LJ, Heeringa SG, Kessler RC, Schoenbaum C, Stein,MB. The Army Study to Assess Risk and Resilience in Servicemembers (Army STARRS). *Psychiatry.* 2014;77:107–119.
3. Ursano RJ, Kessler RC, Stein MB, et al. Risk factors, methods, and timing of suicide attempts among U.S. Army Soldiers. *JAMA Psychiatry.* 2016;73(7):741–749.
4. Ursano RJ, Kessler RC, Stein MB, et al. Suicide attempts in the US Army during the wars in Afghanistan and Iraq, 2004 to 2009. *JAMA Psychiatry.* 2015;72:917–926.

Note: Robert J. Ursano, MD, and Murray B. Stein, MD, MPH, were co-principal investigators; Ronald C. Kessler, PhD, and Steven G. Heeringa, PhD, were site principal investigators; Michael Schoenbaum, PhD, and Lisa Colpe, PhD, MPH, were collaborating scientists; and Kenneth L. Cox, MD, MPH, was a consulting scientist on the Army STARRS project.

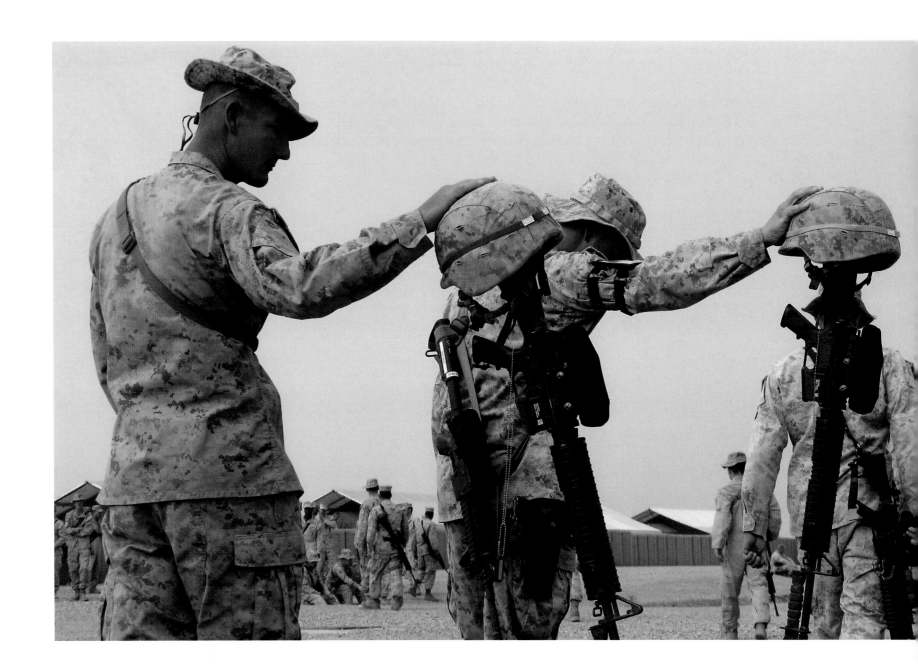

CHAPTER thirty-three

Family and Community Support

STEPHEN J. COZZA, MD; PAULA RAUCH, MD; and MARY KELLER, EDD

THE PROBLEM

THE PROPORTION OF AMERICANS WHO SERVE in our armed forces (less than 1 percent) is smaller than at any prior point in our nation's history. As a result, the families of those who serve often feel that most Americans do not understand the pride, commitment, and sacrifices that accompany military family life.[1] Many families also face the lasting impact of physical injuries and the "invisible wounds" of 21st century combat—chiefly, posttraumatic stress and traumatic brain injury (TBI) (Figure 33.1). Since the start of Operations Enduring Freedom, Iraqi Freedom, and New Dawn, over 52,000 men and women have suffered combat injuries that range from moderately to profoundly impairing. For injured service members and their families, the impact of these injuries continues long after they complete their service.[2]

BACKGROUND

Over the past 14 years of conflict, military healthcare professionals have learned many lessons about family-centered care:

- **Family systems and family-focused approaches matter**. Family members function interdependently. A popular conceptualization of this idea is the ecological systems model, which sees a family as a network of relationships, each of which can positively or negatively influence the other members'

FIGURE 33.1. [*Opposite*] US Marine Memorial Service. A memorial service held at Camp Bastion, Helmand Province, Afghanistan, on April 22, 2008, for two US Marines killed in action, First Sergeant Luke Mercardante and Corporal Kyle Wilks, who were killed by an IED (improvised explosive device) on a convoy from Kandahar Air Field to Camp Bastion on April 15, 2008. Photo by Jim Maceda/NBC NewsWire. Reproduced with permission from Getty Images.

VIGNETTE >> Bill, a 25-year-old former US Army sergeant, was seriously wounded in combat when an improvised explosive device detonated near his vehicle. He was evacuated to Landstuhl, Germany, and then to Walter Reed for definitive care for multisystem trauma, lower leg amputation, traumatic brain injury (TBI), and posttraumatic stress disorder (PTSD). His wife, Anne, 24, was living with their two children, ages 2 and 5, at Fort Campbell, Kentucky. Bill's injuries resulted in prolonged hospitalization, multiple surgeries, repeated family separations, eventual medical discharge from the service, and ultimately, relocation to Minnesota, where his extended family lives. Initially, his mother-in-law could help care for the children. But after Bill's second surgical revision, she was diagnosed with breast cancer and required treatment herself. Bill struggled to get the care he needed, and his daughter had lost her access to special education services when they left Kentucky. Bill and Anne argued frequently over finances and his increased drinking. They were referred to community mental health services after a domestic violence incident required police intervention.

health and well-being. The association between child emotional health and parental health has been well documented in civilian and military families exposed to trauma (Figure 33.2). Because relationships within the family system strongly affect individual members, those caring for service members and veterans with combat injuries must be prepared to engage the entire family.[3] However, at the start of the wars in Iraq and Afghanistan, the Department of Defense (DoD), Department of Veterans Affairs (VA), and civilian healthcare systems were not prepared to recognize and address family needs.

- **Injury recovery occurs in phases.** Recovery from injury sometimes requires months or years of care. This can profoundly affect injured service members and their families. The injury recovery trajectory includes four phases: (1) acute care, (2) medical stabilization, (3) transition to outpatient care, and (4) long-term rehabilitation and recovery.[4] During acute care, injured service members receive lifesaving medical interventions far from their families. Medical stabilization includes continuing and definitive medical/surgical care at tertiary care hospitals such as Landstuhl Medical Center in Germany, San Antonio Military Medical Center in Texas, or Walter Reed National Military Medical Center in Bethesda, Maryland. Family members are likely to learn about their loved ones' injuries early in this phase, but may be able to join them only intermittently. Transition to outpatient care involves activities that prepare families for life outside the hospital setting, including planning for follow-up care and ongoing rehabilitation (Chapter 31). These aspects of care require more family engagement. During rehabilitation and recovery, service members continue to progress in their treatment and adapt to

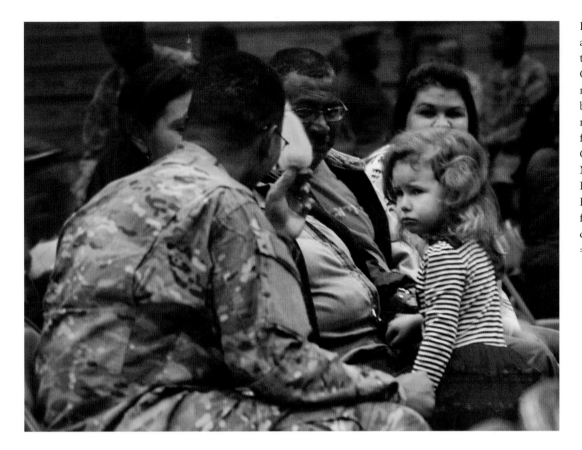

FIGURE 33.2. Specialist Cummings, a human resource specialist assigned to the14th Human Resources Sustainment Center, 1st Theater Sustainment Command, comforts his crying daughter before leaving on a deployment immediately after a deployment ceremony for his unit at the Ritz Epps Fitness Center, Fort Bragg, North Carolina, November 22, 2016. Photo by Private First Class Hubert Delany, 22nd Mobile Public Affairs Detachment. Reproduced from: https://www.dvidshub.net/search/?q=military+families&filter%5Btype%5D=image&view=list&sort=date&page=2.

any longer-term consequences of their injuries (Chapters 28, 29, and 30). During this final phase, military families often transition to new communities and switch to new providers in the VA or the private healthcare system. During and after this transition, complications can occur, recovery may be limited, and additional treatment may be required. Such setbacks can challenge everyone's resilience. Continuity of care may be further complicated by transition to different care facilities, which disrupts community connections and often requires stressful changes in family living arrangements.

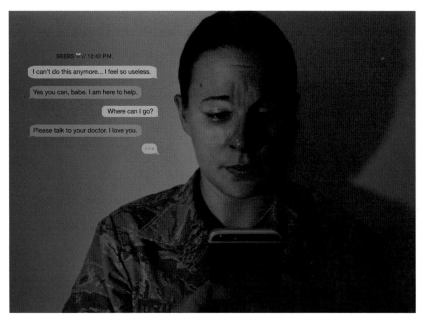

FIGURE 33.3. "I knew depression had taken hold of my life. The illness is common within my immediate family, but I kept these warning signs to myself. I didn't want to appear weak or spineless. I didn't want to be discharged from the military. But that was just the stigma I created for myself." US Air Force photo illustration by Senior Airman Deana Heitzman, November 16, 2016. Reproduced from: https://www.dvidshub.net/image/3003367/reaching-help.

- **Education and communication is paramount**. From the moment military healthcare providers break the news of a service member's injury to the next-of-kin, they must recognize that all members of the patient's multi-generation family will be affected. Engaging family members to address this fact and set the stage for collaborative care will ensure the best support for all involved (Figure 33.3). Every family system is complicated, with pre-existing strengths, challenges, and prior episodes of teamwork or discord. Full assessment of the family system may be deferred until the service member is medically stabilized, but the psycho-social care team needs to consider family dynamics from the start. Psycho-education (a thoughtful and skilled explanation given by informed healthcare providers of the challenges facing patients and their families) is a powerful intervention. Confusion about symptoms, procedures, medications, and emotional response can interfere with coping, while understanding how these factors influence recovery supports coping. Effective communication must continue as the service member's medical situation evolves. Providers should tailor the detail and amount of information they share to each recipient's "need to know" and their "capacity to know."

- A **developmental perspective should be maintained.** When parents are injured, their children's stress adds to ongoing challenges of normal development. Children's reactions vary by age, temperament, and maturity, and a developmental perspective is critical to meeting their needs[4] (Figure 33.4). The emotional trauma of combat injury will be experienced and re-experienced anew for children as they age and their injured parents cope with the injury. Children of all ages may be troubled by injuries that change the parent's cognitive and emotional state. TBI and posttraumatic stress disorder (PTSD) may be particularly upsetting because of the associated difficulties with mood regulation, memory, social activities, and emotional engagement. These changes can profoundly affect the injured service member's parenting capacities. Unless it's properly explained, children may interpret this as a change of affection.

- **Adequate support must be ensured.** Prolonged medical care imposes substantial financial costs. Family coping is enhanced by support for housing, child care, lost spousal wages, and transportation. Otherwise, financial pressure may compound the emotional stress felt by the couple and their dependent children. The military and VA offer some support, while local academic hospitals, community health centers, and a complex web of nonprofits help others. Many families need help to identify these resources.

THE INNOVATION: FAMILY-FOCUSED CARE

Department of Defense

In the last decade, the DoD has recognized the importance of focusing on the entire family to restore and maintain the psychological and physical well-being of wounded, ill, and injured service members.[3] To promote this holistic approach, the military has expanded family access to online support systems, such as MilitaryOneSource (www.militaryonesource.mil), and built up family-centered support on bases, in military medical treatment facilities, and in local communities. Though there are many examples of such initiatives, three stand out:

1. **The Defense Centers of Excellence for Psychological Health and Traumatic Brain Injury**, established in 2007, trains military and civilian behavioral health professionals to provide high-quality, culturally-sensitive, evidence-based behavioral health services to military personnel, veterans, and their families.

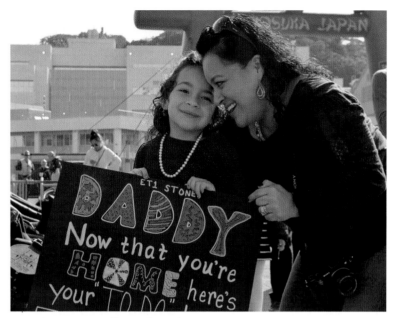

FIGURE 33.4. Family members of Sailors assigned to the Arleigh Burke-class guided-missile destroyer USS *Stethem* (DDG 63) await the ships arrival at Fleet Activities Yokosuka, Japan, November 17, 2016. Photo by Peter K Burghart, Navy Media Content Services. Reproduced from: https://www.dvidshub.net/image/2998652/161117-n-xn177-076.

FIGURE 33.5. [*Opposite*]
"Courage to Care/Courage to Talk"
is a campaign developed by the
Center for the Study of Traumatic
Stress at the Uniformed Services
University of the Health Sciences to
help combat injured families work
together toward recovery.

2. **The Center for Deployment Psychology at the Uniformed Services University**, established in 2006, was created to meet the deployment-related mental and behavioral health needs of military personnel and their families by training behavioral health specialists and more recently, primary care providers, about the population's unique needs.

3. In 2004, the DoD instituted **military family life consultants** (MFLCs) to provide individualized support, in local communities, for behavioral health counseling services. MFLCs are credentialed counselors, social workers, or other mental health professionals. In cooperation with local administrations, MFLCs are assigned in schools that serve many military families.

Department of Veterans Affairs

Coordinating the transition of care after discharge from the military is vitally important. The VA's Office of Veterans Benefits reports that about 25,000 service members separate from the military every month. Though the VA does not have a specific charter to serve families, it has developed specialized hotlines, online tools, and local resources for this purpose. Veterans, providers, and families can access these resources from local Veterans Centers, online, or through mobile Veterans Centers. Relatives of wounded combat veterans are eligible for Veteran Center readjustment counseling services. The VA also provides a special program for veterans' caregivers that includes respite care and other family services and support.

Academic Medical Centers and Community Health Clinics

Academic and community health centers are recognizing and answering the call to serve veterans and their families. Academic medical centers such as the Massachusetts General Hospital, University of California–Los Angeles, Emory, Rush, and New York University have created veteran and family clinics to provide clinical care tailored to the needs of post-9/11 veterans and their families. For example, the Massachusetts General Hospital Home Base Program focuses on treatment for PTSD and TBI. UCLA's Operation Mend offers specialized surgical and psychological care for wounded warriors and support for their families. The Center for the Study of Traumatic Stress at Uniformed Services University of the Health Sciences is an academic center that has conducted research with military children and families to better understand the effects of combat deployment, child maltreatment, combat injury, and military-related bereavement.

New Evidence-Based Family Interventions

Two evidence-informed, family-centered approaches show promise in supporting military child and family health: "Families OverComing Under Stress" (FOCUS)[5] and "After Deployment Adaptive Parenting Tools" (ADAPT).[6] While neither program was specifically designed to address the challenges of combat injury in families, both incorporate trauma-informed strategies to help such families.

Community and School-Based Support

Community-based programs are profoundly important in providing military children and families connections, support, and continuity. Frequent moves and changing schools add to a child's sense of uncertainty and anxiety. If a service member's child was involved in programs such as arts, clubs, or sports, there may be financial or logistical challenges to continuing these activities after their parent's discharge from the service or relocation. Families may need help planning for involuntary transitions, particularly during the stressful time of caring for an injured service member. Local programs, youth organizations, and activities sometimes offer connections and assistance to address these challenges. The National Military Family Association, Blue Star Families, Wounded Warrior Project, and Home Base Program are among the many non-DoD/VA community support programs that serve military families. The Military Child Education Coalition focuses on the unique needs of military-connected children in schools. Its Student-to-Student peer mentorship program is an evidence-informed, publicly recognized student-led support program that helps military children. Also of note, the National Child Traumatic Stress Network offers an array of evidence-based practices for military families.

THE BOTTOM LINE

After 14 years of war, we've learned a lot about the value of partnering with families and stabilizing the family environment of those wounded in combat. This is best done by ensuring access to basic needs, such as housing, education, healthcare, child care, and jobs throughout injury recovery and adjustment; by identifying and promoting services that support family organization, communication, coping, and resilience; and by sustaining systems of support for families who need help over many years[2] (Figure 33.5). In addition, injured service members, veterans, and their families need ready access to knowledgeable and caring civilian providers and evidence-based treatment. This is particularly important when TBI or mental health issues are involved.

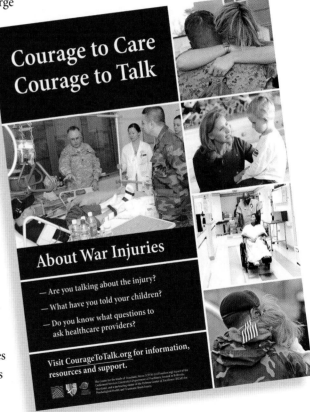

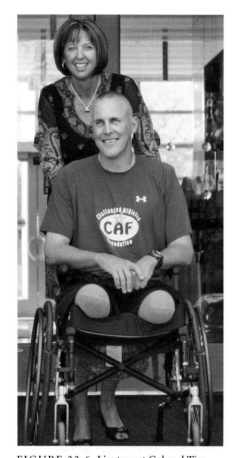

FIGURE 33.6. Lieutenant Colonel Tim Karcher and Alesia Karcher leave a physical therapy session, November 6, 2009, at the Center for the Intrepid in San Antonio and head to the Fisher House, where the former 2nd Squadron, 5th Cavalry Regiment commander is recovering. Reproduced from: https://www.dvidshub.net/image/222795/wounded-warrior-month-road-recovery.

Six strategies are particularly important to assure post-injury family health: (1) maintain a physically safe and structured environment; (2) engage required community resources; (3) develop and share knowledge within and outside the family that builds shared understanding; (4) build a positive, emotionally safe and warm family environment; (5) master and model important interpersonal skills, including problem-solving and conflict resolution; and (6) maintain a vision of hope and optimism for the injured service member, his or her family, and those they love[4] (Figure 33.6).

Notes

1. Cozza SJ, Lerner RM. Military children and families: introducing the issue. *Future Child.* 2013;23(2):3–11.
2. Holmes AK, Rauch PK, Cozza SJ. When a parent is injured or killed in combat. *Future Child.* 2013;23(2):143–162.
3. Wadsworth SM, Lester P, Marini C, Cozza SJ, Sornborger J, Strouse T. Approaching family-focused systems of care for military and veteran families. *Mil Behav Health.* 2013;1:31–40.
4. Cozza SJ. Parenting in military families faced with combat-related injury, illness, or death. In: Gewirtz AH, Youssef AM, eds. *Parenting and Children's Resilience in Military Families.* Heidelberg, Germany: Springer International Publishing; 2016: 151–173.
5. Lester P, Liang LJ, Milburn N, et al. Evaluation of a family-centered preventive intervention for military families: parent and child longitudinal outcomes. *J Am Acad Child Adolesc Psychiatry.* 2016;55(1):14–21.
6. Gewirtz AH, Pinna KL, Hanson SK, Brockberg D. Promoting parenting to support reintegrating military families: after deployment, adaptive parenting tools. *Psychol Serv.* 2014;11(1):31–40.

Additional Resources

Princeton-Brookings Future of Children website. *Military Children and Families.* 2013;23(2). http://futureofchildren.org/publications/journals/journal_details/index.xml?journalid=80. Accessed October 18, 2016.

Uniformed Services University of the Health Sciences, Center for the Study of Traumatic Stress. *Proceedings: Workgroup on Intervention with Combat Injured Families.* Bethesda, MD: USU; 2007. http://www.cstsonline.org/assets/media/documents/CSTS_workshop_intervention_combat_injured_families_web.pdf. Accessed October 19, 2016.

Rauch PK, Muriel AC. *Raising an Emotionally Healthy Child When a Parent is Sick*. New York, NY: McGraw-Hill; 2006.

FOCUS: Family Resilience Training for Military Families website. http://www.focusproject.org/. Accessed October 19, 2016.

University of Minnesota. ADAPT 4U: After Deployment Adaptive Parenting Tools. http://www.cehd.umn.edu/fsos/projects/adapt/about.asp. Accessed October 19, 2016.

Red Sox Foundation and Massachusetts General Hospital. Staying Strong website. http://www.stayingstrong.org. Accessed October 19, 2016.

Red Sox Foundation and Massachusetts General Hospital. Home Base website. http://www.homebase.org/. Accessed October 19, 2016.

Red Sox Foundation and Massachusetts General Hospital. The Training Institute at Home Base website. http://www.homebasetraining.org. Accessed October 19, 2016.

Masten AS. *Ordinary Magic: Resilience Processes in Development*. New York, NY: Guilford Press; 2014.

American Academy of Pedicatrics. Deployment and military medical home resources website. https://www.aap.org/en-us/advocacy-and-policy/aap-health-initiatives/Pages/Deployment-and-Military.aspx. Accessed October 19, 2016.

National Child Traumatic Stress Network. Military and veteran families and children webpage. http://nctsn.org/resources/topics/military-children-and-families. Accessed October 19, 2016.

Other Web-Based Resources

- MilitaryOneSource: www.militaryonesource.mil
- The Defense Centers of Excellence for Psychological Health and Traumatic Brain Injury: http://www.dcoe.mil/
- The Center for Deployment Psychology at the Uniformed Services University: http://deploymentpsych.org/
- Military family life consultants (MFLCs): http://www.militaryonesource.mil/parenting?content_id=269730
- VA Caregiver Support: http://www.caregiver.va.gov/support/support_benefits.asp
- Families OverComing Under Stress (FOCUS): http://www.focusproject.org/
- After Deployment Adaptive Parenting Tools (ADAPT): http://www.militaryfamilies.psu.edu/programs/after-deployment-adaptive-parenting-tools-adapt
- The Military Child Education Coalition: http://www.militarychild.org/
- National Child Traumatic Stress Network: http://www.nctsn.org/

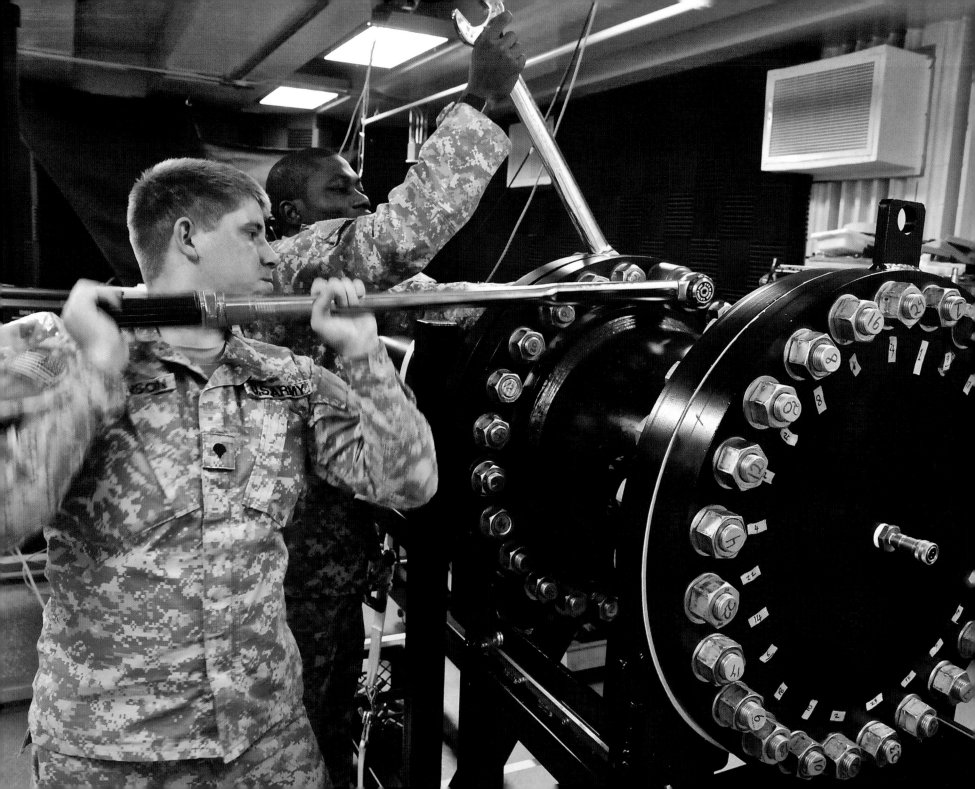

SECTION THREE

Challenges

[*Section Three image*] Specialist Daniel Oladejo (right) and Specialist Peter Johnson, biomedical science technicians with the US Army Institute of Surgical Research, make adjustments to the shock tube at Fort Sam Houston, Texas. The shock tube is a piece of equipment designed to simulate exposure to explosions similar to what Soldiers may encounter while in combat. February 23, 2016. US Army photo by Sergeant Aaron Ellerman, 204th Public Affairs Detachment/Released. Reproduced from: https://www.dvidshub.net/image/2426041/refining-innovation.

CHAPTER thirty-four

Anticipating the Challenges of Potential Battlefields

STEPHEN L. JONES, MD; BRUCE L. GILLINGHAM, MD; and SEAN L. MURPHY, MD

INTRODUCTION

I
N THE FUTURE, OUR MILITARY HEALTH SYSTEM will face distinctly different challenges than it has in the past. As noted in Chapter 6, the measures needed to protect the health of the force are largely determined by the environment in which the conflict occurs, the social and political terrain, and the enemy's capabilities and actions. If we assume the casualty care system that worked well in Iraq and Afghanistan will perform equally well in the next conflict, then we will be ill prepared for a fight that unfolds under vastly different conditions.

THE GLOBAL SECURITY ENVIRONMENT

The world today is increasingly volatile, uncertain, and complex. During 14 years of counterinsurgency campaigns in Iraq and Afghanistan, the United States' readiness to fight a large-scale conventional war has faded. Meanwhile, the capabilities of potential adversaries have grown and American forces no longer enjoy a clear technological advantage on the battlefield.

Foreign terrorist organizations pose an immediate global threat with acts of terrorism, the seizure and holding of territory, and the spread of their violent ideology through social media. Russia's illegal annexation of the Crimea, continued aggression in Ukraine, and threats against Romania, Poland,

and the Baltic nations are a direct challenge to the NATO alliance. North Korea threatens security in northeast Asia with advances in missile technology, weapons of mass destruction, and the potential for a massive artillery barrage of Seoul. Meanwhile, in the contested waters of the South China Sea, a newly assertive China is building artificial reefs with airstrips capable of supporting military aircraft. The signing of an international accord has diminished the immediate threat of a nuclear-armed Iran, but the country continues to export terrorism and actively undermine regional stability. A military confrontation with any of these nations, or an unforeseen crisis in another part of the world, could lead to a vastly different type of conflict than those America fought in Afghanistan and Iraq.

POTENTIAL SCENARIOS

Megacity Conflicts

By the year 2030, over 60 percent of the world's population will live in cities of 10 million people or more.[1] The inhabitants of these "megacities" will be mostly young, well-connected through smart phones, and possessing technical skills, a combination that potentially can make them increasingly dangerous. Although some megacities such as New York, Tokyo, and Seoul have robust infrastructure and stable governments, others lack even basic public health services. Global air travel may trigger epidemics that require military assistance to contain. The environment in megacities is far more complex than the mountains and deserts of Afghanistan and Iraq. Military operations will unfold in multiple domains: below the streets, in buildings, on rooftops, in the air, in space, in cyberspace, and of course in the human domain. The American military's experience in Mogadishu, Somalia, underscores the challenge of mounting military operations in such environments.

Air-Sea Battle

Another ever-present challenge is the potential that Iran or China will attempt to deny freedom of movement through international shipping lanes. Originally, the concept for a conflict of this type was known as an "air-sea battle," but the term has been recently replaced by "anti-access/area denial." The military tactics and procedures devised to respond to such a challenge are entitled the "Joint Concept for Access and Maneuver in the Global Commons."[2] Marked advances in air, land, and sea-based weapons systems have altered the equation for providing medical support in such conflicts. Because the proliferation of anti-ship missiles increases the risk of strikes against hospital ships and other large floating platforms, we must rethink traditional strategies for treating large numbers of casualties, particularly in maritime environments far from shore. Under such conditions, it will be difficult to match the high combat survival rates achieved in our recent Middle East conflicts.

Evolving Terrorism and "New Generation" Warfare

The current fighting in Syria, Iraq, and Ukraine provide insight into evolving terrorist tactics and the Russian "new generation warfare."[3,4] The use of chemical weapons including chlorine and mustard agents by ISIS has been widely reported. The attacks in Paris and Brussels underscore the threat of terrorist attacks at home. Observers in Ukraine report the extensive use of remotely piloted vehicles for real-time targeting with follow-on massed artillery or rocket strikes within minutes. These attacks have employed thermobaric warheads, cluster bombs, scatterable mines, and top-attack munitions that can quickly devastate units. In 2014, a massed rocket strike virtually destroyed two Ukrainian mechanized battalions at Zelenopillya in minutes. Reactive armor, a new auto-loading system, and improved optics make Russian tanks more formidable than those fielded in the past.

In a full-scale conventional conflict against a technologically capable adversary, US casualties will be greater than in recent conflicts. Because modern military operations employ more widely dispersed units than in the past, hospitals in rear areas may be more vulnerable to quick raids by armored forces or infiltrating infantry.

Prolonged Field Care

During Operation Enduring Freedom (OEF) and Operation Iraqi Freedom (OIF), severely injured service members were often whisked from battlefields in Afghanistan or Iraq to definitive care in the United States within three or four days of the original injury. In future conflicts, rapid air evacuation may be impossible due to widespread jamming and targeting of communication systems, enemy anti-aircraft fire, and sophisticated air defense systems. Long distances, such as those commonly encountered in sub-Saharan Africa and the Pacific Ocean, may delay the arrival of evacuation aircraft for hours or days. Under such circumstances, medical teams will need to provide prolonged field care until air or ground evacuation is possible.

Disaggregated Operations

The US military's growing use of small, highly mobile units requires a different approach to medical staffing than in the past. Because it is not feasible to support each unit with a full medical team, we must expand the skills and capabilities of medics, corpsmen, and medical technicians to fill this role. Tablet computers preloaded with appropriate clinical guidelines and decision support tools will help, as will portable ultrasound, point-of-care lab testing, and emerging technologies to control bleeding and treat infection. When communication can be established by satellite, telehealth will allow medics and corpsmen in the field to consult medical specialists in the United States. Someday soon, remotely piloted vehicles may be used to resupply isolated units, and robotic vehicles may be used to retrieve casualties under fire.

Cyber Warfare

In a world that is increasingly reliant on the Internet, extremist groups and state-sponsored hackers can take out the power, water, and information systems that support healthcare facilities. Hackers can already gain access to infusion pumps and reprogram them to deliver fatal doses of medication.[5] In a future military conflict, military healthcare professionals may be forced to operate without the telecommunications, telehealth, and global positioning systems we use to facilitate casualty evacuation and treatment.

Cyber warfare is in its infancy, but it will almost certainly grow in importance and complexity (Figure 34.1). There are already signs that it generates its own set of health consequences. America's cyber warriors routinely encounter graphic audio and video recordings depicting terrorist cruelty. Pilots of unmanned aerial vehicles (drones) frequently witness battlefield trauma, and in the course of carrying out missions may, from time to time, inadvertently inflict civilian casualties. Because both roles engender significant psychological stress, we need to develop more medically integrated operational support than was available in the past.

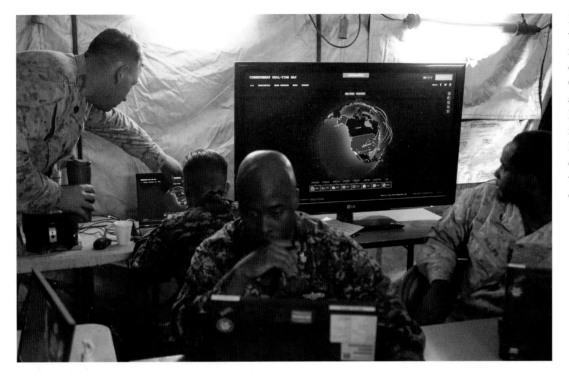

FIGURE 34.1. Marines and Sailors with 553 Cyber Protection Team monitor network activity during a large scale exercise at Marine Corps Air Station Miramar, California, August 22, 2016. 553-CPT is a team of cyber defense specialists with Fleet Cyber Command. Photo by Corporal Garrett White, I Marine Expeditionary Force. Reproduced from: https://www.dvidshub.net/image/2808344/marines-with-mef-strengthen-cyber-defensive-capabilities.

RETHINKING HEALTH SUPPORT

Enabling a Smaller Footprint

To support rapid deployments abroad, all three services are developing lightweight, modular medical units that respond within hours or days rather than weeks or months. Because early-entry forces often do not include field hospitals, these forward resuscitative/surgical teams will need enhanced intensive care and holding capabilities.

Naval operations are increasingly being conducted by individual ships that separate from an amphibious "ready group" on short notice to pursue different objectives. Operating hundreds of miles

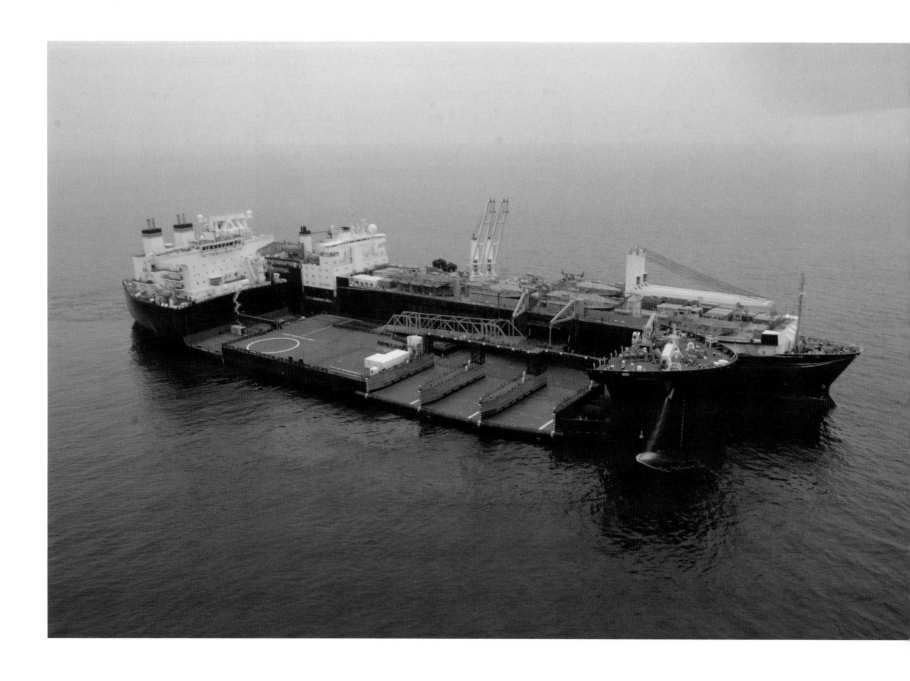

apart in hostile waters, each ship will rely upon an "expeditionary resuscitative surgical system"—a mobile, eight-person surgical team modeled after the Army forward surgical teams that performed so successfully in Iraq and Afghanistan. The Navy is also developing modular medical packages that can be pre-positioned on platforms of opportunity, such as an expeditionary transfer dock (ESD), a highly flexible ship that enables logistics movement from sea to shore to support a broad range of military operations (Figures 34.2 and 34.3).[6]

Optimizing Human Performance

Our technological edge over potential adversaries may be smaller than it once was, but we continue to maintain an advantage in human performance (Chapter 42). To sustain this edge, the US military is supporting research to help service members achieve and maintain a high level of physical and cognitive performance and be resilient in the face of setbacks or injury.

In recent years, the military has recognized that its special operations forces are, in fact, elite athletes. To support these warriors, Special Operations Command has started embedding athletic trainers, clinical psychologists, and sports medicine physicians into its units to optimize their health and promote faster recovery from injury. This approach has proven to be so effective that it is now being rolled out to conventional forces as well.

Recently, the Army and Marine Corps have embraced human performance optimization (Chapter 42) to improve unit-level training of infantry squads.[7] The Navy's "Team Dimensional Training" teaches Soldiers and Marines to maintain awareness of their surroundings and spot tell-tale signs, such as the absence of children in a village, to alert them to an impending attack. A resilience component teaches warfighters to monitor their emotional state and focus on what's important. Squads are also given a framework for conducting after-action reviews to improve their performance and correct any shortcomings.

Envisioning Future Medical Operations

The US military's "Joint Force 2020" describes how the Army, Navy, Air Force, and Marines will work together to quickly respond to crises around the world by conducting operations in air, sea, land, space, and cyber domains.[8] A corollary document, the "Joint Concept for Health Services," describes how the health components of the joint force will support globally integrated operations.[9] Facilitating combined operations will require greater interoperability among the services and our allies. In addition

FIGURE 34.2. [*Opposite*] Maritime prepositioning force ship USNS GYSGT *Fred W. Stockham* (T-AK 3017) and Expeditionary Transfer Dock USNS *Montford Point* (T-ESD 1) perform a "skin-to-skin" maneuver by connecting side-by-side with one another at sea. In this instance, the *Montford Point* acts as a floating pier for a simulated offload. March 13, 2016. US Navy photo by Mass Communication Specialist 3rd Class Madailein Abbott/Released. Reproduced from: https://www.dvidshub.net/image/2463605/mscs-usns-stockham-and-usns-montford-point-perform-skin-skin-maneuver.

FIGURE 34.3. [*Opposite*] A US Marine Corps MV-22B Osprey with Special-Purpose Marine Air-Ground Task Force—Crisis Response—Africa takes off from a runway for Dakar, Senegal, after supporting Operation United Assistance in Monrovia, Liberia, December 4, 2014. US Marine Corps photo by Lance Corporal Andre Dakis/SPMAGTF-CR-AF Combat Camera/Released. Reproduced from: https://www.dvidshub.net/image/1699675/us-marines-complete-two-months-support-ebola-response-west-africa.

to supporting combat operations, military health providers will be periodically tasked with supporting non-combat engagements, such as humanitarian missions (Chapter 5). The recent Ebola crisis in West Africa is one such example. To prepare for these missions, the military is educating selected officers in global health engagement so they will have the necessary knowledge and skills to work effectively with nongovernmental organizations, foreign militaries, and the UN High Commissioner for Refugees in support of humanitarian assistance operations.

CONCLUSION

It is impossible to predict where American forces will next be sent to fight. To protect the health of American forces abroad, our military health system must not only retain the skills and capabilities we developed over the past 14 years of war, we must also preserve our capacity to anticipate and adapt to new threats. The most important lesson learned during OEF and OIF is that we must always be ready to learn, evolve, and overcome.

Notes

1. *The Megacity: Operational Challenges for Force 2025 and Beyond.* Fort Eustis, VA: Army Capabilities Integration Center; 2014. http://pdf.yt/d/FnYX-XA4yCJDwcBW. Accessed October 19, 2016.
2. US Navy website. The air-sea battle concept summary. http://www.navy.mil/submit/display.asp?story_id=63730. Accessed May 25, 2016.
3. Ignatius D. Defeating the Islamic State will be a long war. RealClearPolitics.com. 2016. http://www.realclearpolitics.com/articles/2016/01/19/defeating_the_islamic_state_will_be_a_long_war_129361.html. Accessed May 8, 2016.
4. Karber PA. *"Lessons Learned" From the Russo-Ukrainian War, Personal Observations.* Vienna, VA: The Potomac Foundation; 2015. https://prodev2go.files.wordpress.com/2015/10/rus-ukr-lessons-draft.pdf. Accessed May 8, 2016.
5. US Food and Drug Administration. Vulnerabilities of Hospira LifeCare PCA3 and PCA5 Infusion Pump Systems: FDA safety communication. May 13, 2015. http://www.fda.gov/MedicalDevices/Safety/AlertsandNotices/ucm446809.htm. Accessed May 8, 2016.

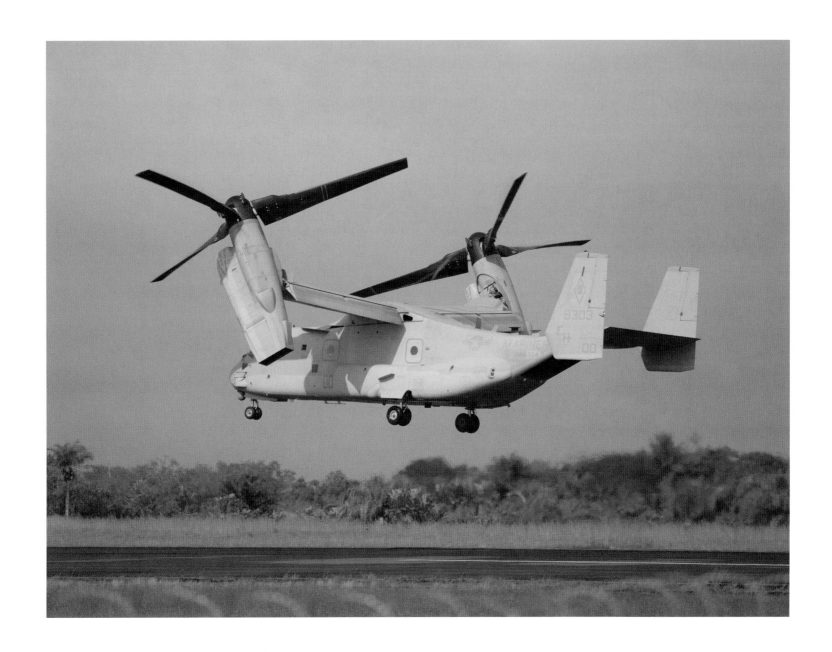

6. US Navy. *CNO's Navigation Plan, 2015–2019.* http://www.navy.mil/cno/docs/140818_cno_navigation_plan.pdf. Accessed May 25, 2016.

7. Wolf R. *Squad Overmatch Tactical Combat Casualty Care (TC3) Study.* Orlando, FL: US Army Program Executive Office: Simulation, Training and Instrumentation; 2015.

8. *Capstone Concept for Joint Operations: Joint Force 2020.* Washington, DC: Joint Chiefs of Staff; 2012. http://www.dtic.mil/doctrine/concepts/ccjo_jointforce2020.pdf. Accessed May 8, 2016.

9. *Joint Concept for Health Services.* Washington, DC: Joint Chiefs of Staff; 2015. http://www.dtic.mil/doctrine/concepts/joint_concepts/joint_concept_health_services.pdf. Accessed May 8, 2016.

Recommended Reading

Murray CK, Jones SL. Army Medical Department at war: healthcare in a complex world. *US Army Med Dep J.* 2016;Apr-Sep:199–208.

CHAPTER thirty-five

Prehospital Trauma Care: The Next Frontier

ROBERT MABRY, MD, and RUSS KOTWAL, MD, MPH

INTRODUCTION

OVER THE PAST 14 YEARS OF WAR, the United States has achieved unprecedented survival rates among casualties arriving alive to combat support hospitals. The key phrase is "arriving alive." No healthcare system can bring the dead back to life. This is why it is essential to provide optimal trauma care at the point of injury, continue it throughout evacuation, and keep injured Soldiers, Sailors, Airmen and Marines alive to reach definitive surgical care (Figure 35.1).

Even with perfect *hospital* care, up to 25 percent of combat deaths in war zones may be preventable.[1] The vast majority of these "potentially preventable" deaths happen on the battlefield, *before* the injured service member reaches a combat support hospital (Figure 35.2). To push combat death rates lower, we must close the gap between what is possible and what is currently delivered in the field, prior to arrival at the closest hospital. This same challenge applies to civilian trauma systems as well. To do this, the Military Health System (MHS) must give prehospital care the same sort of attention it has historically given to in-hospital care.

To save more lives on the battlefield, our front-line healthcare providers—combat medics, corpsmen, and MEDEVAC teams—will need innovative treatments and technologies to control internal bleeding, prevent respiratory failure, and treat other important causes of preventable death. But better technol-

VIGNETTE >> September 2025, 0200 (local time): During a firefight in an urban area of a distant country, Corporal Smith is severely injured by a bullet that penetrates his body armor. Within seconds, sensors embedded in Smith's undergarment detect impending shock. This triggers an alert on the platoon sergeant's heads-up display, indicating that Corporal Smith requires immediate medical evacuation.

The moment Corporal Smith is brought to the platoon's casualty collection point, the combat medic starts transfusing a unit of whole blood, a drug that improves clotting, and a broad-spectrum antibiotic. Using a handheld ultrasound, he confirms internal bleeding. Because Corporal Smith's blood pressure is dropping, the medic makes a small incision and injects a clot-promoting foam into his abdomen. It swiftly stops the bleeding. As Corporal Smith's blood pressure improves, he starts to complain of significant pain. Because other casualties are arriving, the medic hands Corporal Smith a nasal inhaler he can use for pain relief. Its mix of medicines controls pain, preserves blood pressure, and reduces the risk that Corporal Smith will later develop posttraumatic stress disorder.

Due to the difficult urban terrain, the medic requests evacuation by drone. Guided by its global positioning system (GPS) and ground-sensing radar, the drone lands atop a radio beacon placed in a small, walled courtyard in complete darkness. Corporal Smith is loaded aboard and flown to the nearby forward surgical team. En route, telemetry from Corporal Smith's body sensors is relayed to the forward surgical team. Based on the data, Corporal Smith is taken to the operating room the moment he arrives. Total time from injury to surgery: 47 minutes.

ogy, while necessary, is not enough. We must also define and adopt consensus standards for training and treatment, and devise common systems to collect and analyze prehospital data. The MHS should also designate a responsible party to drive improvements.

WHO OWNS BATTLEFIELD MEDICINE?

Today, no senior officer, service, agency, or department "owns" battlefield care—the quintessential function of military medicine.[2] Operationally, battlefield commanders control most prehospital casualty care assets because combat medics, battalion physicians, physician assistants, flight medics, and associated equipment are assigned to their units. However, combat commanders are not experts in far-forward medical care, and they lack the resources to train their personnel to deliver it. Instead, battlefield commanders rely on the Army, Navy, and Air Force medical departments to provide the right personnel, medical training, equipment doctrine, and mix of medical forces.

The service medical departments train and equip combat medical forces and are mainly responsible for providing subsequent in-hospital care. However, they tend to defer day-to-day responsibility for the delivery of battlefield care to line commanders. While sharing responsibility in this way may seem reasonable at first glance, the axiom "when everyone is responsible, no one is responsible" applies. Until the question of "Who owns battlefield medicine?" is resolved, prehospital combat casualty care will remain fragmented and inefficient.

THE UNIQUE DEMANDS OF CARE ON THE BATTLEFIELD

Mastering the skills required to treat troops in garrisons at a medical clinic or hospital is important, but it is very different than treating casualties at the point of injury, much less under fire (Figure 35.3). Likewise, delivering patient care in a modern hospital emergency room, even one located in a busy urban trauma center, is distinctly different than managing a battalion aid station during major combat operations or transporting critically injured Soldiers and Marines in a MEDEVAC helicopter.

Developing Battlefield Medicine Specialists

Over the years, there have been several efforts to define the core competencies of a "board-certified" military physician. But the requirements remain undefined. At a minimum, the US military needs an adequately staffed cadre of physicians with specialized skills in prehospital and operational care. The closest civilian analog are board-certified emergency medicine specialists with subspecialty training and certification in emergency medical services (EMS).

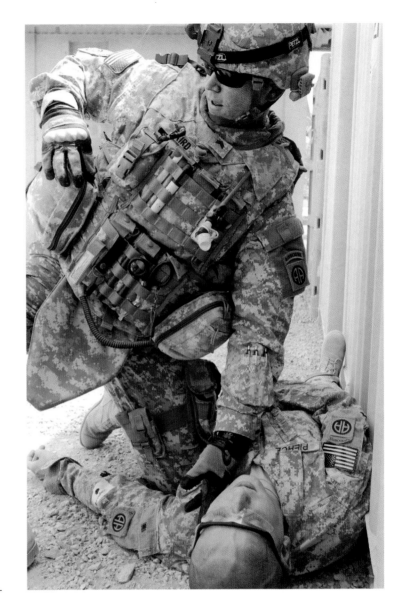

FIGURE 35.1. Sergeant Scott Baird of Pigeon Forge, Tennessee, a medic assigned to the 2nd Battalion, 505th Parachute Infantry Regiment, 3rd Brigade Combat Team, 82nd Airborne Division, Multi-National Division–Baghdad, reaches for his medical pouch during a trauma training exercise at Joint Security Station Loyalty, eastern Baghdad, July 16, 2009. Photo by Sergeant 1st Class Alex Licea, 3rd Brigade Combat Team, 82nd Airborne Division. Reproduced from: https://www.dvidshub.net/image/187959/medics-hone-critical-skills-during-training-exercise.

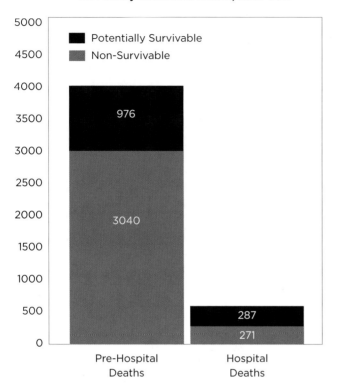

US Military Battlefield Deaths, 2001–2011

■ Potentially Survivable
▦ Non-Survivable

Pre-Hospital Deaths: 976 (Potentially Survivable), 3040 (Non-Survivable)

Hospital Deaths: 287 (Potentially Survivable), 271 (Non-Survivable)

Civilian EMS doctors employ a systems approach to improve prehospital care on the streets of the United States. Military specialists would take a similar approach to improve battlefield care. Although it will be challenging to recruit enough EMS physicians to fill every operational role, the military should clearly define the unique skills required of battlefield healthcare providers so its training can be modified to match. This can best be accomplished by involving clinical experts in prehospital battlefield medicine (Figure 35.4).

Today, the MHS has only a handful of board-certified prehospital care specialists. With few clinical experts to inform senior leaders, it's not surprising that there are no uniform standards for combat casualty care training, equipment, protocols, or procedures across the force, among the services, or even within similar units.

Priorities for Research and Development

Future research efforts should focus on the most important causes of preventable death and disability on the battlefield. Because internal bleeding is currently the leading cause of such deaths,[1] it should be the primary focus of our research efforts (see Chapters 10-12, 16, and 17). To date, several technologies look promising. All are designed to enable medics to slow or temporarily stop internal bleeding, so a casualty can reach the operating room before it's too late.[3,4] Although there is substantial evidence that several emerging technologies are effective, most are not available to our conventional military forces.

Enabling Use of Effective Products

One obstacle is regulatory caution. For example, although freeze-dried human plasma is widely used in Europe, it is not approved for use in

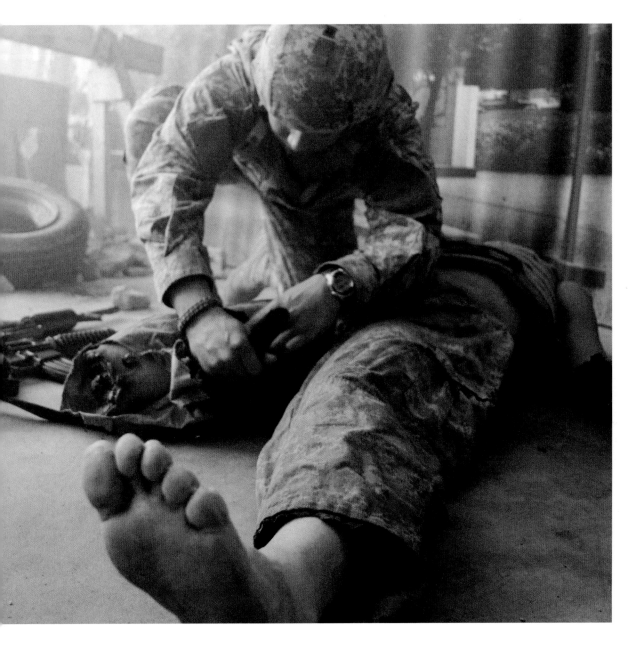

FIGURE 35.2. [*Opposite*] Recent studies of combat deaths have determined that the vast majority of those that are preventable with better trauma care occur at the point of injury or during MEDEVAC, prior to the casualty reaching a forward surgical team or combat support hospital. Thus, efforts to save more lives should focus on improving prehospital care.

FIGURE 35.3. A Soldier from the 252nd Engineer Company, 103rd Engineer Battalion, 213th Regional Support Group, Pennsylvania Army National Guard, applies a tourniquet to a simulated casualty during a Combat Lifesaving Course at Fort Indiantown Gap, Pennsylvania, November 6, 2013. Photo by Staff Sergeant Coltin Heller, 109th Mobile Public Affairs Detachment. Reproduced from: https://www.dvidshub.net/image/1048694/stop-bleeding.

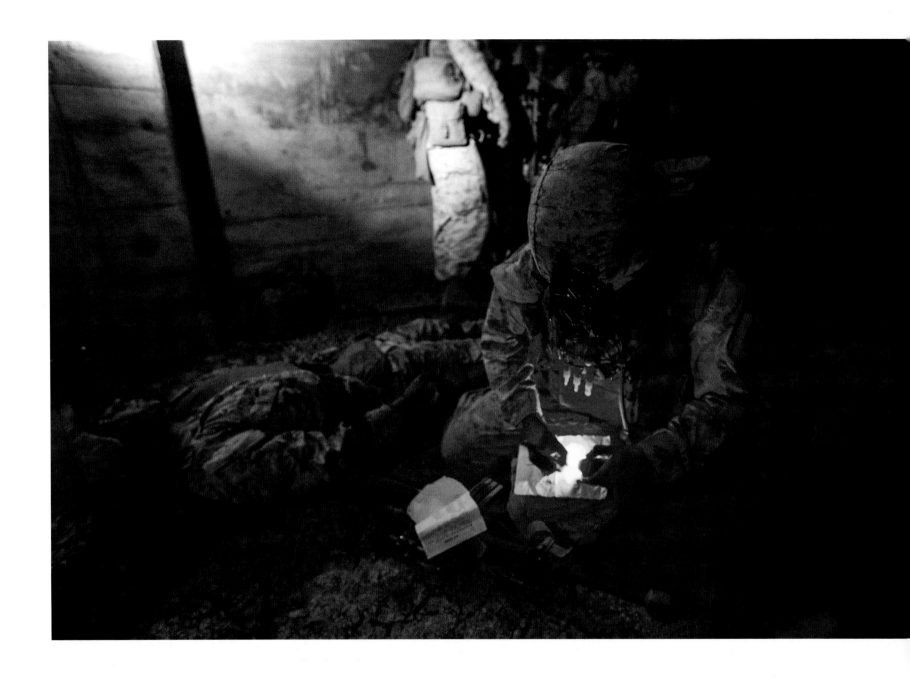

the United States. Currently, it is only available to Special Operations Forces (SOF) under a Food and Drug Administration investigational new drug protocol. Therefore, conventional, reserve, and National Guard units lack access to this treatment. Likewise, donor-to-donor transfusions of fresh whole blood, a mainstay of battlefield care in World War II and Korea, are performed only by SOF medical personnel. US Army flight medics were not allowed to adopt en route blood transfusion protocols until 2012, 11 years into the war (Figure 35.5). Tranexamic acid (Chapter 17) has been used to treat abnormal menstrual bleeding since the 1970s. Although its use is recommended by the Committee on Tactical Combat Casualty Care (CoTCCC, Chapter 11), combat medics employ it unevenly.

Pain control is another target of opportunity. Recently, the CoTCCC, in concert with the American College of Emergency Physicians, endorsed a "triple option analgesia plan" that incorporates the use of (1) fentanyl lozenges (pioneered by the 75th Ranger Regiment and the Army Special Missions Unit); (2) intramuscular ketamine (pioneered by United Kingdom physicians and quickly adopted by US Air Force Pararescue personnel); and (3) standard opiate analgesics such as morphine. This set of options gives medics the flexibility to pick the best approach for each casualty based on blood pressure, level of pain, and other factors.

Despite a clear consensus in the military medical community on the importance of battlefield pain control, the most recent papers on this issue note that less than 40 percent of casualties are getting *any* analgesia at the point of injury.[5] Among those who do, two-thirds are receiving morphine instead of safer alternatives.[6] Going forward, development of better prehospital approaches to reducing bleeding, controlling pain, preventing infection, and perhaps administering medication to block the subsequent development of posttraumatic stress may be as important to improving long-term outcomes as the adoption of modern tourniquets was for reducing preventable deaths in Iraq and Afghanistan[7] (Chapter 18).

Developing New Technologies

Recently, researchers have developed promising techniques to enable prehospital providers to place endovascular or intercavitary devices to plug a shattered blood vessel or slow bleeding from badly damaged solid organs such as the liver, kidney, or spleen (Chapter 37). Examples include resuscitative endovascular balloon occlusion of the aorta (REBOA)[8] and ResQFoam[9] (Arsenal Medical Inc, Water-

FIGURE 35.4. [*Opposite*] A Navy corpsman fills out a tactical combat casualty care card after triaging a patient during a night raid training exercise at Marine Corps Base Camp Pendleton, California, May 19, 2016. US Marine Corps photo by Sergeant Xzavior McNeal, 11th Marine Expeditionary Unit /Released. Reproduced from: https://www.dvidshub.net/image/2625960/night-raid.

FIGURE 35.4. C Company, 6th Battalion, 101st Combat Aviation Brigade, provides rapid response medical evacuation capabilities from five sites across Regional Command South and Regional Command Southwest. The company's UH-60A Black Hawk helicopters are the primary medical evacuation platform. A MEDEVAC crew consists of two pilots, one flight medic, and one crew chief, with additional medical aid provided by a flight surgeon or critical care nurse on selected missions. Standard launch time from notification to wheels-up for an urgent patient is seven to eight minutes. August 28, 2010. Photo by Sergeant 1st Class Sadie Bleistein, 101st Combat Aviation Brigade. Reproduced from: https://www.dvidshub.net/image/313538/101st-combat-aviation-brigade-medevac-company.

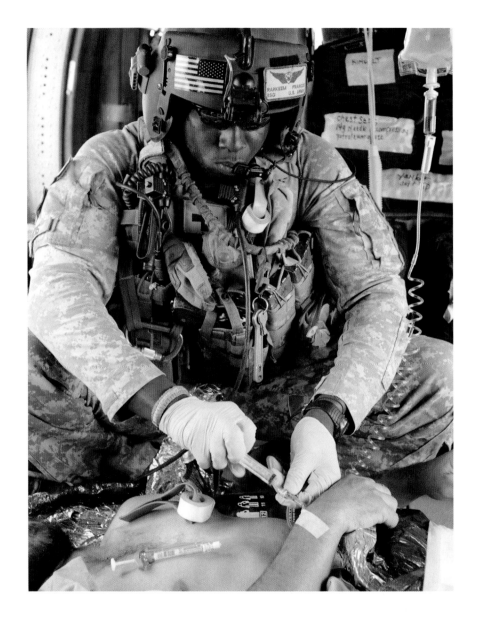

town, MA). REBOA requires inserting a large plastic catheter into the femoral artery, a major blood vessel in the groin. This technically demanding task is difficult to accomplish in a hospital emergency room, and would be even harder on a battlefield. ResQFoam is much simpler. All it requires is making a small incision to inject the material into the abdomen. Another product, XStat (RevMedx Inc, Wilsonville, OR), lets medics inject tiny sponge-like discs coated with an anti-bleeding agent into large, noncompressible wounds. Within seconds, the sponges expand to 10 times their original size, plugging the wound. These and other emerging technologies have great potential, but their use must be guided by clinical leaders, carefully designed protocols, and rigorous training.

Data and Metrics ("You Can't Manage What You Don't Measure")

The importance of data to support decision-making cannot be overstated. Data collection must start at the point of injury to inform both medical and non-medical leaders. The Joint Trauma System (Chapter 8) demonstrates the power of using data to inform clinical practice guidelines, protocols, and procedures, which can then be continuously refined and distributed in near real time. This is also the best way to inform and shape training to help warfighters survive battlefield trauma. Measuring performance improves accountability and helps systems achieve better outcomes. Continuous quality improvement is the only way to steadily reduce and ultimately eliminate preventable battlefield deaths and disability.[10]

CONCLUSION

We cannot afford to forget what we learned at great cost over the past 14 years of war. If we thoughtfully incorporate this knowledge going forward, we can avoid the loss of expertise and insights that followed America's prior wars. Better yet, if we embrace the problem-solving approach the US military applied to such great effect in Iraq and Afghanistan, and make it part of the ongoing work of the MHS, we can steadily improve prehospital battlefield care during the next interwar period and be better positioned to optimize survival in any future war.[11]

Notes

1. Eastridge BJ, Mabry RL, Seguin P, et al. Death on the battlefield (2001-2011): implications for the future of combat casualty care. *J Trauma Acute Care Surg.* 2012;73:S431–S437.

2. Mabry RL, DeLorenzo R. Challenges to improving combat casualty survival on the battlefield. *Mil Med.* 2014;179:477–482.

3. Mabry RL, Apodaca A, Penrod J, Orman JA, Gerhardt RT, Dorlac WC. Impact of critical care trained flight paramedics on casualty survival during helicopter evacuation in the current war in Afghanistan. *J Trauma Acute Care Surg.* 2012;73:S32–S37.

4. Kotwal RS, Howard JT, Orman JA, et al. The effect of a golden hour policy on the morbidity and mortality of combat casualties. *JAMA Surg.* 2016;151:15–24.

5. Shackelford SA, Fowler M, Schultz K, et al. Prehospital pain medication use by U.S. forces in Afghanistan. *Mil Med.* 2015;180(3):304–309. doi: 10.7205/MILMED-D-14-00257.

6. Schauer SG, Robinson JB, Mabry RL, Howard JT. Battlefield analgesia: TCCC guidelines are not being followed. *J Spec Oper Med.* 2015;15(1):85–89.

7. Schauer SG, Bellamy MA, Mabry RL, Bebarta VS. A comparison of the incidence of cricothyrotomy in the deployed setting to the emergency department at a level 1 military trauma center: a descriptive analysis. *Mil Med.* 2015;180:60–63.

8. Biffl WL, Fox CJ, Moore EE. The role of REBOA in the control of exsanguinating torso hemorrhage. *J Trauma Acute Care Surg.* 2015;78:1054–1058.

9. Chang JC, Holloway BC, Zamisch M, Hepburn MJ, Ling GS. ResQFoam for the treatment of non-compressible hemorrhage on the front line. *Mil Med.* 2015;180:932–933.

10. Eastridge BJ, Mabry RL, Blackbourne LH, Butler FK. We don't know what we don't know: prehospital data in combat casualty care. *US Army Med Dep J.* 2011:Apr-Jun:11–14.

11. National Academies of Sciences, Engineering, Medicine. *A National Trauma Care System: Integrating Military and Civilian Trauma Systems to Achieve Zero Preventable Deaths After Injury.* Washington, DC: National Academies Press; 2016. http://www.nationalacademies.org/hmd/Reports/2016/A-National-Trauma-Care-System-Integrating-Military-and-Civilian-Trauma-Systems.aspx. Accessed July 11, 2016.

CHAPTER thirty-six

Pushing Past the Limits: Strategies to Advance Resuscitation and Recovery

MATTHEW J. MARTIN, MD; HASSAN ALAM, MD; and JEREMY PERKINS, MD

FUTURE BATTLEFIELD, 2030

AN INFANTRY SQUAD PREPARES FOR A DISMOUNTED PATROL through an area of insurgent activity. Before departing, they enter a tent marked "Battle-Prep." The Soldiers have a narrow armband with a digital monitor placed around their right upper arms. While checking their weapons, body armor, and protective clothing, each Soldier drinks a small vial of liquid that boosts their tolerance to blood loss, protects their tissue against stress and inflammation, and enables the brain, heart, and other vital organs to tolerate reduced oxygen delivery for longer periods of time.

During the patrol, an improvised explosive device blast injures several squad members. Medics swiftly apply tourniquets and hemostatic dressings to stop external bleeding. Freeze-dried plasma, reconstituted with water, is intravenously administered to three injured Soldiers. The most severely injured one also receives an injection that slows his metabolism by 90 percent and modulates his body's inflammatory response.

Once the casualties reach a nearby forward surgical team, they receive biosynthesized red blood cells and platelets that don't require cross-matching. After the most severely injured Soldier undergoes damage-control surgery, he is given a reversal agent that slowly brings him out of his temporary state of "suspended animation." None of the injured Soldiers dies or suffers shock-related organ damage.

THE CHALLENGE

This scenario might read like science fiction, but many of the described advances are either already in the field or in various stages of research and development. The military is applying lessons learned in Iraq and Afghanistan to improve battlefield management of hemorrhage. These include widespread use of tourniquets (Chapter 10), topical hemostatic agents (Chapter 12) and tranexamic acid (Chapter 17), and balanced resuscitation with blood products rather than overzealous crystalloid infusion (Chapter 16). Several strategies to control non-compressible truncal bleeding have recently been introduced or are in development (Chapter 37).

Although these results are impressive, much work remains. Nearly 90 percent of combat trauma deaths occur before the patient reaches a fixed medical facility.[1] Nearly a quarter of these deaths are potentially preventable with optimal prehospital care (Chapters 11 and 35). Those who reach a medical facility alive have a 90 to 95 percent chance of survival. However, many of those who later die succumb to complications of severe hemorrhage.[2]

Figure 36.1 summarizes many of the concerns and limitations we face in countering battlefield deaths. Massive bleeding and organ impairment often progress rapidly. Critically injured troops often require blood products that are currently unavailable in the field, or they require surgical interventions that must be promptly performed (ie, started within "the golden hour" of trauma care). Maintaining adequate stocks of human-donor blood products in a war zone is inef-

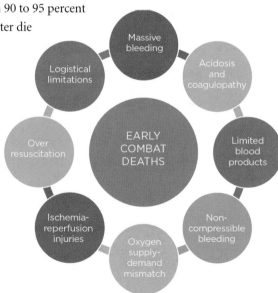

It seems that there will always be a surgery of war. This will contribute as much to progress as war itself. "

Harvey Graham

1939

ficient, expensive, and logistically difficult; it also carries a small but measurable risk of triggering a transfusion reaction or inadvertently transmitting a blood-borne disease (eg, hepatitis, HIV). Even when resuscitation is successful, reestablishing blood flow to badly damaged tissues can trigger a cascade of harmful or even fatal effects, known as "ischemia-reperfusion injury."

OXYGEN SUPPLY VERSUS DEMAND

This challenge of treating battlefield casualties can be explained in terms of addressing a life-threatening imbalance of oxygen demand and supply. "Supply" is a function of how well the lungs are working and how much blood is available to carry oxygen to the body's vital organs and tissues. "Demand" is determined by how much oxygen is needed by the brain, heart, and other vital organs, and how well these organs and various body tissues can tolerate lack of oxygen due to reduced blood flow. To date, nearly all of the advances in treating life-threatening hemorrhage have focused on improving the *supply* side of oxygen delivery: stop bleeding, replace lost blood through transfusion of blood products and clotting factors, and maintain an adequate level of oxygen in the blood. While bleeding control remains an important priority for research, next-generation advances in combat casualty care will also address the demand side of the equation (Figure 36.2). If novel therapies can temporarily reduce the dependence of the brain, heart, and other organs on high levels of oxygen delivery, it may enable injured warfighters to survive otherwise deadly injuries.

CURRENT AND PENDING INNOVATIONS

Freeze-Dried Plasma
Plasma is the liquid component of blood. It contains thousands of proteins, growth factors, buffers, antibodies, hormones, and enzymes.

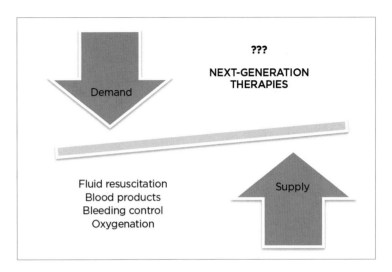

FIGURE 36.1. [*Opposite*] Concerns and limitations in countering battlefield deaths.

FIGURE 36.2. [*Top*] Supply and demand in advances in treating life-threatening hemorrhage.

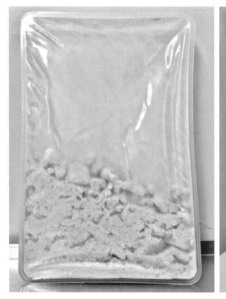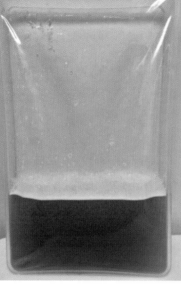

FIGURE 36.3. Freeze-dried plasma in powdered form (left) and reconstituted (right).

FIGURE 36.4. [*Opposite*] Biopharming process diagram.

There is ample evidence that early administration of plasma not only restores lost blood volume but also protects various cells and organs.

Fresh-frozen plasma is extremely effective, but it requires frozen storage, must be thawed before administration, and requires careful type- and cross-matching before it can be infused. This makes it impractical for battlefield use. Most of these limitations can be overcome by converting plasma into a freeze-dried, shelf-stable product.[3,4] Moreover, freeze-dried plasma can be stored for years and is easily reconstituted with sterile water when needed (Figure 36.3).

Surprisingly, freeze-drying is not a new technology. Freeze-dried plasma was widely used during the Second World War, but it fell out of favor in the 1970s due to concerns about hepatitis (and later, HIV) because it was made from plasma pooled from many donors. Modern manufacturing has solved this problem by using plasma from single donors who are carefully screened for communicable diseases.

Freeze-dried plasma is approved for clinical use in Europe, and it is carried by NATO troops and some American Special Operations units in Afghanistan. However, because it is not approved by the Food and Drug Administration (FDA) for use in the United States, most American units cannot use it. FDA approval would allow it to benefit US military forces as well as patients in civilian trauma centers.

Cryopreserved and Freeze-Dried Platelets

Platelets are another important blood product that reduces bleeding. Unfortunately, it has a shelf life of only seven days at 20°C to 24°C. This presents a difficult logistical problem for combat casualty care. Cryopreserved platelets (CPPs), stored in a special preservative solution, allow platelets to be stored for at least two years at -20 °C to

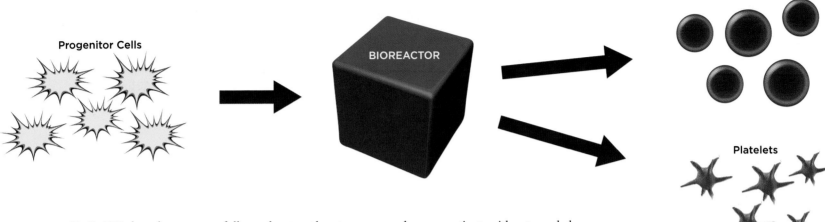

Progenitor Cells

BIOREACTOR

Red Blood Cells

Platelets

-80 °C. CPPs have been successfully used to treat heart surgery and cancer patients with extremely low platelet counts.[5–7] They are currently used in Europe, but the FDA has not yet approved them for use in the United States.

Researchers have also studied freeze-dried platelets. They retain much of their clotting capability, although other functions are lost during the freeze-drying process.[8,9] They also have a shorter shelf life than cryopreserved platelets. Further advances in freeze-drying may improve the function of these platelets when they are reconstituted from powder form. Hopefully, advances in CPPs and freeze-dried platelets will enable far-forward surgical teams to carry and use platelets.

Blood "Pharming"

This term describes the artificial production of blood cells outside the human body. The goal is to produce safe and effective blood products without human donors. Theoretically, blood pharming could produce large quantities of universally compatible blood products on demand.[10] The products would be created in "bioreactors" that generate the desired cell types (red blood cell, platelet, etc; Figure 36.4).[11] In 2007, the Defense Advanced Research Projects Agency provided startup funding to develop this concept. While this technology is not yet available, it has the potential to revolutionize transfusion therapy. In time, bioreactors might be scaled down and simplified to the point that they could become part of a combat support hospital's standard equipment.

Blood Substitutes

The primary function of red blood cells is to deliver oxygen to tissues. The protein that enables red blood cells to do this is hemoglobin. Over the last few decades, several pharmaceutical companies have tried to synthesize blood substitutes from chemically modified human or animal hemoglobin. The idea is appealing because a successful blood substitute could restore blood volume and enhance oxygen delivery without the logistical challenges of infusing banked red blood cells. Unfortunately, the results to date are disappointing. The first clinical trials of blood substitutes produced unacceptable side effects. A safe and effective blood substitute would be a major advance.

Advanced Hemostatic Agents

Soon after the terror attacks of September 11, 2001, the Department of Defense funded successful efforts to develop hemostatic (clot-promoting) wound dressings (Chapter 12). Since then, several products have entered the market. The current challenge is figuring out how to stop bleeding from sites in the body where a tourniquet can't be applied, such as a damaged artery or vital structure in the chest or abdomen. Efforts are underway to develop agents that can slow or stop this type of bleeding. Promising ideas include a self-expanding foam to treat abdominal injuries; a variety of vascular occlusive balloons (Chapter 37); special devices that apply pressure to blood vessels in the groin or abdomen; and a device that injects small, rapidly expanding hemostatic sponges into the cavity of a gunshot wound.[12-14]

Ischemic Preconditioning

Ischemia, the interruption of blood flow to an organ or tissue for prolonged periods of time, is very harmful. But it now appears that brief, controlled periods of ischemia followed by reperfusion can make the body more resistant to longer interruptions of blood flow.[15,16] Interestingly, these changes can be induced by brief periods of controlled ischemia in a remote tissue bed, such as the arm, not just in the area that later suffers injury. Perhaps someday this simple technique may be used to boost the body's tolerance to ischemia. However, we need more studies to determine the effectiveness, optimal method, and timing of ischemic preconditioning.

Immunomodulation

Sometimes severe injuries with blood loss trigger widespread inflammation, which can compound damage to cells and organs. We now know that humans respond differently to trauma based on their genes and how various proteins in their cells respond to shock. Once we better understand how these cellular changes occur, we may be able to design effective ways to protect against shock and its consequences. For example, we now know that administering large volumes of crystalloid intravenous fluid (once a mainstay in trauma care) can do more harm than good, while giving fresh whole blood and plasma is protective. In the future, we may be able to tailor treatments to prevent or reverse harmful physiological events (Chapter 38).

"Suspended Animation"

One of the most interesting and forward-thinking areas of research involves finding a way to dramatically reduce the body's need for oxygen so the body can better tolerate major bleeding. The ultimate extension of this idea would be to engender a temporary state of "suspended animation" that could buy time for surgeons to correct an otherwise fatal injury.[17] Although we are not close to achieving suspended animation, several research efforts are underway.

Potential Impact

In a landmark paper on causes of battlefield deaths, Colonel (Retired) Brian Eastridge estimated that one in four combat deaths are potentially preventable.[1] Most of these deaths were due to uncontrolled bleeding or bleeding-related complications. This observation prompted an unprecedented effort to develop a variety of devices, products, and procedures to slow or stop bleeding in the battlefield (Chapter 4). The next giant leap in combat casualty care may come from enhancing the body's ability to tolerate blood loss and other low-flow states. This may enable warfighters to overcome injuries that were previously considered non-survivable.

If one or more of these technologies works out, civilians will benefit as much as service members. Rural hospitals are generally not well supplied with blood products. The ability to keep freeze-dried products on hand, and one day have a blood pharming machine, would markedly enhance their capability to stabilize severely injured patients before transferring them to a regional trauma center. Emergency medical service units could administer lifesaving medications to trauma and cardiac arrest victims during transport to definitive care. Perhaps one day rescuers responding to a mass casualty event will be able to use one or more of the products envisioned in this chapter to decrease preventable deaths and save more severely injured victims. If and when this happens, it will be due in no small part to the painstaking work of Department of Defense-funded laboratories and military research networks.

Notes

1. Eastridge BJ, Mabry RL, Seguin P, et al. Death on the battlefield (2001-2011): implications for the future of combat casualty care. *J Trauma Acute Care Surg.* 2012;73(6 Suppl 5):S431–437.

2. Martin M, Oh J, Currier H, et al. An analysis of in-hospital deaths at a modern combat support hospital. *J Trauma.* 2009;66:S51–60; discussion S60–61.

3. Martinaud C, Ausset S, Deshayes AV, Cauet A, Demazeau N, Sailliol A. Use of freeze-dried plasma in French intensive care unit in Afghanistan. *J Trauma.* 2011;71:1761–1764; discussion 1764–1765.

4. Shuja F, Shults C, Duggan M, et al. Development and testing of freeze-dried plasma for the treatment of trauma-associated coagulopathy. *J Trauma.* 2008;65:975–985.

5. Barnard MR, MacGregor H, Ragno G, et al. Fresh, liquid-preserved, and cryopreserved platelets: adhesive surface receptors and membrane procoagulant activity. *Transfusion.* 1999;39(8):880–888.

6. Daly PA, Schiffer CA, Aisner J, Wiernik PH. Successful transfusion of platelets cryopreserved for more than 3 years. *Blood.* 1979;54(5):1023–1027.

7. Schiffer CA, Aisner J, Wiernik PH. Clinical experience with transfusion of cryopreserved platelets. *Br J Haematol.* 1976;34(3):377–385.

8. Fischer TH, Bode AP, Parker BR, et al. Primary and secondary hemostatic functionalities of rehydrated, lyophilized platelets. *Transfusion.* 2006;46(11):1943–1950.

9. Johnson L, Coorey CP, Marks DC. The hemostatic activity of cryopreserved platelets is mediated by phosphatidylserine-expressing platelets and platelet microparticles. *Transfusion.* 2014;54(8):1917–1926.

10. Figueiredo C, Blaszczyk R. Genetically engineered blood pharming: generation of HLA-universal platelets derived from CD34+ progenitor cells. *J Stem Cells.* 2014;9(3):149–161.

11. Zeuner A, Martelli F, Vaglio S, Federici G, Whitsett C, Migliaccio AR. Concise review: stem cell-derived erythrocytes as upcoming players in blood transfusion. *Stem Cells.* 2012;30(8):1587–1596.

12. Rago AP, Sharma U, Sims K, King DR. Conceptualized use of self-expanding foam to rescue special operators from abdominal exsanguination: percutaneous damage control for the forward deployed. *J Spec Oper Med.* 2015;15(3):39–45.

13. Biffl WL, Fox CJ, Moore EE. Re: REBOA and catheter-based technology in trauma. *J Trauma Acute Care Surg.* 2015;79(1):175.

14. DuBose JJ, Scalea TM, Brenner M, et al. The AAST prospective Aortic Occlusion for Resuscitation in Trauma and Acute Care Surgery (AORTA) registry: data on contemporary utilization and outcomes of aortic occlusion and resuscitative balloon occlusion of the aorta (REBOA). *J Trauma Acute Care Surg.* 2016;81:409–419.

15. Przyklenk K, Whittaker P. Remote ischemic preconditioning: current knowledge, unresolved questions, and future priorities. *J Cardiovasc Pharmacol Ther.* 2011;16(3-4):255–259.

16. Tapuria N, Kumar Y, Habib MM, Abu Amara M, Seifalian AM, Davidson BR. Remote ischemic preconditioning: a novel protective method from ischemia reperfusion injury—a review. *J Surg Res.* 2008;150(2):304–330.

17. Safar PJ, Tisherman SA. Suspended animation for delayed resuscitation. *Curr Opin Anaesthesiol.* 2002;15(2):203–210.

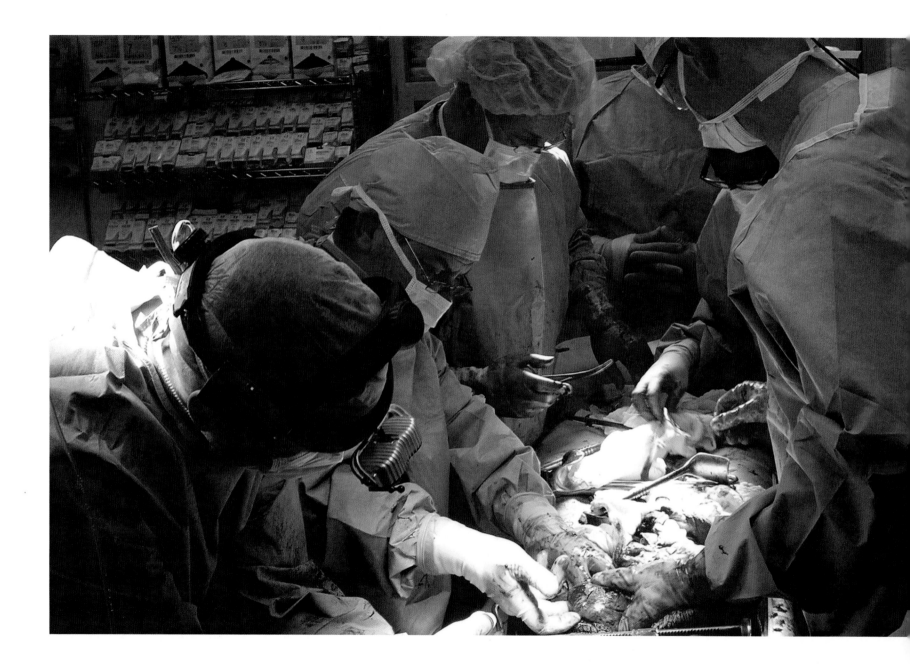

CHAPTER thirty-seven

Endovascular Control of Bleeding

JOSEPH J. DUBOSE, MD, and TODD E. RASMUSSEN, MD

BRINGING A NEW TOOL TO THE FIGHT

NON-COMPRESSIBLE BLEEDING REMAINS one of the greatest challenges to trauma care in war zones and civilian settings. While use of tourniquets has dramatically improved outcomes for extremity injuries (Chapter 10), it is far more difficult to control severe bleeding from damaged organs and blood vessels inside the torso. The traditional way surgeons attempt to stop catastrophic bleeding in the torso is by cutting open the chest or abdomen, and using one or more vascular clamps or applying direct pressure to squeeze the aorta enough to stop blood from flowing further downstream (Figure 37.1). This technique preserves blood flow to vital "upstream" organs, such as the brain, heart, and lungs, but stops blood from traveling further "downstream" to the abdomen, pelvis, and legs. This buys precious time for surgeons to make emergency repairs to damaged blood vessels and organs before the clamp is released and blood flow is restored.

Emergency thoracotomy is generally considered a procedure of last resort, and for good reason. Performing it can cause substantial bleeding and often results in long-term complications such as wound infection, nerve or tissue damage, or complications caused by prolonged interruption of blood flow to important organs in the abdomen and pelvis.

Seeking faster and less invasive ways to control life-threatening internal bleeding, surgeons have turned to endovascular techniques ("endovascular" means "inside the blood vessel"). Generally, the proce-

FIGURE 37.1.
[*Opposite*] Trauma surgical team at work conducting resuscitative thoracotomy and emergent laparotomy.

VIGNETTE >> Afghanistan, 2010. In a firefight with enemy forces, a 28-year-old coalition warrior suffered a serious gunshot wound to his torso. The MEDEVAC helicopter team that flew him to the closest combat support hospital placed a breathing tube in his windpipe and pushed intravenous fluids and blood products en route. Despite these measures, his blood pressure was dangerously low. Recognizing the Soldier was on the verge of death, surgeons took him straight to the operating room for an emergency thoracotomy. They swiftly entered his chest, cross-clamped his aorta, and rapidly explored his abdomen (Figure 37.2). This revealed the extent of damage. The bullet had shattered the left lobe of his liver,

punched holes through his transverse colon, damaged the tail of his pancreas, and disrupted his left kidney beyond repair (Figure 37.3).

Working as rapidly as they could, the surgeons removed the Soldier's left kidney, cut out the damaged section of colon, and packed his liver to in an effort to stop the bleeding. Despite their best efforts, the patient worsened and soon progressed to cardiopulmonary collapse. Although the team did everything they could to save him, including open cardiac massage and intra-cardiac injections of adrenalin, they were unsuccessful.

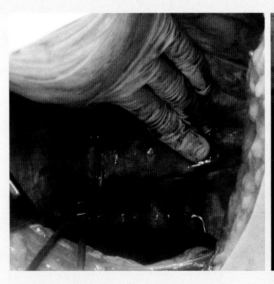 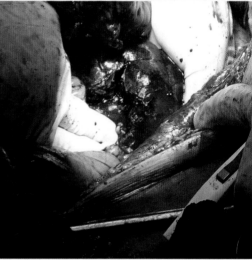

FIGURE 37.2.
[*Left*] Left thoracotomy showing clamp control of the distal thoracic aorta.

FIGURE 37.3.
[*Right*] High-grade renal injury requiring nephrectomy.

dure involves inserting a large needle into the right or left femoral artery at the junction of the patient's leg and groin, and then sliding a plastic sheath into the artery. Once the sheath is in place, doctors remove the needle and thread a long plastic catheter through the sheath upstream into the aorta. Once the catheter is in the right position, doctors inflate a balloon at the tip of the catheter to block blood from flowing downstream while repairs to damaged abdominal and pelvic organs and blood vessels are made.

The version of this technique that has attracted the most attention to date is termed "resuscitative endovascular balloon occlusion of the aorta" or REBOA. Like the surgical technique of emergency thoracotomy and cross-clamping of the aorta, REBOA is intended to temporarily stop blood flow to the lower half of the body while allowing blood flow to continue to the heart, brain, and lungs (Figure 37.4). A major benefit of REBOA is that it can be done quickly and much less invasively than cutting open the patient's chest to mechanically clamp the aorta.

REBOA has already been shown to reduce the risk of death from ruptured aortic aneurysm—a life-threatening condition in which the aorta literally springs a leak. Now, doctors are examining its use for treating life-threatening bleeding from damaged organs and non-compressible blood vessels in the lower chest, abdomen, or pelvis.[1-7]

REBOA has many potential benefits. Because skilled physicians can quickly thread a catheter into the femoral artery, it does not require immediate access to an operating suite. Using REBOA soon after

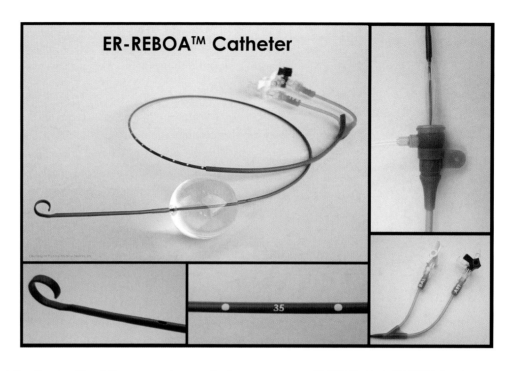

FIGURE 37.4. ER-REBOA catheter (Pryor Medical Devices, Arvada, CO). This integrated device does not require wire exchange, features external catheter markings that can be used to facilitate appropriate depth of placement, and possesses a distal arterial monitoring port for utilization. Image courtesy of Prytime Medical, Inc (www.prytimemedical.com).

injury can limit total blood loss and allow rescuers to infuse blood, plasma, and platelets to support the patient's heart and brain while preparing for major surgery. Because REBOA is much less traumatic than an emergency thoracotomy, it entails fewer complications and may offer the patient better odds of survival.

REBOA also has limits. While most surgeons and emergency physicians possess the basic skills to perform the technique, doing it quickly and with reasonable safety requires additional training and familiarity with the procedure. If blood flow to the lower half of the body is interrupted for too long, the patient can suffer widespread organ damage. Placement of a sheath in the femoral artery for lengthy periods of time requires constant vigilance to detect bleeding at the puncture site or clotting around the sheath that could shut off the blood supply to the affected leg.

IMPACT

In one recent study by the United Kingdom (UK) Joint Theatre Trauma Registry, researchers examined patients who had indications for REBOA after combat injuries. The researchers noted that one in five severely injured UK combat casualties had a focus of hemorrhage in the abdomen or pelvic junctional region that was potentially treatable with REBOA. Most of them bled to death before reaching surgery.[4] Based on these findings, the authors suggested the UK military explore use of REBOA to gain rapid control of bleeding and resuscitate patients during medical evacuations. In the civilian sector, a similar approach could help temporarily control bleeding from various forms of life-threatening trauma, including blunt and penetrating abdominal injuries and severe pelvic fractures.

The continued evolution of endovascular technologies promises to further simplify REBOA so it may be performed as soon as possible after injury. New devices may provide smaller diameter solutions and other innovations that make the REBOA easier and safer to do in austere environments and even in prehospital settings. This might significantly improve outcomes of severe, non-compressible hemorrhage in both military and civilian settings.

NEXT STEPS

Although REBOA is the endovascular technique that has garnered the most attention to date, it is not the only endovascular technique for treating life-threatening bleeding. Another experimental technique, known as "selective aortic arch perfusion," or SAAP, involves threading an endovascular catheter into the aorta and inflating it the same way doctors perform REBOA. However, instead of simply blocking blood flow, a SAAP catheter allows doctors to infuse medications and blood products into the aorta above the balloon so they reach the patient's heart and brain. This capability might be helpful in cases of extreme low blood pressure or cardiac arrest.[7] Another technique involves using a catheter to slide an endovascular stent into place. Once the stent is opened inside a torn or damaged blood vessel, it may slow or stop bleeding from the tear in the vessel wall while preserving downstream blood flow to important organs and tissues. While these techniques differ in certain respects, all offer promising ways to gain rapid control of bleeding from non-compressible vessels.

CHANGING THE FUTURE

In this chapter's vignette, had REBOA been available at the time the coalition warrior arrived at the combat support hospital, a surgeon or emergency room doctor familiar with the technique could have quickly performed the procedure. As soon as downstream blood flow was blocked by inflating the balloon, the bleeding in the Soldier's abdomen would have stopped. This could have prevented him from further deteriorating as he underwent damage control surgery (Chapter 15). At the end of surgery, the balloon would be slowly deflated and removed, while surgeons carefully watched the patient for further bleeding. Then, he would have been MEDEVACed a second time to a regional hospital, and soon thereafter flown by Critical Care Air Transport Team to Landstuhl, Germany, and from there to the United States.

The difference in the two scenarios? Early control of bleeding. By avoiding the need for an emergency thoracotomy, the patient would have required fewer blood products. Most importantly, he might have avoided sliding into irreversible shock and, soon thereafter, cardiovascular collapse. Hopefully, in the future REBOA and procedures like it will enable more military and civilian victims of massive trauma to survive their injuries.

Notes

1. Stannard A, Eliason JL, Rasmussen TE. Resuscitative endovascular balloon occlusion of the aorta (REBOA) as an adjunct for hemorrhagic shock. *J Trauma.* 2011;71:1869–1872.

2. Brenner ML, Moore LJ, DuBose JJ, et al. A clinical series of resuscitative endovascular balloon occlusion of the aorta for hemorrhage control and resuscitation. *J Trauma Acute Care Surg.* 2013;75:506–511.

3. Morrison JJ, Ross JD, Houston R 4th, Watson JD, Sokol KK, Rasmussen TE. Use of a resuscitative endovascular balloon occlusion of the aorta in a highly lethal model of noncompressible torso hemorrhage. *Shock.* 2014;41:130–137.

4. Morrison JJ, Ross JD, Rasmussen TE, Midwinter MJ, Jansen JO. Resuscitative endovascular balloon occlusion of the aorta: a gap analysis of severely injured UK combat casualties. *Shock.* 2014;41:388–393.

5. Brenner M. REBOA and catheter-based technology in trauma. *J Trauma Acute Care Surg.* 2015;79:174–175.

6. Biffle WL, Fox CJ, Moore EE. The role of REBOA in the control of exsanguinating torso hemorrhage. *J Trauma Acute Care Surg.* 2015;78:897–903; discussion 904.

7. Manning JE, Ross JD, McCurdy SL, True NA. Aortic hemostasis and resuscitation: preliminary experiments using selective aortic arch perfusion with oxygenated blood and intra-aortic calcium coadministration in a model of hemorrhage-induced traumatic cardiac arrest. *Acad Emerg Med.* 2016;23(2):208–212. doi: 10.1111/acem.12863.

CHAPTER thirty-eight

Optimizing Surgical Outcomes with Biomarker-Based Decision-Making

ERIC ELSTER, MD, and ARNAUD BELARD, MBA

BRINGING A NEW TOOL TO THE FIGHT

TODAY, SURGICAL MANAGEMENT of complex battle-injured patients (and complex surgical patients in America's civilian hospitals) largely depends on the surgeon's experience and judgment, coupled with limited laboratory testing. Relying on judgment alone disposes a surgeon to various biases, with foreseeable consequences, including potential undertreatment of some patients (who subsequently have bad outcomes), and overtreatment of others (leading to needless additional surgery, an increased risk of perioperative complications, and higher costs). With time and experience, clinical judgment improves, but it can never be ideal.

Military surgeons in Afghanistan and Iraq faced these dilemmas daily while treating wounded service members. Common complications after operating on combat injuries include wound dehiscence (failure of the wound to stay closed after its edges are sewn together or a skin graft is applied) and development of complex bacterial or fungal infections (Chapter 27). Both problems lead to lengthy delays to definitive wound closure, increased pain, nutritional setbacks, higher costs, and possible further loss of function if an amputation level has to be raised to save a service member's life.

Fortunately, the odds for patients may soon improve. Recently, Department of Defense and civilian researchers identified promising panels of biomarkers (ie, biological signals indicating the presence

FIGURE 38.1. [*Opposite*] Improving clinical outcomes and resource utilization through the implementation of clinical decision support tools. "Big data" refers to all available patient-specific medical data (eg, clinical, lab, biomarker, radiology images).

of disease or infection) and devised mathematical models that can markedly improve the accuracy of surgical diagnoses and improve the management of complex combat wounds. Through these clinical decision support tools (CDSTs), surgeons in the future should be able to achieve better outcomes at lower cost, benefitting civilian and military patients alike.

CLINICAL DECISION SUPPORT TOOLS IN CRITICAL CARE: THE FUTURE IS NOW

Spurred by two influential National Academy of Medicine (NAM) reports, *To Err is Human*[1] and *Crossing the Quality Chasm*,[2] the healthcare industry began to embrace CDSTs about a decade ago. Recently, another NAM "quality chasm" report, titled *Improving Diagnosis in Health Care*,[3] called for the healthcare sector to accelerate adoption and deployment of CDSTs. But adoption has been slow.

CDSTs are broadly defined as computer applications that analyze data to help surgeons and other healthcare providers make better treatment decisions. These "active knowledge" systems analyze huge amounts of clinical data to generate patient-specific advice. CDSTs can take many forms and are already being used across the healthcare landscape to enhance patient safety, reduce medical errors, optimize treatment, and improve outcomes. Such tools include the National Surgical Quality Improvement Program Risk Calculator, which predicts the risk of postoperative complications, and the Acute Physiology and Chronic Health Evaluation (APACHE) score, which assesses the severity of illness for adult patients admitted to intensive care units. Although helpful, these predictors rely on limited physiological data to generate broad risk predictions.

Nowhere is the accuracy and timeliness of diagnoses and clinical decisions more important than in surgical management and critical care, where making correct decisions directly impacts the odds of recovery or death. Using a patient's biomarkers to drive the timing and nature of treatment is an example of "precision medicine," which tailors an individual's treatment to their personal biology and physical characteristics, as opposed to estimating the best course of management based on clinical judgment and population-level data. In surgical care, employing a personalized approach means using biomarkers and other clinical data that signal the patient's physical status to determine the optimal time to operate or perform other interventions. This reduces the risk of an incorrect diagnosis, suboptimal care, and, as a result, poor outcomes and higher costs.

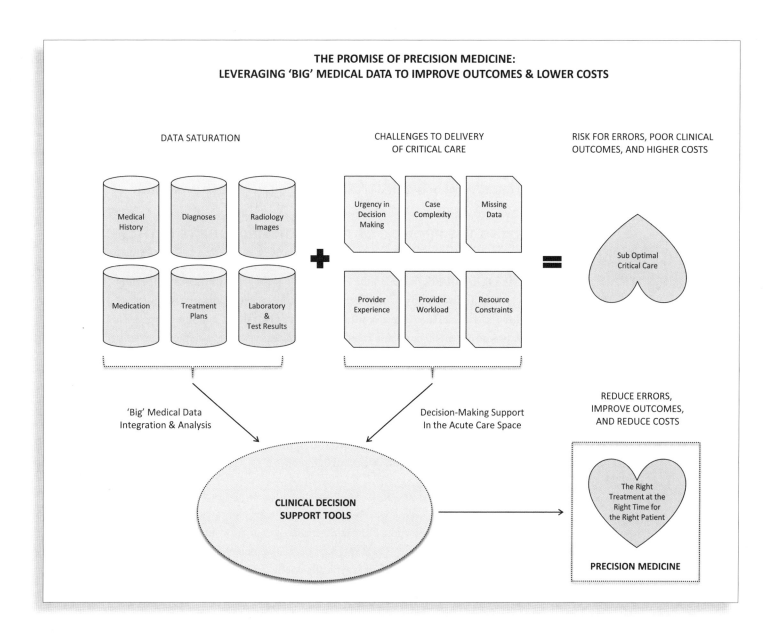

THE PROMISE OF PRECISION MEDICINE:
LEVERAGING 'BIG' MEDICAL DATA TO IMPROVE OUTCOMES & LOWER COSTS

DATA SATURATION

CHALLENGES TO DELIVERY
OF CRITICAL CARE

RISK FOR ERRORS, POOR CLINICAL
OUTCOMES, AND HIGHER COSTS

Medical History

Diagnoses

Radiology Images

Medication

Treatment Plans

Laboratory & Test Results

Urgency in Decision Making

Case Complexity

Missing Data

Provider Experience

Provider Workload

Resource Constraints

Sub Optimal Critical Care

'Big' Medical Data Integration & Analysis

Decision-Making Support In the Acute Care Space

REDUCE ERRORS, IMPROVE OUTCOMES, AND REDUCE COSTS

CLINICAL DECISION SUPPORT TOOLS

The Right Treatment at the Right Time for the Right Patient

PRECISION MEDICINE

CDSTs therefore have the potential to produce better care at lower cost through accurate, patient-specific diagnoses and interventions. In an era dominated by data saturation, which can increase the risk of diagnostic errors, CDSTs are designed to leverage and interpret all available medical data to support complex decision-making (Figure 38.1).

The use of CDSTs in emergency departments and acute surgical units has thus far been limited to routine analysis of clinical, physiological, and laboratory data. More advanced use of biomarker panels to enhance the predictive power of clinical algorithms remains infrequent. Leveraging all available medical data to derive truly individualized diagnoses and therapies is the next step.

REALIZING THE PROMISE OF PRECISION MEDICINE IN CRITICAL CARE

If precision medicine using CDSTs is done right, it should enable military surgeons and other healthcare providers to deliver the right care to the right patient at the right time. This is the goal of the Surgical Critical Care Initiative (SC2i),[4] a consortium of federal and non-federal entities established to develop biomarker-driven CDSTs to improve the treatment of critically ill and injured patients. Starting with legacy data from over 300 combat-wounded patients, this research collaboration, which is based at the Uniformed Services University of the Health Sciences in Bethesda, Maryland, is enrolling patients across several military and civilian trauma centers and leveraging a growing bank of aggregated clinical and biomarker data to develop clinical decision support models.

Currently, SC2i is focusing on two challenges important to combat surgeons: (1) identifying patients at increased risk of developing invasive fungal wound infections, and (2) timing the closure of traumatic amputations to minimize the risk of wound dehiscence.

1. **Invasive fungal wound infections.** Confronted with a surge of invasive fungal infections during Operation Enduring Freedom, SC2i spearheaded the development of a CDST to help identify and treat this serious complication. Fungal infections of combat wounds are a dreaded complication, traditionally associated with a higher risk of death (~8 percent in the combat wounded), suffering, and disability. Managing this disease typically entails an increased likelihood of bacterial co-infections, serial surgeries to remove dead and diseased tissue, and amputation revisions.

2. **Closing complex wounds.** A second model that uses clinical and biomarker data from patients is being developed to predict the optimal time to close complex wounds from combat or civilian trauma. Grounded in research on datasets from civilian as well as military patients, this CDST model is expected to reduce wound dehiscence rates to 5 percent from the current rate of 15 percent. Achieving this goal will produce multiple benefits, including decreased pain, fewer complications, better outcomes, and lower net costs. It should also increase the likelihood that a severely injured warfighter can eventually return to duty.

HOW CLINICAL DECISION SUPPORT TOOLS BENEFIT THE MILITARY HEALTH SYSTEM

Over the recent conflicts, the military has significantly reduced battlefield death rates by improving vehicles, body armor, and other protective equipment (Chapter 9); point-of-injury care (including use of tourniquets and other techniques of Tactical Combat Casualty Care, Chapters 10 and 11); and systems such as MEDEVAC, Critical Care Air Transport Teams, and the Joint Trauma System (Chapters 8, 13, 23, and 25). The higher battlefield survival rates these innovations produced challenged military surgeons, critical care nurses, and other healthcare providers to rapidly improve their capacity and skill at treating severely injured service members who would not have reached the hospital alive in earlier conflicts. During Operations Enduring Freedom, Iraqi Freedom, and New Dawn (OEF/OIF/OND), the surgical management of these patients was largely informed by the surgical team's clinical experience, backed by pattern recognition. The last 14 years of conflict produced substantial numbers of critically wounded service men and women, many of whom sustained systemic polytrauma, mangled extremities, and/or traumatic amputations from blasts.[5] The result was surgical complication rates of 15 to 20 percent, similar to those seen in contemporary civilian hospitals and surgical populations.[6] Future deployment of CDSTs should help military surgeons better manage such injuries.

Return to function of severely wounded service members has been a US military priority since World War II. But only half the survivors in the recent conflicts returned to duty because so many suffered severe extremity injuries. We believe applying precision medicine to their operative and postoperative management will boost this figure and contribute to more efficient stewardship of healthcare resources in combat zones and worldwide. Every dollar spent on healthcare comes out of the Department of

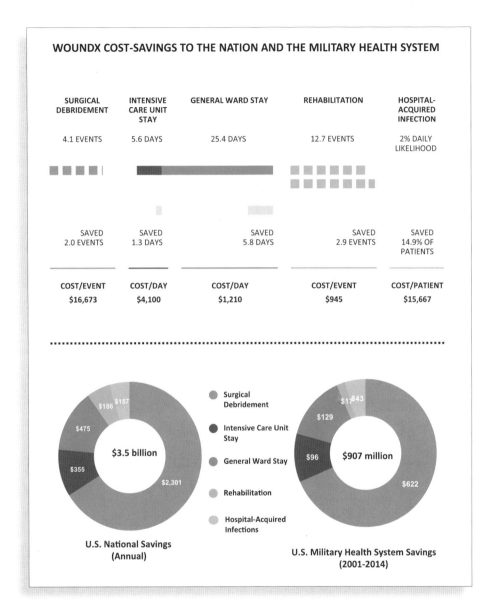

WOUNDX COST-SAVINGS TO THE NATION AND THE MILITARY HEALTH SYSTEM

SURGICAL DEBRIDEMENT	INTENSIVE CARE UNIT STAY	GENERAL WARD STAY	REHABILITATION	HOSPITAL-ACQUIRED INFECTION
4.1 EVENTS	5.6 DAYS	25.4 DAYS	12.7 EVENTS	2% DAILY LIKELIHOOD
SAVED 2.0 EVENTS	SAVED 1.3 DAYS	SAVED 5.8 DAYS	SAVED 2.9 EVENTS	SAVED 14.9% OF PATIENTS
COST/EVENT $16,673	COST/DAY $4,100	COST/DAY $1,210	COST/EVENT $945	COST/PATIENT $15,667

$3.5 billion

- Surgical Debridement
- Intensive Care Unit Stay
- General Ward Stay
- Rehabilitation
- Hospital-Acquired Infections

$186 $157 $475 $355 $2,301

U.S. National Savings (Annual)

$907 million

$17 $43 $129 $96 $622

U.S. Military Health System Savings (2001-2014)

Defense's budget to support our forces. The cost of treating complex extremity injuries incurred during OIF and OEF was so substantial, it accounted for 65 percent of total inpatient resource spending and 64 percent of projected disability costs. In the future, CDSTs may play a pivotal role in improving outcomes *and* reducing healthcare costs.

In a pilot test, the SC2i developed a robust evaluation of the potential cost savings associated with correctly timing the closure of complex traumatic extremity wounds, whether sustained in combat or on America's highways.[7] The estimate was based on a thorough medical and public policy review of 200 peer-reviewed articles and reports, and a survey of 24 US hospitals. Based on the findings, widely implementing CDSTs could substantially reduce the need for repeated surgeries and shorten the average hospital stay. Had this tool been available early during OEF/OIF (from 2001 to 2004), it might have saved the Military Health System (MHS) more than $870 million (Figure 38.2). Achieving comparable savings in the much larger civilian sector could amount to $3.4 billion saved annually, or roughly $50,000 per patient. This illustrates the power of improved clinical decision making.

FIGURE 38.2. Resource impact of implementing a clinical decision support tool for timing of wound closure using WounDX (DecisionQ, Arlington, VA).

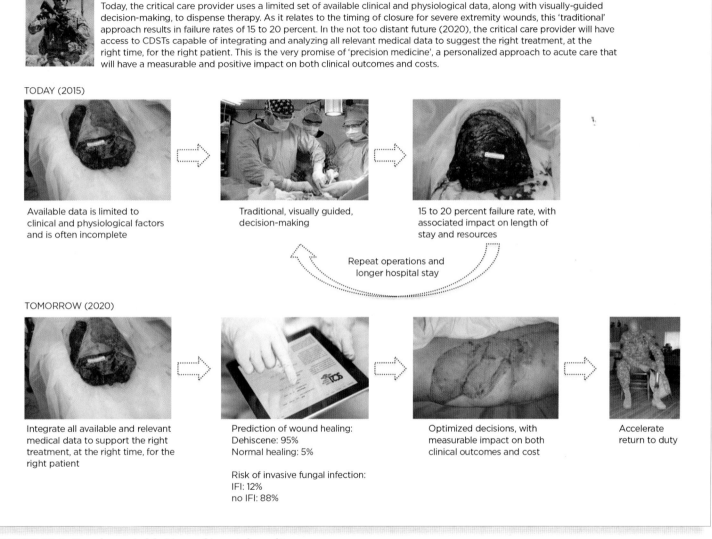

Clinical Decision Support Tools and Combat Casualty Care: Realizing the Promise of Precision Medicine on the Battlefield

Today, the critical care provider uses a limited set of available clinical and physiological data, along with visually-guided decision-making, to dispense therapy. As it relates to the timing of closure for severe extremity wounds, this 'traditional' approach results in failure rates of 15 to 20 percent. In the not too distant future (2020), the critical care provider will have access to CDSTs capable of integrating and analyzing all relevant medical data to suggest the right treatment, at the right time, for the right patient. This is the very promise of 'precision medicine', a personalized approach to acute care that will have a measurable and positive impact on both clinical outcomes and costs.

TODAY (2015)

Available data is limited to clinical and physiological factors and is often incomplete

Traditional, visually guided, decision-making

15 to 20 percent failure rate, with associated impact on length of stay and resources

Repeat operations and longer hospital stay

TOMORROW (2020)

Integrate all available and relevant medical data to support the right treatment, at the right time, for the right patient

Prediction of wound healing:
Dehiscene: 95%
Normal healing: 5%

Risk of invasive fungal infection:
IFI: 12%
no IFI: 88%

Optimized decisions, with measurable impact on both clinical outcomes and cost

Accelerate return to duty

FIGURE 38.3. Complex surgical decision-making—today and tomorrow.

THE FUTURE OF CRITICAL CARE IN THE MILITARY

For the past 15 years, the NAM has mapped out an evolving vision for 21st century medicine that rests on the delivery of precise, safe, and cost-effective care. Next-generation CDSTs, processing ever-growing amounts of clinical data on individual patients, may play a decisive role in fulfilling the vision of precision medicine.

The MHS has a unique mission: to provide lifesaving point-of-injury and surgical critical care to those injured in combat. Using CDSTs that can intelligently interpret biomarker panels and other medical data to improve clinical decisions, the MHS will be able to deliver better care at significantly lower costs.

Today, the surgical treatment of 19-year-old Soldiers with severe blast injuries relies on traditional, visually-guided judgment. We know from recent experience that this approach is less effective and more expensive than data-driven decision-making. As early as 2020, we hope military critical care providers will be able to use robust machine-learning CDSTs to integrate all relevant physical, physiological, and biological data to reach an informed diagnosis and map a highly personalized plan of treatment. Hopefully, warriors treated in this manner will be more likely to recover, successfully rehabilitate, and return to duty (Figure 38.3).

American service members in harm's way deserve the best medical and surgical care American medicine can provide (Figure 38.4). Using comprehensive patient data to develop a personalized course of treatment can improve care and reduce healthcare costs. Recognizing the potential power of this approach, the federal government has made precision medicine a priority.[8] The Department of Defense is

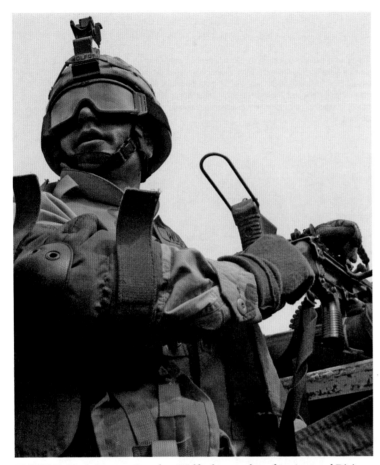

FIGURE 38.4. Sergeant Jonathan Wolford, a member of 1st Armored Division, checks on the crew of his armored personnel carrier during an improvised explosive device sweep in northern Baghdad, February 7, 2005. Photo by Sergeant Matthew Wester, 100th Mobile Public Affairs Detachment. Reproduced from: https://www.dvidshub.net/image/4144/sgt-jonathan-wolford-checks-crew.

uniquely positioned to harness precision medicine and CDSTs to improve the care and outcomes of combat-wounded patients.

Notes

1. Kohn LT, Corrigan JM, Donaldson MS, eds. *To Err is Human: Building a Safer Health System.* Washington, DC: National Academies Press; 2000.

2. Institute of Medicine, Committee on Quality of Health Care in America. *Crossing the Quality Chasm: A New Health System for the 21st Century.* Washington, DC: National Academies Press; 2001.

3. Balogh EP, Miller BT, Ball JR, eds. *Improving Diagnosis in Health Care.* Washington, DC: National Academies Press; 2015.

4. Uniformed Services University of the Health Sciences. Surgical Critical Care Initiative (SC2i) website. http://www.sc2i.org. Accessed October 24, 2016.

5. US Department of Defense. Casualty report website. http://www.defense.gov/casualty.pdf. Accessed October 19, 2016.

6. Forsberg JA, Potter BK, Wagner MB, et al. Lessons of war: turning data into decisions. *EBioMedicine.* 2015;2:1235–1242. doi: 10.1016/j.ebiom.2015.07.022. eCollection 2015.

7. Uniformed Services University of the Health Sciences. Surgical Critical Care Initiative (SC2i) reports. http://www.sc2i.org/research/reports. Accessed 24 October 24, 2016.

8. The White House. Precision medicine initiative website. http://www.whitehouse.gov/precision-medicine. Accessed October 19, 2016.

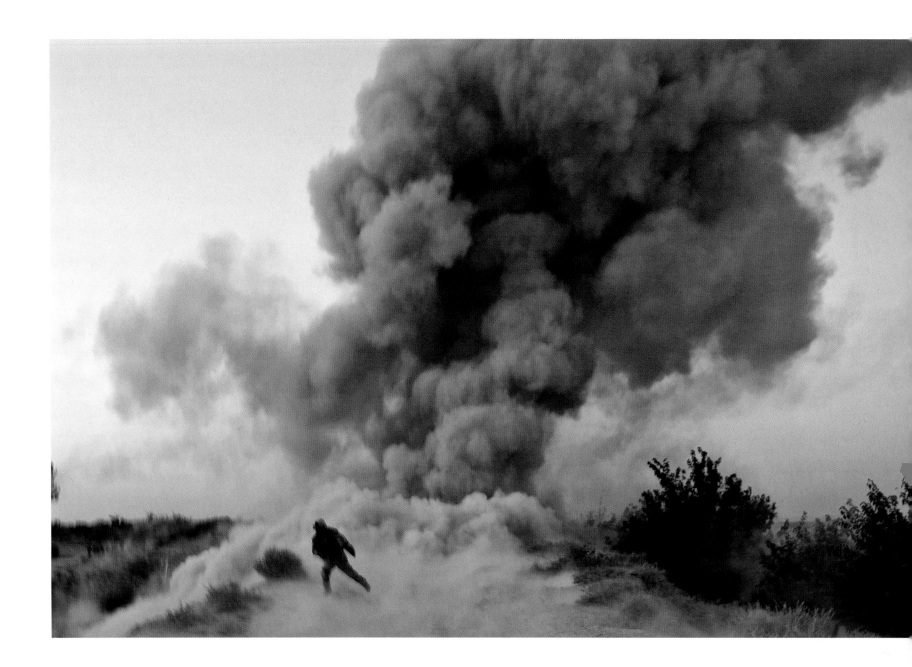

CHAPTER thirty-nine

Neuroscience

ALICIA T. CROWDER, PHD; JAMIE GRIMES, MD; and REGINA C. ARMSTRONG, PHD

THE PROBLEM OF TRAUMATIC BRAIN INJURY

ETWEEN 2001 AND 2015, MORE THAN 333,000 American service members sustained a traumatic brain injury (TBI).[1] The vast majority of these injuries—more than 80 percent—were mild. Nine percent were moderate brain injuries, and 2.4 percent were severe. One-fifth of these TBIs were related to deployment or injuries sustained in combat (Figure 39.1). The rest occurred in the United States as a result of car or motorcycle crashes, training accidents, sports-related concussions, or other off-duty incidents.

In most cases, a mild TBI resolves quickly without lasting consequences. But some brain injuries—particularly those caused by blasts combined with the intense physiological and psychological stress of combat—can produce complex, overlapping symptoms such as poor concentration, sleep disruption, fatigue, and headaches, as well as persistent problems with vision, balance, and hearing.[2] In addition, there is growing concern that sustaining several mild TBIs, or a single moderate or severe TBI, may increase a person's risk of later developing an early-onset neurodegenerative disease such as chronic traumatic encephalopathy or dementia.[3]

FIGURE 39.1. [*Opposite*] A US Marine of the 2nd Marine Expeditionary Brigade runs to safety moments after an improvised explosive device blast in Garmsir district of Helmand Province in Afghanistan on July 13, 2009. Two US Marines were killed. Manpreet Romana/AFP/Getty Images. Reproduced with permission from Getty Images.

FIGURE 39.2. [*Opposite*]
Map depicting the location and staffing of US military concussion care centers (CCCs) in Afghanistan, 2011–2012.

CJOA-A: Combined Joint Operating Area–Afghanistan
CRCC: concussion restorative care center
CSCC: concussion specialty care center
OT: occupational therapy
RC: Regional Command

Photograph courtesy of the Defense and Veterans Brain Injury Center.

MEETING THE TRAUMATIC BRAIN INJURY CHALLENGE

Victims of moderate and severe TBI require meticulous clinical care. This is difficult to provide in far-forward settings. Evaluation and treatment of mild TBIs in combat zones is challenging as well due to the variability of symptoms and the well-known tendency of combat troops to deny or minimize their symptoms in order to return to their units. While the desire to not let their teammates down is laudable, an inappropriate return-to-duty decision can put the injured service members and their unit at risk of further harm due to impaired thinking or function.

To improve the accuracy, consistency, and outcomes of TBI evaluation and treatment in combat zones, the Department of Defense (DoD) initiated a comprehensive research program during Operations Enduring Freedom and Iraqi Freedom (OEF/OIF) to improve the care of warfighters. It dramatically changed how warfighters are screened, evaluated, diagnosed, and treated in combat zones. Important developments included devising new guidelines for examining and treating patients at the point of injury and throughout their medical evacuation to combat support hospitals (CSHs), and the creation and distribution of evidence-based guidelines and clinical pathways to improve subsequent care. To advance TBI evaluation and treatment, the US military launched a sophisticated research program with DoD scientists and collaborating civilian partners in hopes of identifying important mechanisms of brain injury, and using these findings to create useful countermeasures to protect brain cells from damage and promote rapid and long-lasting recovery.

INITIAL IMPROVEMENTS IN CARE

In the early years of OIF/OEF, the services did not coordinate their approaches to TBI care. This began to change when the US Army Central Command established the Joint Trauma System (JTS) in 2004 (Chapter 8). Initially, the JTS focused on improving casualty care from the point of injury to a CSH in Iraq or Afghanistan and from there via Critical Care Air Transport Team flights to Landstuhl, Germany, or the United States (Chapter 25). Over time, data collection was expanded to include care at major military hospitals and Department of Veterans Affairs (VA) facilities in the United States. This regular process of collecting and analyzing data—from the point of injury through to definitive care—directly led to several important advances, including the adoption of patient management guidelines for deploying neurosurgeons (Chapter 19).

To identify service members with TBI, senior DoD leadership mandated a standardized approach to evaluating, treating, and tracking anyone who potentially suffered a concussion in Afghanistan. This laid the groundwork for event-based screening. To ensure that no one is missed, anyone involved in an event that might produce TBI, such as being in close proximity to an explosion, had to be evaluated. Those who quickly recovered were swiftly returned to duty, but those who did not received further care. This process reduced unnecessary medical transports while ensuring that those who were harmed got early treatment. Beginning in 2009, service members received standardized neurological assessments for suspected TBI, such as the Military Acute Concussion Evaluation (MACE) and concussion management algorithms.[4,5]

To consistently deliver this guideline-driven approach, the US military established five concussion care centers in forward operating bases close to areas of sustained combat in Afghanistan. Patients who needed a higher level of care than these centers could provide were MEDEVACed to concussion specialty care centers located at Bagram and Kandahar Air Fields. Over six months in 2011, the Army's four concussion care centers cared for 825 injured warfighters. The average stay was two to three days, and return-to-duty rates ranged from 94 to 100 percent. The Marine Corps center in southern Afghanistan treated over 800 warfighters, 92 percent of whom returned to duty (Figure 39.2).

Because moderate or severe TBI can cause life-threatening complications or lasting disability, these patients were transported to the CSH, and from there to higher levels of care. To ensure optimal treatment at the point of injury, combat medics, corpsmen,

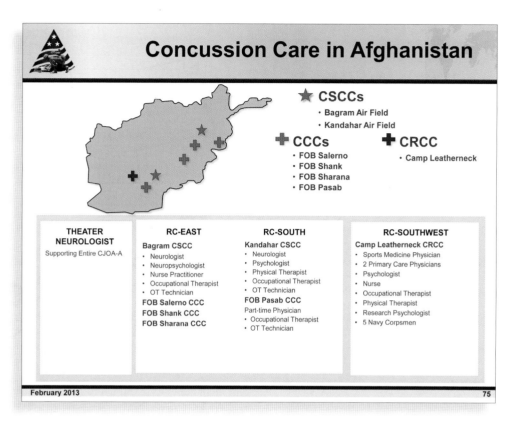

Concussion Care in Afghanistan

★ **CSCCs**
- Bagram Air Field
- Kandahar Air Field

✚ **CCCs**
- FOB Salerno
- FOB Shank
- FOB Sharana
- FOB Pasab

✚ **CRCC**
- Camp Leatherneck

THEATER NEUROLOGIST	RC-EAST	RC-SOUTH	RC-SOUTHWEST
Supporting Entire CJOA-A	**Bagram CSCC** • Neurologist • Neuropsychologist • Nurse Practitioner • Occupational Therapist • OT Technician **FOB Salerno CCC** **FOB Shank CCC** **FOB Sharana CCC**	**Kandahar CSCC** • Neurologist • Psychologist • Physical Therapist • Occupational Therapist • OT Technician **FOB Pasab CCC** Part-time Physician • Occupational Therapist • OT Technician	**Camp Leatherneck CRCC** • Sports Medicine Physician • 2 Primary Care Physicians • Psychologist • Nurse • Occupational Therapist • Physical Therapist • Research Psychologist • 5 Navy Corpsmen

February 2013   75

FIGURE 39.3.

Map of military traumatic brain injury treatment centers in the United States, 2016. Blue facilities are in operation; red facilities are planned or under construction.

ISC: Intrepid Spirit Center
NICoE: National Intrepid Center of Excellence

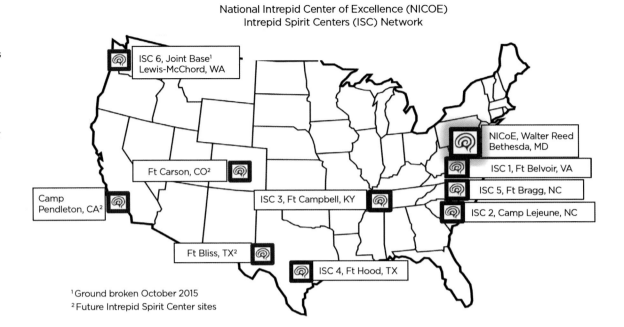

National Intrepid Center of Excellence (NICOE)
Intrepid Spirit Centers (ISC) Network

ISC 6, Joint Base[1] Lewis-McChord, WA

NICoE, Walter Reed Bethesda, MD

Ft Carson, CO[2]

ISC 1, Ft Belvoir, VA

Camp Pendleton, CA[2]

ISC 3, Ft Campbell, KY

ISC 5, Ft Bragg, NC

ISC 2, Camp Lejeune, NC

Ft Bliss, TX[2]

ISC 4, Ft Hood, TX

[1] Ground broken October 2015
[2] Future Intrepid Spirit Center sites

and flight crews were trained to follow evidence-based guidelines developed by military TBI specialists. Once these casualties reached a CSH, they received prompt evaluation, supportive care, and an immediate computed tomography scan. If the scan revealed a surgically treatable problem, a neurosurgeon was promptly involved. If life-threatening brain swelling developed (a common complication of TBI), a decompressive hemicraniectomy might be performed (Chapter 19).

Surviving a moderate to severe TBI is only the first step on the road to recovery. To help warfighters recover as much function as possible, substantial resources were put into improving hospital care and rehabilitation (Chapter 29). During the first decade of OEF and OIF, the DoD and VA created a national network of treatment centers and programs in military and VA hospitals (Chapter 29, Figure 29.1). Today, the Department of Defense is advancing research and augmenting the care of wounded warriors and veterans with TBI and other injuries through a national network of Intrepid Spirit Centers, anchored by the National Center of Excellence in Bethesda, Maryland (Chapter 29 and Figure 39.3).

ADVANCING BRAIN INJURY TREATMENT

TBI is an enormously complex problem. Over the past 40 years, major universities, federal agencies, and pharmaceutical companies have repeatedly tried and failed to develop an effective drug to treat TBI. To date, no one has succeeded.

Given the substantial impact of TBI and posttraumatic stress disorder (PTSD) on the US military, Congress has invested significant resources to advance medical research and development. In 2007, it appropriated $900 million for these conditions—two-thirds to improve clinical care and one-third for basic and applied research. In addition, the John Warner National Defense Authorization Act of 2007 directed DoD to mount the first-ever longitudinal study of the effects of OIF/OEF-related TBI on service members and their families. The Military Health System supports several organizations with complementary missions. Their efforts are closely aligned with the knowledge and capability gaps identified by the JTS:

- The **Defense and Veterans Brain Injury Center (DVBIC).** Previously called the Defense and Veterans Head Injury Program, this was the first DoD Center of Excellence to integrate specialized TBI care, research, and education in military treatment facilities and the VA healthcare system at 16 sites across the nation. Today, DVBIC supports expert healthcare providers, research assistants, and educators in a national network of affiliated medical treatment facilities across the DoD and VA.

- The **National Intrepid Center of Excellence (NICoE).** Part of Walter Reed National Military Medical Center in Bethesda, Maryland, NICoE was established through a partnership between the DoD, the Intrepid Fallen Heroes Fund, and the American public. NICoE focuses on complex TBI patients, defined as service members who have sustained a mild TBI and have compounding physical or behavioral health problems that are difficult to treat.

TARGETING TRAUMATIC BRAIN INJURY

By late 2009, the ongoing impact of traumatic brain injury (TBI)/concussive injuries on US and coalition forces was undeniably profound. Despite significant investments in research to develop prevention and treatment options, senior military leaders were increasingly frustrated with the lack of definitive treatment protocols.

At a Pentagon meeting led by General Pete Chiarelli, then vice chief of staff of the Army, and General James F. Amos, then assistant commandant of the Marine Corps, I was directed to devise a campaign plan to address the growing problem of TBI and its adverse impact on military readiness. Acting on their orders, I convened a meeting at a Silver Spring, Maryland, hotel with a small group of subject matter experts to determine a way ahead for managing these injuries. Attendees including senior scientists, clinicians, and medical operations specialists from both the Department of Defense (DoD) and several interagency organizations.

The product of this two-day meeting was a set of consensus clinical algorithms for the early recognition and care of concussive injuries. These event-driven protocols and associated training programs were quickly released to the force. Initial training was conducted at Fort Campbell with the 101st Airborne Division (Air Assault). When the "Screaming Eagles" were subsequently deployed to Afghanistan, they quickly implemented the newly-adopted TBI protocols. The division also established several concussive care centers (CCCs) for injured troops. The Marine Corps also participated in the preparatory training and established their own concussion restorative care center in Kandahar province (see Figure 39.2).

Two years later, while serving as the US forces surgeon general in Afghanistan in 2011–2012, I witnessed firsthand the benefits of standardized TBI training, clinical protocols, and CCCs. By this time, TBI prevention, recognition, and treatment protocols were widely implemented across the DoD. Additionally, deployed medical providers at remote locations could virtually connect with specialists during "TBI Tuesday" telemedicine sessions (see Chapter 24).

This technology enabled rapid professional interaction and expert consultation, becoming invaluable to improving patient care.

The development and operationalization of a standardized, evidence-based approach to TBI training and treatment showed immediate positive effects on force readiness. In a letter to Admiral Mike Mullen, chairman of the Joint Chiefs of Staff, then Major General John Campbell, 101st commanding general, proclaimed that the TBI training had improved his unit's health and avoided "more than 4,000 unnecessary evacuations" from the theater of operations.

Soon after we implemented our protocols, the National Football League, the NCAA, and other organizations reached out to DoD experts for assistance in creating similar policies to address concussive injuries in sports. As a result, our experience with TBIs on the battlefield has changed the culture of recognition and treatment, whether the injury occurs in combat, during a civilian motor vehicle crash, or on a sports field. This is a direct result of actions taken by military healthcare providers, military health researchers, and compassionate senior military leaders.

Richard W. Thomas, MD, DDS
President, Uniformed Services University of the Health Sciences
Previously, Director, Healthcare Operations, Defense Health Agency

- **The Center for Neuroscience and Regenerative Medicine (CNRM).** Also located in Bethesda, Maryland, on the campus of the Uniformed Services University of the Health Sciences, CNRM is a partnership between the university, Walter Reed, and the National Institutes of Health. It focuses on basic, translational, and clinical research to develop advanced diagnostics and new treatments for TBI, particularly those caused by blasts.

- **The US Army Medical Research and Materiel Command (MRMC).** Located at Fort Detrick, Maryland, the MRMC ensures that the DoD's research funding decisions address the military's priority needs. Working through various joint program committees, MRMC staff maintains close contact with military medicine experts in operational medicine, neurology, surgical critical care, rehabilitation, and other disciplines to address a wide range of military health problems, including TBI. MRMC research is performed at a wide range of laboratories and medical centers, including DoD facilities, civilian trauma centers, academic and university laboratories, and other sites. To minimize overlaps, MRMC coordinates its efforts with those of other federal agencies and congressionally directed medical research programs (Chapter 4).

MILITARY-CIVILIAN PARTNERSHIPS

Overarching guidance for DoD research comes from the TBI National Research Action Plan. Begun as an executive order in 2012, this plan directs the DoD, VA, National Institutes of Health, and Centers for Disease Control and Prevention to "improve the coordination of agency research into these conditions and reduce the number of affected men and women through better prevention, diagnosis, and treatment for TBI and PTSD."[6] The plan has guided several research consortia (listed below) to address major barriers to progress. Each program is linked with a variety of partner organizations that can be found on the websites listed at the end of the chapter.

- **TBI End Points Development Initiative.** Funded through the DoD as a collaborative effort with the US Food and Drug Administration, this program seeks to develop sensitive and specific ways to detect and classify different forms of TBI.

- **Chronic Effects on Neurotrauma Consortium.** This joint DoD-VA effort is dedicated to studying the long-term consequences of mild TBI in service members and veterans. The consortium is building a foundation to understand chronic symptoms and how to improve rehabilitation.

- **The NCAA–DoD Grand Alliance.** This DoD-supported prospective project with the National Collegiate Athletic Association and the military service academies is monitoring the incidence of mild TBI and return-to-play indicators after mild TBI in male and female college athletes.

- **Transforming Research and Clinical Knowledge in TBI (TRACK-TBI).** This research consortium's goals include creating a large, high-quality TBI database that collects clinical, imaging, genomic, proteomic, biomarker, and outcome data. TRACK-TBI is funded through the National Institutes of Neurological Disorders and Stroke and the DoD.

LONG-TERM OBJECTIVES

Devise Better Pathways of Care

The three services are combining best practices in a joint TBI pathway of care to optimize warfighter outcomes through the consistent delivery of evidence-based treatment. Just as the JTS advanced general trauma care in Iraq and Afghanistan, the TBI pathway of care will foster systematic communication and feedback to continue to improve treatment.

Improve Data Sharing

Centralizing TBI research data accelerates progress through data aggregation, secondary analysis, and comparative effectiveness research. The Federal Interagency Traumatic Brain Injury Research informatics system was established in 2011 by the DoD and the National Institutes of Health as a secure, centralized data repository.

Define the Neuroanatomy and Pathophysiology of Traumatic Brain Injury

A large body of evidence suggests that combat TBI and civilian TBI differ significantly. Understanding the pathophysiology of military TBI is critical to improving its prevention, diagnosis, and treatment.

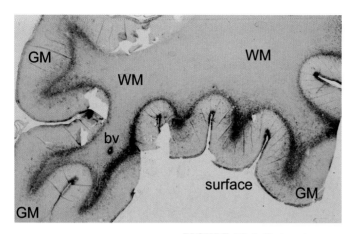

FIGURE 39.4. Postmortem human brain tissue section showing distinctive pattern of astroglial scarring (brown in cells) along white matter (WM) junctions with gray matter (GM), around blood vessels (bv), and along the surfaces of the brain. Photograph courtesy of Dr. Daniel Perl, Center for Neuroscience and Regenerative Medicine Neuropathology Core.

Brains must be examined after death to identify the underlying pathophysiology and inform efforts to improve imaging and biomarker measurement in living patients. To advance this work, the DoD established a brain tissue repository within the CNRM to study the damage that can occur during military service. This team recently published a landmark study that found, for the first time, a distinctive pattern of damage in the brains of service members who suffered TBI/PTSD after exposures to blasts (Figure 39.4).[7]

Develop Better Diagnostic Tests

Future advances in TBI care hinge on evolving objective scientific efforts to refine the classification, diagnosis, prognosis, treatment, and outcome criteria of TBI. For example, circulating molecules in blood samples might reflect the extent of injury or measure effectiveness of promising therapies.[8] Likewise, advanced high-resolution brain imaging using a variety of technologies may enable clinicians to see patterns of cell damage too subtle to be detected with less sophisticated tools (Figure 39.5).

Develop Effective Treatments

Despite promising pre-clinical data and, in a few instances, encouraging pilot studies in humans, every major drug trial conducted by industry and academic research teams to date has failed. To avoid a similar fate, the DoD research programs described above are systematically advancing capabilities that should increase the odds of success. One noteworthy collaboration is a partnership between researchers at the Uniformed Services University and Dr. Stanley Prusiner, a Nobel Prize-winning brain researcher at the University of California, San Francisco, who first hypothesized a link between tau, an abnormal protein that damages brain cells prions, and subsequent development of chronic traumatic encephalopathy (CTE).[9] Working together, they are screening and testing promising agents to prevent CTE by blocking accumulation of tau in brain cells.

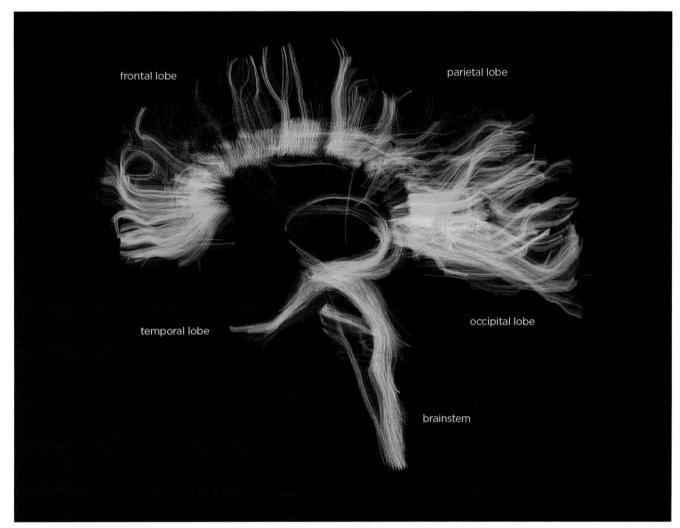

FIGURE 39.5. Magnetic resonance imaging scan with advanced diffusion imaging to follow nerve fiber tracts in human brain. Photograph courtesy of Dr. Dzung Pham, Center for Neuroscience and Regenerative Medicine Image Processing Core.

CONCLUSION

The conflicts in Afghanistan and Iraq have stimulated important advances in brain injury care, and many more are under development. As the military's TBI research continues, it will be important for researchers to recognize and respect the problem's immense complexity, and thoughtfully pursue promising leads. A "quick fix" won't work. Hopefully, in the not-too-distant future, the investments made in in TBI research will pay off, and this condition will no longer be a major cause of death and disability among troops and civilians worldwide.

Notes

1. Defense and Veterans Brian Injury Center. DoD numbers for traumatic brain injury worldwide – totals. http://dvbic.dcoe.mil/files/tbi-numbers/DoD-TBI-Worldwide-Totals_2000-2015_Q1-Q4_March-30-2016_v1.0_2016-04-14.pdf. Accessed July 12, 2016.

2. Halbauer JD, Ashford JW, Zeitzer JM, Adamson MM, Lew HL, Yesavage JA. Neuropsychiatric diagnosis and management of chronic sequelae of war-related mild to moderate traumatic brain injury. *J Rehabil Res Dev.* 2009;46(6):757–796.

3. Daneshvar DH, Goldstein LE, Kiernan PT, Stein TD, McKee AC. Post-traumatic neurodegeneration and chronic traumatic encephalopathy. *Mol Cell Neurosci.* 2015;66(Pt B):81–90. doi: 10.1016/j.mcn.2015.03.007. Epub 2015 Mar 7.

4. Brain Trauma Foundation. *Guidelines for Field Management of Combat-Related Head Trauma.* New York, NY: BTF; 2005.

5. Badjatia N, Carney N, Crocco TJ, et al. Guidelines for prehospital management of traumatic brain injury, 2nd edition. *Prehosp Emerg Care.* 2007;12 Suppl 1:S1–52. https://braintrauma.org/uploads/04/13/Prehospital_Guidelines_2nd_Edition_2.pdf. Accessed November 6, 2016.

6. Department of Defense, Department of Veterans Affairs, Department of Health and Human Services, Department of Education. *National Research Action Plan: Responding to the Executive Order Improving Access to Mental Health Services for Veterans, Service Members and Military Families (August 31, 2012).* Washington, DC: DoD, VA, DHHS, ED; August 2013. https://www.whitehouse.gov/sites/default/files/uploads/nrap_for_eo_on_mental_health_august_2013.pdf. Accessed December 16, 2016.

7. Shively SB, Horkayne-Szakaly I, Jones RV, Kelly JP, Armstrong RC, Perl DP. Characterisation of interface astroglial scarring in the human brain after blast exposure: a post-mortem case series. *Lancet Neurol.* 2016;15:944–953. doi: 10.1016/S1474-4422(16)30057-6.

8. Balakathiresan N, Bhomia M, Chandran R, Chavko M, McCarron RM, Maheshwari RK. MicroRNA let-7i is a promising serum biomarker for blast-induced traumatic brain injury. *J Neurotrauma.* 2012;29(7):1379–1387. doi: 10.1089/neu.2011.2146. Epub 2012 Apr 13.

9. Prusiner SB. Biology and genetics of prions causing neurodegeneration. *Annu Rev Genet.* 2013; 7:601–623. doi: 10.1146/annurev-genet-110711-155524. https://www.ncbi.nlm.nih.gov/pmc/articles/PMC4010318/. Accessed November 6, 2016.

Recommended Reading

Hinds SR 2nd, Livingston SR. Traumatic brain injury clinical recommendations: impact on care and lessons learned. *US Army Med Dep J.* 2016;Apr–Sep:97–101.

Web Resources

- Defense and Veterans Brain Injury Center (DVBIC): http://dvbic.dcoe.mil/
- National Intrepid Center of Excellence (NICoE): http://www.wrnmmc.capmed.mil/NICoE/SitePages/index.aspx
- Center for Neuroscience and Regenerative Medicine (CNRM): https://www.usuhs.edu/cnrm
- US Army Medical Research and Materiel Command (MRMC): https://ccc.amedd.army.mil/Pages/default.aspx
- TBI End Points Development Initiative: https://tbiendpoints.ucsf.edu/
- Chronic Effects of Neurotrauma Consortium: https://cenc.rti.org/
- NCAA–DoD "Grand Alliance": http://www.careconsortium.net/
- Transforming Research and Clinical Knowledge in TBI (TRACK-TBI): https://tracktbi.ucsf.edu/
- TBI Pathway of Care: http://www.dcoe.mil/blog/14-12-17/DVBIC_Director_Explains_TBI_Pathway_of_Care.aspx
- Federal Interagency Traumatic Brain Injury Research informatics system (FITBIR): https://fitbir.nih.gov/

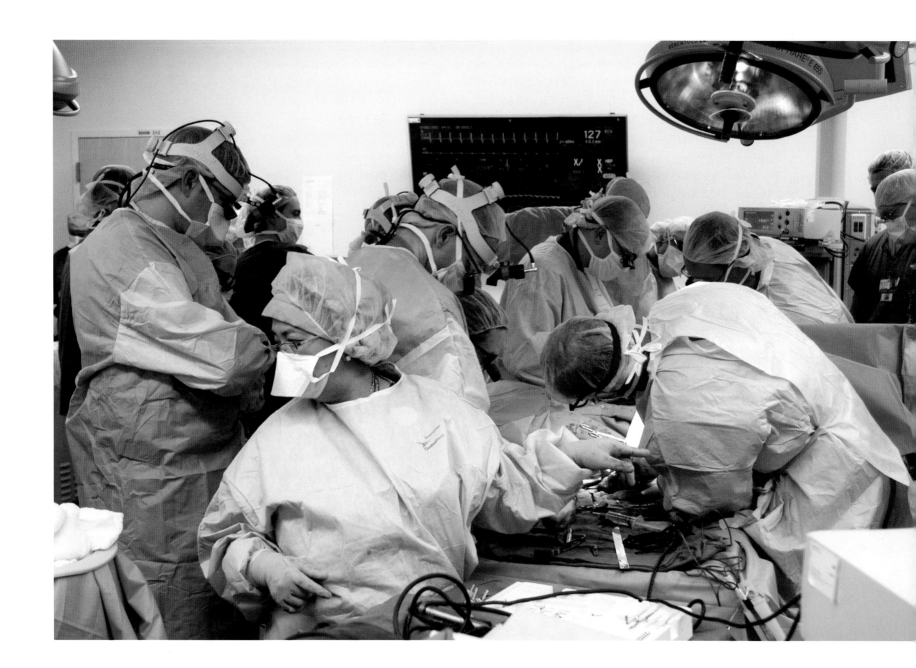

CHAPTER forty

Applying Regenerative Medicine to Battlefield Injuries

ATHONY ATALA, MD; JONATHAN FORSBERG, MD, PHD; and KAREN RICHARDSON

INTRODUCTION

THANKS TO ADVANCES IN BODY ARMOR, battlefield evacuation, and medical care, more US service members are surviving combat injuries than ever before. However, blasts and high-energy projectiles can inflict wounds so devastating that those who survive face daunting odds of recovering productive lives. Blast injuries can damage multiple tissues, including skin, muscle, nerve, blood vessels, and bone, and can involve severe bacterial and environmental contamination. Our surgical and medical responses to these patients often fall short. We need a new treatment paradigm, in which regenerative medicine could play a central role.

Regenerative medicine takes advantage of the body's natural healing ability to restore or replace damaged tissue. A multidisciplinary field, regenerative medicine brings together scientists from molecular biology, genetics, cell biology, physiology, pharmacology, biomaterials, and nanotechnology to collaboratively develop therapies that repair, replace, or literally regrow damaged tissue and even whole organs. Once considered science fiction, regenerative medicine is becoming a clinical reality. The Department of Health and Human Services has hailed the field as the "next evolution of medical treatments,"[1] and doctors have already implanted specially engineered bone, cartilage, skin, cornea, blood vessels, vaginas, and segments of the urinary tract into patients.[2]

[*Opposite*] Surgeons perform a double-arm transplant on US Army Sergeant Brendan Marrocco at Johns Hopkins Hospital in Baltimore, December 18, 2012. Marrocco, 26, lost all four limbs to an explosively formed projectile in Iraq in 2009. The Armed Forces Institute of Regenerative Medicine funded research to advance the techniques that made the surgery possible. US Army photo courtesy of Johns Hopkins Hospital/Released. Reproduced from: https://www.dvidshub.net/image/ 823929/double-amputee.

Congress and the Department of Defense (DoD) are funding research to apply regenerative medicine to battlefield injuries. DoD is the second largest federal funder of such research, providing almost $253 million (or about 9 percent of all federal investment in regenerative medicine) in fiscal years 2012 through 2014.[3] Much of the DoD's research is done by the Armed Forces Institute of Regenerative Medicine (AFIRM). AFIRM is an interdisciplinary network that includes the Army, Navy, Office of Naval Research, Air Force, National Institutes of Health, Veterans Administration, and DoD.[4] AFIRM's team, which is currently working on 60 projects, includes many of the country's leading regenerative medicine researchers. AFIRM is a "results-focused" program that funds scientific research and requires discoveries to be tested and compared so the most promising therapies can be rapidly advanced to clinical trials (see Chapter 4).

RESTORING FUNCTION TO SEVERELY TRAUMATIZED LIMBS

Improvements in body armor, which shields the chest, back, and abdomen, have enabled more warfighters to survive their injuries, but their limbs remain exposed. Typically, limb injuries include loss of muscle, connective tissue, and bone, as well as significant damage to the nerves that control limb movement. There is also a risk of developing compartment syndrome, a complication that impairs blood flow, further damages nerves, and can lead to muscle death—all of which increase the odds of amputation.

To counter these problems, AFIRM researchers are investigating treatments ranging from cell and drug therapy to tissue engineering and rehabilitation, hoping to help wounded service members regain as much function as possible after severe limb injuries (Chapter 26). A project that uses cells from a patient's own bone marrow to regenerate limb tissue has shown promising results in a pilot study and will soon be expanded to a clinical trial within AFIRM. Several teams are focusing on regenerating damaged peripheral nerves that control limb movement. Another team is developing a cell therapy to treat compartment syndrome. In addition, researchers are working to bioengineer small blood vessels in the lab that can be implanted by surgeons to reconstruct severely damaged limbs.

Of course, not all damaged limbs can be saved. For some amputee patients, the skin that covers their residual stump is not tough enough to withstand the pressure and friction of a prosthesis. To address this problem, military and civilian AFIRM researchers graft skin cells from patients' palms and feet to create a "tougher" skin. This technology, currently being tested in humans, could one day help amputees worldwide.

Another technique under development is to attach a prosthesis directly to the skeleton. This process, called osseointegration, could benefit hundreds of patients with amputations who are wheelchair-bound because they cannot tolerate a traditional, socket-based prosthesis. When metal protrudes from the skin, infection is the most common complication. However, researchers at the Wake Forest Institute for Regenerative Medicine, along with US military researchers at the Naval Medical Research Center, are working to reduce the risk of infection by engineering a better skin interface or by coating the entire prosthesis in living, durable tissue. This technology could be applied to patients who are consider-ing osseointegration, or have undergone osseointegration as an alternative to traditional socket-based prostheses.

FACIAL AND SKULL INJURIES

In Iraq and Afghanistan, head and neck injuries accounted for nearly 30 percent of all battle injuries.[5] These injuries are especially debilitating because the face is so essential to perceptions of who we are and how we relate to others. Restoring form and function to the face and skull can dramatically improve quality of life, emotional health, and job opportunities.

These injuries are hard to repair because they require replacement tissues such as bone, nerve, blood vessels, fat, and muscle. A variety of projects are underway to address this challenge, from "bio-printing" replacement bone with 3D printers to regenerating facial nerves and muscle. An AFIRM team is devel-oping an antibiotic-releasing porous material that can temporarily replace missing bone in patients with severe facial and skull injuries. The material can help prevent infections that often lead to multiple operations. Another treatment developed by AFIRM researchers that will soon be evaluated is designed to be a readily available, off-the-shelf material with properties similar to fat tissue. It can help recon-struct missing tissue without having to transfer fat from other parts of the patient's body.

SKIN REGENERATION FOR BURN VICTIMS

Doctors treat about 500,000 burns in the United States each year, with medical costs approaching $2 billion annually. Burn patients face multiple challenges, including infection, a tendency for burns to expand in size and severity during the first few days, and the possibility that the patient lacks enough unburned skin to graft onto their wounds. Imperfect healing can result in excessive scarring that leads to disfigurement and contractures.

AFIRM research aims to overcome these challenges and deliver treatments that will improve the outcomes of burned warriors and civilians alike. Projects with the potential to reduce scarring include a novel small molecule and topical application of a cholesterol-lowering medication. For skin regeneration, one team is developing a stem cell dressing, and another aims to "paint" healing tissue directly onto burn wounds. These treatments, which attempt to promote formation of new skin tissue, could help patients avoid the need for painful skin grafts, which involve covering the burn with unburned skin that is surgically removed from another part of the patient's body (Chapter 20).

NEW TREATMENTS TO PREVENT REJECTION OF FACE AND HAND TRANSPLANTS

Vascularized composite allograft (VCA) transplants are a new category of transplant donations regulated under the nation's organ procurement system. This category includes hand, limb, and face transplants from deceased donors. Unlike transplants of major organs such as the heart and kidney, which are life-or-death matters, VCA transplants are infrequently performed because of the significant side effects of anti-rejection medications, including an increased risk of cancer.

AFIRM researchers are working to develop treatments to ensure that the body does not reject implanted tissue. If they are successful, it will enable more wounded service members to take advantage of these life-changing procedures. The goal of this research is to develop strategies that regulate—rather than suppress—the immune system in ways that allow the body to tolerate implanted tissue. To meet this goal, research teams are evaluating the potential of stem cells derived from bone marrow, cord blood, fat, and other sources as treatments. These cells have natural abilities to modulate the immune response.

AFIRM teams are also exploring ways to assess the health of the transplanted tissue. If we can detect problems early enough, we may be able to act to prevent rejection. Several promising anti-rejection treatments are being assessed in clinical studies of hand and face transplantation open to US service members. Lessons learned through this program may be applied to other types of transplantation.

RECONSTRUCTION OF THE GENITAL AND URINARY ORGANS AND LOWER ABDOMEN

Pelvic injuries resulting from improvised explosive device blasts are often extensive. They often result in permanent urinary and fecal incontinence, loss of sexual function, and infertility. Current methods for repairing genitourinary tissue are far from perfect. When the urethra (the tube that carries urine out of the body) is surgically reconstructed with similar tissue taken from another part of the body, the rebuilt tube can become scarred and narrow. The result is pain, bleeding, and difficulty urinating.

AFIRM teams are working to bioengineer replacement tissue that can be used in reconstructive procedures to repair damaged bladder, urine tube, penile, and testicular tissue. In addition, a project is under way to restore penile function using a combination of stem cell injections and low-energy shock wave therapy. Also, 3D bio-printers are being used in an effort to recreate functioning testicular tissue that can be implanted to produce the male hormone testosterone and even sperm, providing function similar to a normal organ.

AN EXCITING FUTURE

DoD-sponsored regenerative medicine research has the potential to transform treatments offered by a wide range of specialties, from orthopedics and rehabilitation to transplant and burn surgery. Someday soon, surgeons may use bioengineered tissues to replace bone defects, repair damaged skulls, preserve residual limb length, heal burns, and even replace some severely damaged organs. Many of these treatments are already being evaluated in clinical trials. Some have already been commercialized. Work of this sort has the potential to change regenerative medicine from science fiction to reality, benefitting our troops and civilians alike.

Notes

1. US Department of Health and Human Services. *2020: A New Vision—A Future for Regenerative Medicine.* Washington, DC: HHS; January 2005.

2. Orlando G, Soker S, Stratta RJ. Organ bioengineering and regeneration as the new Holy Grail for organ transplantation. *Ann Surg.* 2013;258:221–232.

3. US Government Accountability Office. *Regenerative Medicine: Federal Investment, Information Sharing and Challenges in an Evolving Field.* Washington, DC: GAO; June 2015. GAO-15-553. http://www.gao.gov/products/GAO-15-553. Accessed October 19, 2016.

4. Armed Forces Institute of Regenerative Medicine website. http://www.afirm.mil/. Accessed October 19, 2016.

5. Owens BD, Kragh JF Jr, Wenke JC, Macaitis J, Wade CE, Holcomb JB. Combat wounds in operation Iraqi Freedom and Operation Enduring Freedom. *J Trauma.* 2008;64:295–299.

CHAPTER forty-one

In-Theater Research: Optimizing the Combat Environment to Continue to Advance the State of the Science

LISA OSBORNE, PHD; M. MARGARET KNUDSON, MD; and JOHN HOLCOMB, MD

THE CHALLENGE

MILITARY MEDICAL PERSONNEL STRIVE TO PROVIDE the highest level of care in every setting where they serve. Solid on-the-ground research is crucial to this effort. Historically, wars produce significant advances in medical care, and this is particularly evident in the last 15 years of conflict with the development of the Joint Trauma System (Chapter 8). Data-driven medical advances require scientific rigor and systematic evaluation of outcomes, which isn't easy in combat environments. The last coordinated research program amid combat operations was during Vietnam (40 years ago), and the process for ethical research activities has changed dramatically since then.[2]

When Operation Iraqi Freedom began in March 2003, there was no mechanism to ethically conduct and receive regulatory approval for research projects in combat areas. Therefore, individual providers created small clinical data sets while deployed in an attempt to review outcomes and evaluate care. As the war progressed, it became clear that a coordinated human protections research program was needed to protect privacy and to ensure that ethical standards of conducting research (known as the Belmont principles) were upheld.[3]

VIGNETTE >> Northeastern Iraq, 2007. Specialist Andrew Harriman was the first medic on the scene when a flatbed truck carrying 30 Soldiers blew up after tripping an anti-tank mine. Harriman deployed all 11 available tourniquets, saving many lives including one Soldier with triple amputations. Later that same year, Harriman himself suffered a gunshot wound when trying to board a Chinook helicopter. He was left to tend to his own wound, a severed bone and artery in his lower leg. By applying his own tourniquet, designed to be self-deployed, Harriman was able to stop the bleeding long enough to be transported by MEDEVAC helicopter to a combat support hospital for definitive care, thus saving his life (Figure 41.1).[1]

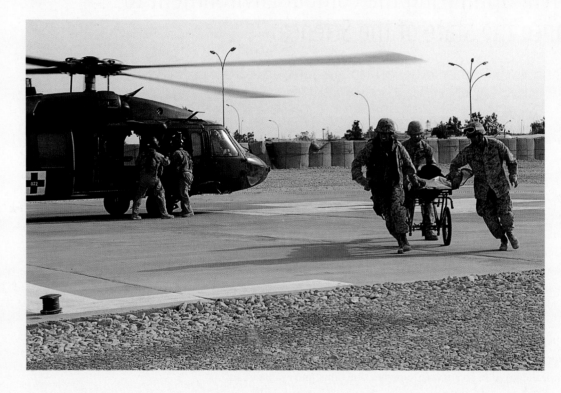

FIGURE 41.1.
Marines and Sailors with Al Asad Surgical, 1st Marine Logistics Group, work with the Army's 82nd Medical Company to provide expedient medical care and transportation for an injured Marine, March 22, 2006, at Al Asad Air Base, Iraq. Reproduced from: https://www.dvidshub.net/image/17491/navy-docs-focus-keeping-marines-iraqis-alive.

Developing a human research protection program for the combat setting is historically important. To establish this program, it was necessary to identify a way to review and oversee projects, and to identify individuals in the combat zone who would have official authority for these processes. As the Iraq war continued, research requirements expanded into Afghanistan and Kuwait. This landmark effort demonstrates that it's possible to conduct ethically sound research in theater, and emphasizes the commitment of military medical personnel in upholding the same high standards of research conduct and protections that are observed in the United States.

With the Human Protections Program in place in 2005, leaders developed a team of forward deployed US Army personnel to facilitate the review and conduct of research in theater. Since a mature trauma system requires research, the US Army Institute of Surgical Research developed the process and coordinated the selection and training of the teams sent to the combat zones.[4] These teams, working in combination with Navy and Air Force personnel, became the Joint Combat Casualty Research Team (JC2RT) (Figure 41.2). Working in regions where the US military "footprint" was fairly large—for instance, on the big NATO base in Kandahar—the team expanded as the number of research projects increased. Ultimately, 16 teams rotated into theater, conducting a wide variety of research projects.

LESSONS LEARNED

We've learned important lessons about the feasibility of conducting research in combat settings.[5] Due to austere conditions and constrained resources, only studies that would add to the knowledge base of care in a deployed setting should be conducted. Studies must be well designed and fully specified for conduct

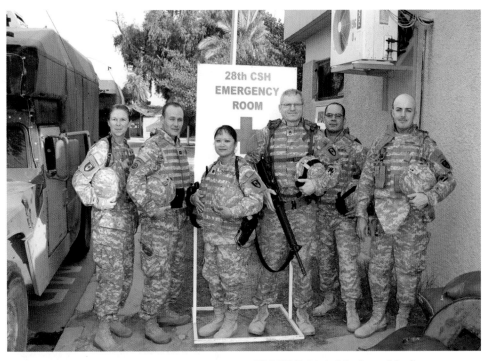

FIGURE 41.2. Members of the first Deployed Combat Casualty Research Team attached to the 28th Combat Support Hospital, located at Ibn Sina Hospital in Baghdad, Iraq. From left to right: First Lieutenant Michelle Littrel (research nurse), Captain Aaron Hildebrand (research nurse), Lieutenant Colonel Veronica Thurmond (deputy director), Staff Sergeant Timothy Wallum (noncommissioned officer-in charge), Captain Mario Rivera (research nurse), and Major Jeremy Perkins (director).

FIGURE 41.3. The Shock Trauma Platoon, operating with the Forward Resuscitative Surgical System, treated 40 service members and 10 civilians wounded in action, providing emergency treatment, stabilizing the patients, and forwarding them to higher echelons of care. Taqaddum, Iraq, February 25, 2005. Reproduced from: https://www.dvidshub.net/image/5955/shock-trauma-platoon.

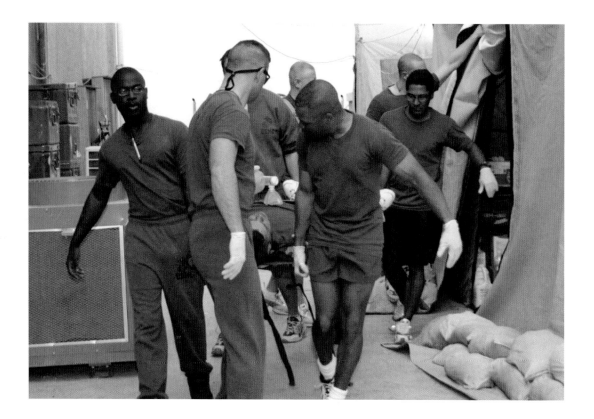

in combat regions. Exhaustion and limited resources can hamper the ability to develop such protocols. Unfortunately, protocols written by persons unfamiliar with the unique aspects of combat environments are generally fraught with feasibility issues, and often logistically impossible.[6] Therefore, recently deployed members are among the most successful in preparing research protocols that address timely topics with feasible methods.

Another important lesson is that the most scientifically rigorous study designs are difficult to conduct in theater because human research protection regulations require patients to sign informed consent forms before entering a study. It is difficult to obtain this consent from severely injured persons in emergency settings, and therefore most protocols performed in combat zones focused on collecting data, rather than intervening with treatment or mediciation.[6] In civilian emergency settings, a family member (or legally authorized representative) can grant informed consent. In combat settings, it's impossible to notify family members in time to obtain such consent (Figure 41.3).

Human research protection regulations protect patients, but they also can create hurdles. A good example is the inability to conduct research with devices or drugs still awaiting approval in the combat setting (Chapter 35). There are efforts to enable the Food and Drug Administration to approve these projects.[7] Such legislation would provide the opportunity to properly evaluate medical devices and potentially expedite the development of lifesaving monitoring equipment.

CONSIDERATIONS FOR THE FUTURE

The future of research in combat settings will depend on the Joint Theater Trauma System. Battlefield conditions and logistics of the past may not translate to future conflicts. For instance, if future conflicts involve a smaller footprint or prolonged evacuation times, planners must determine the best place to house researchers. Distant locations may require different methods of collecting data. Refining ways to remotely gather data such as vital signs with ruggedized devices is a priority.

IMPACT

The beneficiary of any war is medicine. Every conflict spurs advances in trauma care. The research teams in Iraq, Afghanistan, and Kuwait contributed to an ever-decreasing mortality rate on the battlefield.[2] Civilian medicine absorbs these lessons. For example, the liberal use of tourniquets in Iraq and Afghanistan saved many lives and limbs (see Chapter 10). Researchers and doctors highlight these important medical lessons at major medical meetings and through prompt publication in journals distributed worldwide.

We have noted barriers to conducting research on the battlefield. Civilians face challenges too, especially for funding. The Department of Defense is the major funder for investigations in trauma care, through its Combat Casualty Care Research Program (see Chapter 4). However, this is not enough, because advances in combat casualty care benefit victims of US street violence just as much as those injured on battlefields. The National Institutes of Health, which funds most healthcare research, should make trauma a priority. To prepare for this, the newly formed Coalition for National Trauma Research is identifying areas that are equally important in civilian and military trauma. This effort will be greatly enhanced by the formal partnership between the Department of Defense's Military Health System and the American College of Surgeons. These collaborations will guarantee that lessons learned on the battlefield are not lost for the next generation and that trauma care continues to advance in our country even as we confront increasingly severe natural and manufactured disasters.

Notes

1. Collier R. Wartime advances in trauma care are coming back to help civilians. *Ottawa Citizen*. January 2, 2015. http://ottawacitizen.com/health/men/wartime-advances-in-trauma-care-come-back-to-help-civilians. Accessed December 31, 2015.

2. Pruitt BA Jr, Rasmussen TE. Vietnam (1972) to Afghanistan (2014): the state of military trauma care and research, past to present. *J Trauma Acute Care Surg*. 2014;77:S57-65.

3. Brosch, LR, Holcomb JB, Thompson JC, Cordts PR. Establishing a human protection program in a combatant command. *J Trauma*. 2008;64;S9–13.

4. Blackbourne LH, Baer DG, Eastridge BJ, et al. Military medical revolution: military trauma system. *J Trauma Acute Care Surg*. 2012;73:S388-94.

5. McManus JG, McClinton A, Morton MJ. Ethical issues in conduct of research in combat and disaster operations. *Am J Disaster Med*. 2009;4:87–93.

6. Hatzfield JJ, Childs JD, Dempsey MP, et al. Evolution of biomedical research during combat operations. *J Acute Care Surg*. 2013;2:S115–S119.

7. The 21st Century Cures Act. July 2, 2015. http://docs.house.gov/billsthisweek/20150706/CPRT-114-HPRT-RU00-HR6.pdf. Accessed December 16, 2015.

CHAPTER forty-two

Human Performance Optimization

PATRICIA A. DEUSTER, PHD, MPH, and FRANCIS G. O'CONNOR, MD, MPH

INTRODUCTION

WARRIORS—ACTIVE DUTY, RESERVE, AND NATIONAL GUARD—as well as the families that sustain them are the most valuable assets of the Department of Defense (DoD). This makes their health and welfare essential to our national security. The heavy operational demands of the past 14 years, which for most families involved multiple deployments with limited down time in between, substantially strained our armed forces. It also strained troops' spouses, children, parents, and others close to them.

Recognizing the burden of frequent deployments, the DoD examined its approach to maintaining and improving human performance, resilience, well-being, and health. In 2006, a pivotal conference at the Uniformed Services University of the Health Sciences made it clear that the heavy demands our nation was placing on its warriors and their families were threatening their capacity to respond. The military needed a new framework to meet its operational needs without degrading the health and resilience of the Soldiers, Marines, Sailors, and Airmen it sends into harm's way, and the families that sustain them (Figure 42.1).

In response, the DoD embraced two concepts: human performance optimization (HPO) and total force fitness (TFF).[1] Both ideas recognize that service members' health and well-being depend not only on the individuals, but also on their families, the communities that support them, and the units that rely on their service. Today, the terms "HPO" and "TFF" are widely embraced as cornerstones of a strong, effective, and efficient military community, and are ingrained in the DoD as a holistic concept.

BACKGROUND

HPO, the idea that Soldiers' health and resilience are important for their success on the battlefield, is not new. Over the centuries, wise military leaders have emphasized many of these concepts, just in different words. Table 42.1 summarizes selected human performance efforts over the past 150 years.

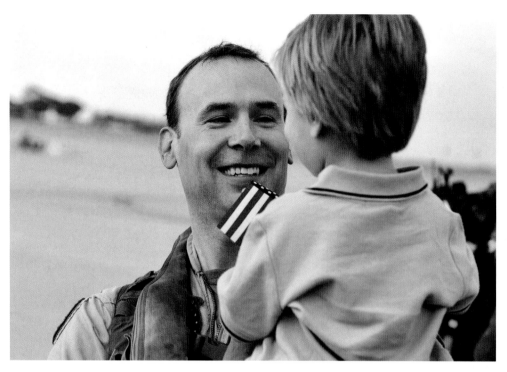

FIGURE 42.1. Navy pilot Jeff McGrady greets his son upon return from deployment, San Diego, March 19, 2011. US Navy photo by Mass Communication Specialist Seaman Benjamin Crossley/Released.

HPO emerged as a key concept in DoD doctrine in 2006, after a report by the Office of Net Assessment, the DoD's in-house think tank, challenged the department to look at how it prepares service members for the demands of modern and future battlefields.[2] In June of that year, Uniformed Services University's Consortium for Health and Military Performance (CHAMP) hosted a workshop called Human Performance Optimization: An Evolving Charge to the Department of Defense. The workshop's proceedings were subsequently published in a special issue of the journal *Military Medicine*.[1]

Viewed in hindsight, this workshop represented a tipping point in how the DoD views individual and family health and its importance for mission success. The recognition that warfighters (and particularly, members of special operations forces) are elite athletes stimulated efforts to optimize each service member's physical and psychological health (Figure 42.2), and strengthen family resilience. One result was the establishment of the Human Performance Resource Center (HPRC),[3] which provides warfighters and their families with practical tips on everything from improving their health and fitness to objective information on the pros and cons of various dietary supplements. Today, the value of HPO is widely recognized within the US military, regardless of the terms used to describe it (Table 42.2).

TOTAL FORCE FITNESS: HUMAN PERFORMANCE OPTIMIZATION ON A GRAND SCALE

Three years after CHAMP hosted the first HPO workshop, it was tasked by the Office of the Chairman of the Joint Chiefs of Staff (CJCS) to host a second workshop aimed at developing a holistic framework for enhancing the overall fitness of the force. This 2009 effort led to the creation of the TFF model (Figure 42.3). The CJCS quickly published formal instructions (found on the HPRC's website[4]) that extended the concept of "physical fitness" to include body, mind, social, and spiritual domains. It also created a comprehensive and holistic framework to support, integrate, and guide service-specific and joint efforts to promote health, enhance the resilience of service members and their families, and improve the efficiency and effectiveness of our armed forces (Figure 42.4).

The TFF framework is designed to keep service members and their families resilient and flourishing under the demanding conditions of military life, from training to deployment, during sustained military operations, and through their return and reintegration at home. In many respects, TFF and HPO are synergistic: HPO provides a framework for optimizing *individual* health and human performance, while TFF defines the desired end state for the *total force*. Together they establish a culture of fitness and health that ensures readiness,

TABLE 42.1. Historical efforts that should be considered human performance opportunities

1870	A French Army officer and military theorist, Ardant du Picq, stated, "The man is the first weapon of battle. Let us study the soldier, for it is he who brings reality to it."[1]
1866	US Army Major Jonathan Letterman, MD, stated that "the leading idea, [for the medical corps] which should be constantly kept in view, is to strengthen the hands of the Commanding General by keeping his Army in the most vigorous health, thus rendering it, in the highest degree, efficient for enduring fatigue and privation, and for fighting."[2]
1933	US Army General (then Colonel) George S. Patton wrote, "Wars may be fought with weapons, but they are won by men. It is the spirit of the men who follow and of the man who leads that gains the victory."[3]
1946	US Army General Dwight D. Eisenhower said, "Guns and tanks and planes are nothing unless there is a solid spirit, a solid heart, and great productiveness behind it."[4]
1987	US Army Special Forces Colonel (Retired) John Collins developed the Special Operations Forces five truths, including "Humans are more important than hardware and their quality is more important than quantities."[5]

1. Castro CA, Adler AB. Optempo: effects on soldier and unit readiness. *Parameters*. 1999;Autumn:86–85.
2. Opening the Army Medical School. *J Am Med Assoc*. 1893;21(21):773–774.
3. Patton GS. Mechanized forces. *Cavalry J*. 1933;42:5–8.
4. Eisenhower DD. Speech to Economic Club of New York. Presented at: Economic Club of New York; November 20, 1946; New York, NY.
5. Collins JM. US Special Operations: personal opinions. *Small Wars J*. December 13, 2008. http://smallwarsjournal.com/jrnl/art/us-special-operations-personal-opinions. Accessed October 25, 2016.

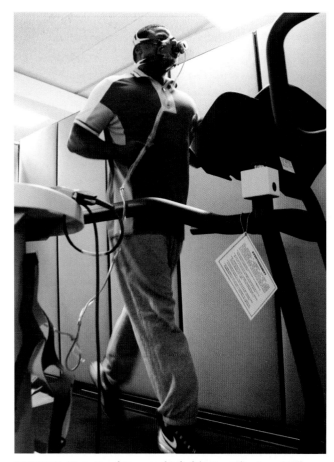

FIGURE 42.2. Daryl Stevens, chief of the Fort Bliss Army Wellness Center, William Beaumont Army Medical Center, demonstrates a volume of oxygen (VO2), or maximal oxygen uptake, test, which measures how efficient your body is with oxygen while you exercise. August 2, 2016. Photo by Marcy Sanchez, William Beaumont Army Medical Center Public Affairs Office (https://www.dvidshub.net/image/2808314/awc-offers-common-sense-approach-improving-health).

promotes resilience, and maintains the strength of our service members and the families and communities that sustain them (Figure 42.5).

TFF can be conceptualized as a web of healthy relationships that contribute to optimal family, community, and unit well-being. However, any assessment of TFF must be context-specific, because teams, units, families, and communities may be effective at certain tasks but ineffective at others. For example, a military unit may accomplish its mission while deployed, but lose its cohesion, fitness, and health after returning from deployment and reintegrating with its supporting community.

THE IMPORTANCE OF SOCIAL FITNESS

The TFF framework encompasses eight mind–body domains (see Figure 42.3). Although all are important, social fitness may be most critical.[5] This finding was underscored in a 2013 RAND report, *Social Fitness and Resilience: A Review of Relevant Constructs, Measures, and Links to Well-Being.*[6] The report identified social support as a key influencer of individual and unit resilience. Social fitness is equally important for family, peer, and community well-being—key signatures of strong military culture and operational success.

THE HUMAN PERFORMANCE OPTIMIZATION DEMANDS/RESOURCE MODEL

Military life requires service members to perform highly demanding tasks, sometimes with little or no notice. To enhance their ability to succeed, the demands/resources model was developed as an organizing framework for HPO.[7,8] The left panel of Figure 42.6 shows how resources and demands interact to influence performance outcomes.[9] Between deployments, service members draw on multiple resources (eg, individual, family, community, and external environment) to rest, recover, and meet personal, community, and organizational demands. Performance is best when individual, family, and external resources match or exceed these demands.

The right panel of Figure 42.6 summarizes factors that serve as resources or demands. Although some are intrinsic to the individual (eg, built-in, wired), others are situation-dependent. For example, a healthy family life is a valuable source of strength and resilience, but chronic or escalating family discord can place substantial strain on a service member and ultimately compromise his or her performance. The DoD offers numerous resources to help warfighters and their families identify and mitigate demands.

Mental techniques and down time are valuable resources. Herzog and Deuster[10] described two specific mental skills that can improve performance and augment psychological fitness: (1) goal-setting and (2) mental imagery to rehearse technical, tactical, and strategic aspects of the task. High-performing athletes often use these techniques.

Mindfulness is another technique that growing numbers of athletes and service members are using to enhance their resilience, improve performance, and preserve their overall health.[11] Although many definitions for mindfulness have been put forward, its key concept is the conscious cultivation of self-awareness to understand what is going on internally (eg, emotions, thoughts, responses) and externally (in the individual's surrounding physical and social environment) (Figure 42.7).

Equally important, service members must be given sufficient time for rest and recovery, and educated to take advantage of it when available. Otherwise, chronic sleep deprivation due to mission tempo, excessive stress, or poor decisions will significantly impair health and ultimately compromise performance.[12,13]

TABLE 42.2. Terms related to military performance optimization

- **Human performance optimization (HPO).** The process of applying knowledge, skills, and emerging technologies to improve and preserve the capabilities of military personnel to execute essential tasks.
- **Performance enhancement.** Optimizing and enhancing every system to the fullest degree possible before deployment.
- **Performance sustainment.** Sustaining performance at pre-deployment levels during deployment.
- **Performance restoration.** Restoring or returning performance to pre-deployment levels after deployment.
- **Human performance modification (HPM).** Actions ranging from the use of "natural" materials, such as caffeine or khat as a stimulant, to the application of nanotechnology as a drug delivery mechanism or an invasive brain implant. (Human Performance Modification: Review of Worldwide Research with a View to the Future. Washington, DC: National Academies Press; 2012.)
- **Total force fitness (TFF).** Framework for understanding, assessing, and maintaining the fitness of the armed forces. The TFF framework consists of eight distinct domains (medical/dental, nutritional, social, behavioral, environmental, psychological, spiritual, and physical).

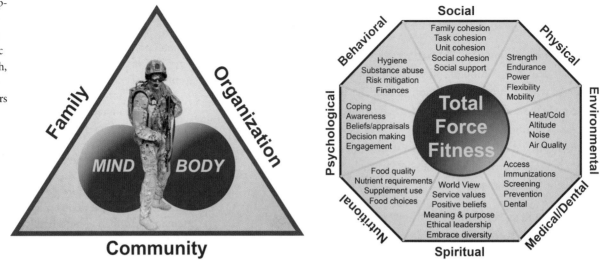

FIGURE 42.3. The conceptual framework of total force fitness and its eight domains; an effort to promote a holistic view for optimizing the health, fitness, readiness, and performance of our service members and their families.

HPO is designed to help service members and their families balance the demands of the mission with their personal goals. If the competing and sometimes conflicting demands of family and work (ie, the mission) are not understood and reconciled, they can negatively impact performance to the point that they threaten achievement of the unit's goals.

MAKING A DIFFERENCE NOW AND IN THE FUTURE

HPO and TFF are informing efforts to strengthen the health of the total force (Table 42.3), but considerable work remains. Future efforts may include writing TFF into policy as a requirement; implementing environmental changes to military installations and surrounding communities that promote health and well-being; instituting effective musculoskeletal injury-prevention programs from the moment of enlistment through training, deployment, and reintegration; and expanding the translation and sharing of HPO practices throughout the DoD.

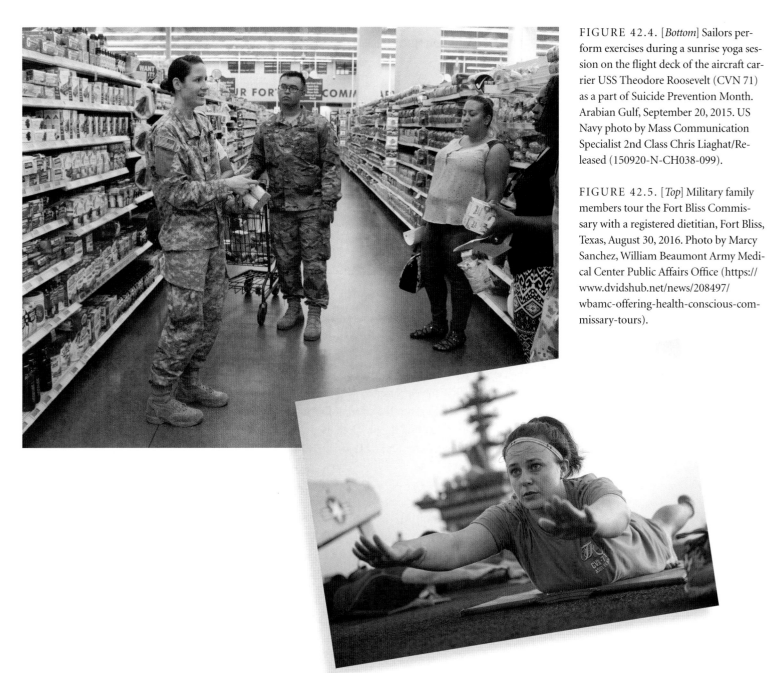

FIGURE 42.4. [*Bottom*] Sailors perform exercises during a sunrise yoga session on the flight deck of the aircraft carrier USS Theodore Roosevelt (CVN 71) as a part of Suicide Prevention Month. Arabian Gulf, September 20, 2015. US Navy photo by Mass Communication Specialist 2nd Class Chris Liaghat/Released (150920-N-CH038-099).

FIGURE 42.5. [*Top*] Military family members tour the Fort Bliss Commissary with a registered dietitian, Fort Bliss, Texas, August 30, 2016. Photo by Marcy Sanchez, William Beaumont Army Medical Center Public Affairs Office (https://www.dvidshub.net/news/208497/wbamc-offering-health-conscious-commissary-tours).

FIGURE 42.6. A brief description of the human performance optimization demand/resources model (left) and an outline of the multiple, competing, and interacting individual, family, and other factors that contribute to performance outcomes (right).

FIGURE 42.7. [*Opposite*] A master resilience trainer performance expert (rear) with the Fort Hood Comprehensive Soldier and Family Fitness Program follows Soldiers with 1st Squadron, 3rd Cavalry Regiment, as they conduct a foot patrol during field training exercises, December 10, 2013. He is assessing the Soldiers' use of the stress management skills they learned during a 10-hour classroom course that focused on breathing techniques, mental agility, and energy control. Photo by Sergeant Ken Scar, 7th Mobile Public Affairs Detachment (https://www.dvidshub.net/image/1138542/csf2-program-instructers-train-3rd-cavalry-regiment-troops-performance-enhancement).

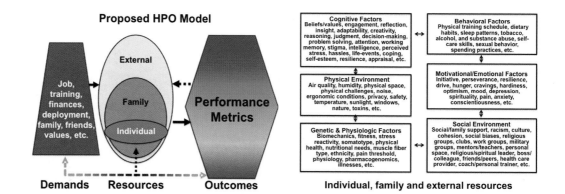

SUMMARY

The high and sustained tempo of combat operations over the past 14 years led the US military to embrace a new paradigm to achieve and sustain individual, family, and unit fitness. The resulting concepts, HPO and TFF, are widely embraced today. They reflect the understanding that the military's most valuable resource is not its weapons systems or technology, but its people: warfighters, support personnel, and their families. In an era characterized by two long wars rather than a short, intense conflict, HPO and TFF have promoted a culture of health, fitness, and resilience that has benefitted not only individual warfighters, but the entire military community. These efforts are designed to assure a ready force capable of meeting the physical, mental, and emotional challenges of current and future military operations, whenever and wherever they occur.

Notes

1. Deuster PA, O'Connor FG, Henry KA, et al. Human performance optimization: an evolving charge to the Department of Defense. *Mil Med.* 2007;172:1133–1137.

2. Russell A, Bulkley B, Grafton C. *Human Performance Optimization and Military Missions: Report for the Director, Office of Net Assessment.* McLean, VA: Science Applications International Corporation; 2005: 10–12, 92–101.

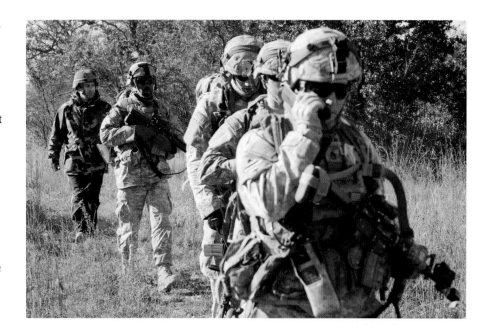

3. Human Performance Resource Center website. www.hprc-online.org. Accessed October 25, 2016.

4. Human Performance Resource Center. Total force fitness arena articles. hprc-online.org/total-force-fitness/total-force-fitness-articles. Accessed October 25, 2016.

5. Castro CA, Adler AB. Optempo: effects on soldier and unit readiness. *Parameters.* 1999;Autumn:86–85.

6. McGene J. *Social Fitness and Resilience: A Review of Relevant Constructs, Measures, and Links to Well-Being.* Santa Monica, CA: RAND Corp; 2013. http://www.rand.org/pubs/research_reports/RR108.html. Accessed October 25, 2016.

7. Bakker AB, Demerouti E, Euwema MC. Job resources buffer the impact of job demands on burnout. *J Occup Health Psychol.* 2005;10:170–180.

8. Demerouti E, Bakker AB, Nachreiner F, Schaufeli WB. The job demands-resources model of burnout. *J Appl Psychol.* 2001;86:499–512.

9. Deuster PA, Grunberg NE, O'Connor FG. An integrated approach for special operations. *J Spec Oper Med.* 2014;14:86–90.

10. Herzog TP, Deuster PA. Performance psychology as a key component of human performance optimization. *J Spec Oper Med.* 201;14:99–105.

11. Deuster PA, Schoomaker E. Mindfulness: a fundamental skill for performance sustainment and enhancement. *J Spec Oper Med.* 2015;15:93–99.

12. Hartzler BM. Fatigue on the flight deck: the consequences of sleep loss and the benefits of napping. *Accid Anal Prev.* 2014;62:309–318.

13. Rajaratnam SM, Howard ME, Grunstein RR. Sleep loss and circadian disruption in shift work: health burden and management. *Med J Aust.* 2013;199:S11–15.

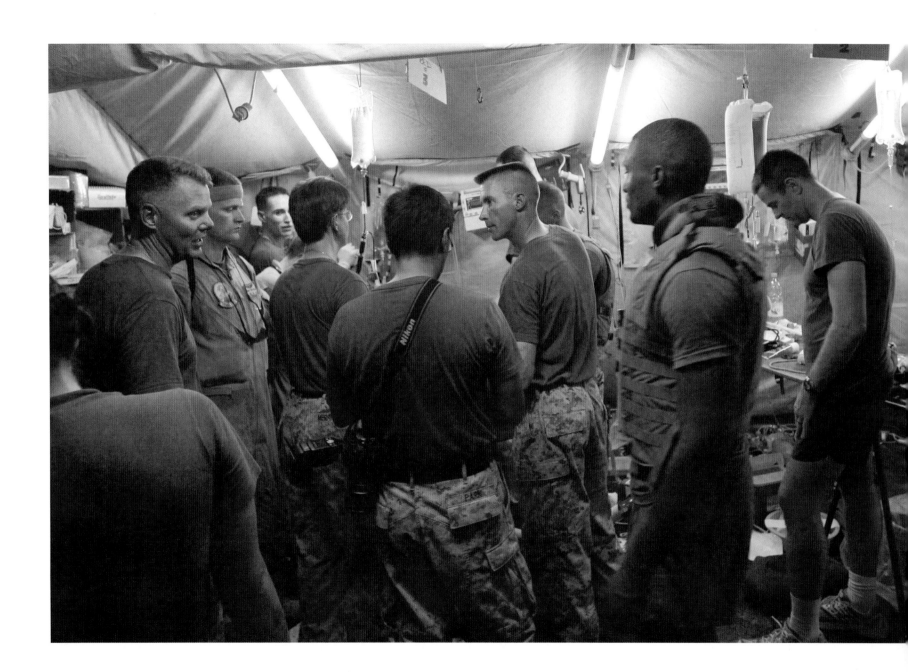

CHAPTER forty-three

Beyond the Battlefield: Civilian-Military Trauma Collaboration

JOHN H. ARMSTRONG, MD; M. MARGARET KNUDSON, MD; and DAVID B. HOYT, MD

INTRODUCTION

AS THE TEMPO OF WAR INCREASED IN 2003, civilian surgeons watched as their military colleagues (active duty and reservists) left their regular surgical practices in the United States and deployed to Iraq and Afghanistan. What is unique to military surgeons is that they must not only be skilled at performing the surgical procedures done in civilian hospitals, but they must also be ready to deploy on short notice to care for grievously wounded service men and women around the globe (Figure 43.1).

Civilian surgeons are also highly skilled, but they are not trained to work in combat zones. Fortunately, there was another way that the civilian trauma surgery community could help. With the permission of the US military, selected civilian trauma surgeons flew to Germany to work alongside their military colleagues at the US Army's Landstuhl Regional Medical Center (LRMC), the initial receiving point for severely wounded service men and women during Operations Enduring Freedom (OEF) and Iraqi Freedom (OIF) (Chapter 25). At the height of these conflicts, the daily influx of casualties from Iraq and Afghanistan transformed LRMC into one of the world's busiest trauma centers, where severely injured warriors received stabilizing care before moving on for more definitive surgery in the United States (Figure 43.2).

FIGURE 43.1. [*Opposite*] Al Anbar Province, Iraq: Naval medical personnel treat wounded service members who just arrived at Camp Taqaddum's main surgical facility for emergency surgery. More extensive care is provided later at one of the combat surgical hospitals in Baghdad or Balad. July 26, 2006. Photo by 1st Lieutenant Robert Shuford, 1st Marine Logistics Group. Reproduced from: https://www.dvidshub.net/image/18657/navy-medical-unit.

FIGURE 43.2. Members of the 455th Expeditionary Aeromedical Evacuation Squadron and the Contingency Aeromedical Staging Facility assist patients inside Landstuhl Regional Medical Center, Germany, March 22, 2013. US Air Force photo by Senior Airman Chris Willis. Reproduced from: https://www.dvidshub.net/image/897640/after-battle-flying-icu.

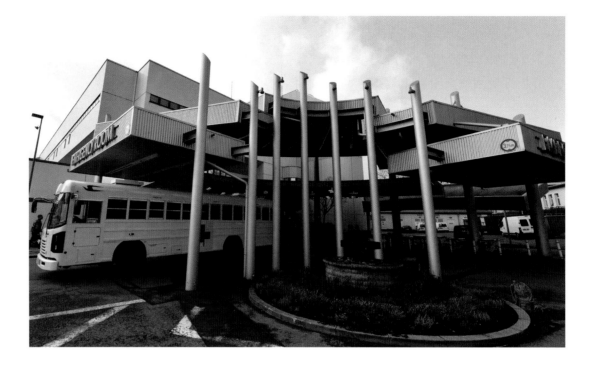

Three professional surgical societies worked with the Department of Defense to create the "Senior Visiting Surgeon" program.[1] Each surgeon volunteered his or her time, and their airfare and base lodging were financially supported by their sponsoring surgical society. Over the course of eight years, 146 vascular and 66 trauma surgeons—among them some of our nation's most renowned surgical leaders—worked alongside their military counterparts at LRMC. Civilian orthopedic surgeons and neurosurgeons participated as well. In addition to bolstering surgical staffing at LRMC, the program facilitated the exchange of clinical information, accelerated scientific discovery, and engendered camaraderie between the military and civilian surgical communities (see "Ensuring the Future of Military Trauma Care").

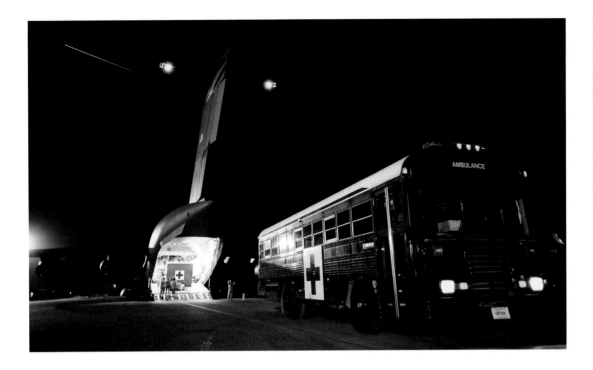

FIGURE 43.3. An ambulance bus from the Contingency Aeromedical Staging Facility prepares to unload ambulatory and litter-bound patients onto a C-17 Globemaster III at Joint Base Balad, Iraq, November 27, 2008. Photo by Senior Airman Jason Epley, 332nd Air Expeditionary Wing. Reproduced from: https://www.dvidshub.net/image/131955/contingency-aeromedical-staging-facility-airmen-move-warriors-out-theater.

SHARED LESSONS

Combat casualty care during the wars in southwest Asia has demonstrated the value of the exchange of ideas between civilian and military trauma communities: military surgeons have adopted best practices developed in the civilian sector and refined them for military use, while civilian surgeons have learned innovative techniques pioneered on the battlefield and adapted them for civilian use. Six lessons from this information exchange are highlighted.

1. **Care as a system.** One of the most valuable concepts borrowed from the civilian sector is that trauma care is an integrated system that spans a continuum of care from the point of injury to stabilization in non-trauma hospitals, definitive care at designated trauma centers, and expert

ENSURING THE FUTURE OF MILITARY TRAUMA CARE

Over the past 15 years, America's military health system (MHS) completely reengineered its approach to trauma care, pushing rates of survival from battlefield wounds to levels not previously seen in the history of warfare. When the enemy adapted by boosting the force and lethality of its improvised explosive devices, we adapted too, making further gains in battlefield survival (see Chapter 8, Figure 8.3).

As we developed and refined new techniques, we shared them with our civilian colleagues. From Tucson to Boston to Orlando and throughout the United States, medical teams are improving emergency care of civilians wounded in mass casualty events by applying lessons learned in Afghanistan and Iraq.

Today, the military-civilian collaboration that grew out of the crucible of war is fostering a strong and growing partnership between the MHS and leading civilian hospitals and clinical organizations. Civilian healthcare leaders are helping us improve our day-to-day operations, advance value-based healthcare, and create innovative solutions to new and emerging challenges. For example, in 2015, when the MHS conducted a comprehensive review of its safety, quality and access practices, Drs. Peter Pronovost, Brent James, and Janet Corrigan, as well as other leaders in quality and safety, provided us with invaluable assistance. The Institute of Healthcare Improvement helped us identify best practices.

One of the most challenging dilemmas facing the MHS is determining how to keep finely honed skills sharp between deployments. With the notable exception of San Antonio Military Medical Center, few stateside military hospitals participate in their community's trauma care network. As a result, their trauma caseloads are a fraction of that encountered in a typical wartime combat support hospital.

To keep the skills of military surgical staff current, the Army, Navy and Air Force rotate key personnel to a handful of civilian trauma centers around the country. Two years ago, Dr. Jonathan Woodson, then assistant secretary of defense (health affairs) established a formal MHS strategic partnership with the American College of Surgeons to expand educational opportunities, assure proficiency and currency, promote systems-based practice, and advance trauma care research.

Going forward, we need to broaden these partnerships so that not just physicians, but also nurses, medical enlisted technicians, and entire emergency care teams benefit from civilian "tours of duty." One way to do this is to increase the number of military hospitals that participate in civilian trauma systems. Another is to rotate teams of military healthcare providers to understaffed public and community hospitals that provide high volumes of complex trauma care.

The more closely military and civilian trauma teams work together, the faster we'll learn together. When civilian surgical leaders from the United States flew to Landstuhl, Bagram, and other combat hospitals to operate alongside military surgeons, they not only taught our doctors valuable skills, they learned from us as well.

Today, America faces a growing array of threats around the world. For the US military, complacency is not an option. After 15 years of war, our MHS knows what it takes to win. We will do everything necessary to keep that edge.

Vice Admiral Raquel Bono, MD
Director, Defense Health Agency
Falls Church, Virginia

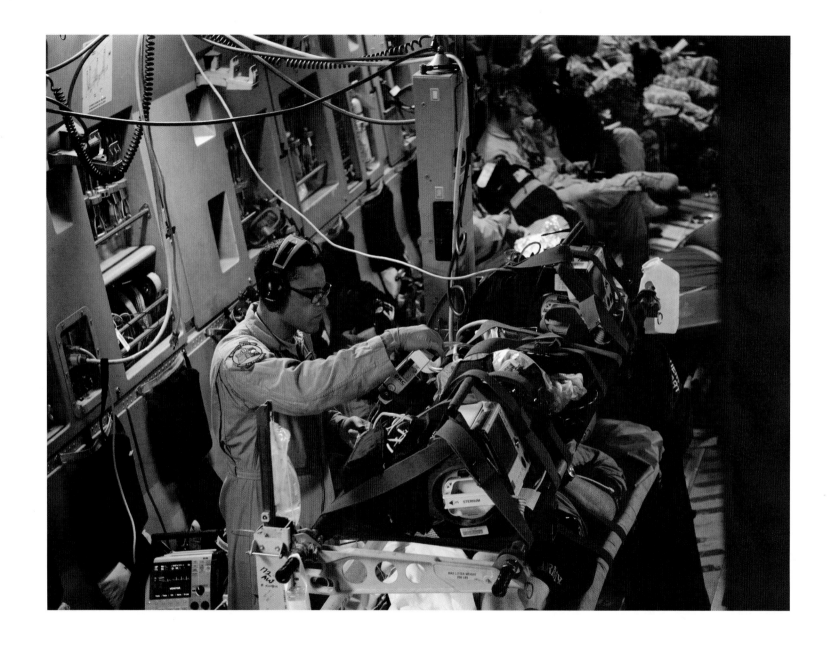

rehabilitative care afterward.[2] The military version extended this comprehensive approach to combat casualty care 10,000 miles away by creating a far-flung but seamless network enabled by medically managed patient movement: MEDEVAC from the field to forward surgical teams, then to combat support hospitals, followed by intercontinental evacuation by US Air Force Critical Care Air Transport Teams (CCATTs)—"intensive care units in the sky" (Figures 43.3 and 43.4).

2. **Use of a trauma registry.** Civilian trauma systems widely use trauma registries to document care and identify opportunities for improvement. Early on in OEF and OIF, military medical leaders adopted and extended this practice to create the Joint Trauma Registry[3] (Chapter 8). The registry has been essential for data-driven performance improvement to save more lives from severe injury.

3. **Standardization of skills.** To ensure that everyone in a trauma resuscitation team is working from the same playbook, the American College of Surgeons Committee on Trauma (ACS-COT) devised the Advanced Trauma Life Support (ATLS) course. Offered to surgeons and non-surgeons alike, this practical, hands-on course has been offered nationwide since 1980. Because nearly all deploying US military surgeons and physicians are trained in ATLS, they were able to work together "down range" using a common clinical framework. In 2014 alone, 24 military ATLS sites provided 122 courses to 1,519 physicians and 290 physician extenders.[4] Recently, with the concurrence of the ACS-COT, military surgeons created a new version of the course, ATLS-OE (Operational Emphasis), which is augmented for combat casualty care (Figure 43.5).

4. **Point-of-injury care.** Civilian surgery gave ATLS to the military, and the military has given Tactical Combat Casualty Care (TCCC) to the civilian world. As noted in chapter 11 of this book, TCCC emphasizes prompt control of life-threatening bleeding through immediate application of tourniquets, hemostatic dressings, and other lifesaving measures. Today, TCCC is used by police SWAT teams, wilderness rescue teams, and a growing number of urban emergency medical services. Some of the skills have been used by civilian bystanders as well. In the first chaotic moments after the Boston Marathon bombings, several bystanders applied makeshift tourniquets and other techniques to treat life-threatening bleeding. The concept of civilian engagement has been enthusiastically embraced by the Hartford Consensus, a group of civilian healthcare leaders seeking to teach the public how to

FIGURE 43.4. [*Opposite*] First Lieutenant Eric Rodriguez, 379th Expeditionary Aeromedical Evacuation Squadron nurse, checks on a patient's medical equipment during an evacuation flight to Landstuhl Regional Medical Center, Germany, April 25, 2012. US Air Force photo by Staff Sergeant Nathanael Callon/Released. Reproduced from: https://www. dvidshub.net/image/790961/c-17-globemaster-iii-medical-evacuation-flight-mission.

FIGURE 43.5. [*Opposite*]
US Navy Commander William Dutton, left, Advanced Trauma Life Support (ATLS) instructor, conducts hands-on training to a class of multinational military medical personnel aboard the Military Sealift Command hospital ship USNS Mercy (T-AH 19), July 21, 2014. US Navy photo by Mass Communication Specialist 3rd Class Justin W. Galvin/Released. Reproduced from: https://www.dvidshub.net/image/1474532/medical-trauma-related-courses-rimpac-2014.

control bleeding following mass casualty and rampage shooter events. The principles were highlighted in 2016 by the federal government's "Stop the Bleed, Save a Life" initiative and the ongoing American College of Surgeons "Stop the Bleed" campaign.[5]

5. **Damage control principles.** Damage control surgery, first developed in civilian trauma centers, was quickly adopted and expanded by military surgeons operating in Iraq and Afghanistan (Chapter 15). Military trauma surgeons, in turn, took the lead in developing the complimentary practice of "balanced resuscitation," which involves infusing a mix of blood, platelets, and clotting factors to reduce bleeding and sustain life (Chapter 16). These techniques, combined with strict maintenance of normal temperature and other lifesaving measures, were brought back to the United States by military trauma professionals who transitioned to civilian practice.

6. **Videoconferencing.** Used by some US trauma systems to promote quality improvement, videoconferencing was adopted on a global scale by the military health system. This enabled trauma case conferences to link healthcare providers in Afghanistan, Iraq, Germany, and the United States to review case management from the point of injury forward to damage control surgery in theater, CCATT transport to LRMC, and subsequently definitive surgical care in a major stateside hospital such as Walter Reed National Military Medical Center or San Antonio Military Medical Center. Through this mechanism, military trauma care providers across the continuum of care shared and learned best practices, identified bottlenecks, corrected potential deficiencies in care, and learned how well their patients did. These conferences reinforced the reality that in trauma care, optimal outcomes depend on a well-organized team effort, even when the concept of "team" extends over 10,000 miles.[1]

NEW CHALLENGES

Typically, the high level of technical skills, knowledge, and teamwork required to deliver optimal casualty care ebbs in peacetime, then slowly recovers during the first months or years of war. In past conflicts, this resulted in less optimal care, and a higher rate of preventable deaths, in the early stages of each war. OEF and OIF followed this pattern. Our challenge is to learn from the past so we do not repeat the same mistakes.

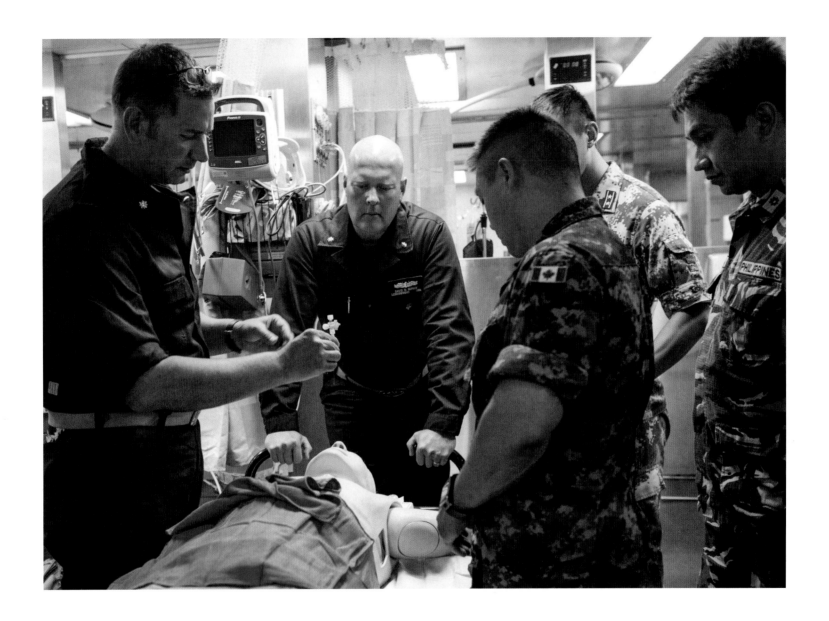

To sustain readiness and ensure that future military providers deploy with the right knowledge and skills, many military medical experts are promoting the idea that every deploying healthcare professional first be required to demonstrate mastery in TCCC and ATLS-OE. This will provide a common language for the care of combat-injured patients.

Other Department of Defense efforts include the Emergency War Surgery Course, which is based on the *Emergency War Surgery Manual*.[6] Both the course and manual codify standards and guidelines for effective combat casualty care. Other advances include the development and rapid dissemination of clinical practice guidelines from the war zones in Iraq and Afghanistan; the widespread use of portable ultrasound to detect bleeding in the chest or abdomen; and a host of service-specific and local courses developed by interested military trauma professionals. One of these military courses serves as the basis for the American College of Surgeon's newest trauma skills course, Advanced Surgical Skills for Exposure in Trauma (ASSET).

Unfortunately, too much of the preparation for deployment remains service-specific and often comes right before deployment. A joint, tri-service curriculum might better prepare military health professionals to work together on inter-service and interdisciplinary teams, but currently each service dictates their own requirements.[7]

Optimal outcomes in trauma depend on regular practice. Currently, only three military treatment facilities are designated trauma centers, and only two (San Antonio Military Medical Center and Madigan Army Medical Center in Tacoma, WA) are allowed to treat civilians. This limits peacetime exposure to critically ill and injured patients. To compensate, each service has established bilateral partnerships with civilian trauma centers: Jackson Memorial Hospital, Miami (Army); Los Angeles County/University of Southern California Medical Center, Los Angeles (Navy); and Baltimore Shock Trauma, the University of Cincinnati, and St. Louis University (Air Force). These partnerships enable military trauma surgeons and selected staff members to gain vital skills by practicing side-by-side with civilian colleagues. While blast injuries are rarely encountered in civilian trauma centers, other types of trauma are, including gunshot wounds, complex fractures, and both blunt and penetrating traumatic brain injuries. Moreover, working in a busy trauma center bolsters team skills.[8]

These partnership programs are useful, but they are insufficient to ensure that all military providers remain current in their skills. In addition, the current training experiences are service-specific. If the military's large medical centers were allowed to participate in their region's trauma system and accept civilian trauma patients, it could make a big difference.

PREPARING FOR THE FUTURE TODAY

Preserving readiness to treat combat casualties cannot be left to chance. It requires a planned and structured approach to education and training that promotes the development and maintenance of individual and team skills. Based on the successful military-civilian cooperation of the past decade, conditions are ideal to establish a more formal collaboration to sustain and increase excellence between wars. The Military Health System Strategic Partnership with the American College of Surgeons codifies this collaboration.[9] Established in October 2014, it has the following aims:

• Develop a standardized, validated training curriculum that includes essential technical and team skills necessary for surgical care in combat zones, disasters, or a humanitarian crisis.

• Sustain a joint trauma system to support care in future conflicts.

• Develop and support a combat casualty care research program in the civilian sector.

• Extend surgical quality expertise from the American College of Surgeons to the military health system by creating a military quality consortium.

Sustaining the readiness of the military health system during peacetime will not only save more lives at the start of the next conflict, it will also help thousands of civilian trauma patients. Civilian trauma care has greatly benefitted from lessons learned in wartime, including advances in blood transfusions, aeromedical evacuation (Figure 43.6), burn care, vascular trauma care, and treatment of other life-threatening injuries. As noted in the recent report on trauma care produced by the National Academies of Science, Engineering, and Medicine, civilian and military researchers should work together to improve trauma care in both civilian and military domains with the goal of achieving "zero preventable

FIGURE 43.6. US civilian aeromedical units grew out of the US military's experience with MEDEVAC helicopters in Korea and Vietnam. The PennStar Flight program (pictured) operates six helicopters, all staffed by expert pilots, critical care flight nurses, and flight paramedics. It performs critical care transports between medical centers, and responds "on-scene" to treat and transport victims with severe trauma from car crashes and other incidents. Photograph courtesy of Dr. C. William Schwab; reproduced with permission from Penn Medicine.

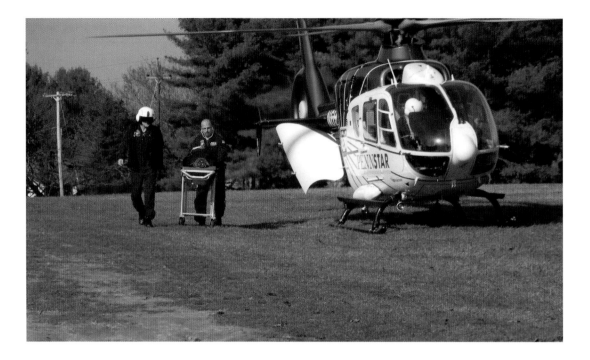

deaths after injury."[10] Because American service members know they will receive the world's best care if wounded, they are more confident when entering the fight. Thus, our nation's military health care system serves as a force multiplier for success on the battlefield.[11]

Notes

1. Knudson MM, Evans TW, Fang R, et al. A concluding after-action report of the Senior Visiting Surgeon Program with the United States Military at Landstuhl Regional Medical Center, Germany. *J Trauma Acute Care Surg.* 2014;76:878–883.

2. Knudson MM. When peace breaks out: The 42nd American Association for the Surgery of Trauma Fitts Oration. *J Trauma Acute Care Surg.* 2016;82(1):10-17.

3. Eastridge BJ, Costanzo G, Jenkins D, et al. Impact of joint theater trauma system initiatives on battlefield injury outcomes. *Am J Surg.* 2009;198:852–857.

4. Personal correspondence, ATLS program office, American College of Surgeons, February 2, 2016.

5. Jacobs LM, Joint Committee to Create a National Policy to Enhance Survivability from Intentional Mass Casualty Shooting Events. The Hartford Consensus III: implementation of bleeding control. *Bull Am Coll Surg.* 2015;100:20-26.

6. *Emergency War Surgery, 4th US Revision.* Fort Sam Houston, TX: Office of The Surgeon General, Borden Institute; 2013.

7. Schwab CW. Winds of war: enhancing civilian and military partnerships to assure readiness. *J Am Coll Surg.* 2015;221:235–254.

8. Remick KN, Elster E. Combat surgeon readiness: partnering during war and peace. *J Trauma Acute Care Surg.* 2016:81(5)Suppl:S72-S74.

9. Knudson MM, Elster EE, Woodson J, Kirk G, Turner P, Hoyt DB. a shared ethos: the military health system strategic partnership with the American College of Surgeons. *J Am Coll Surg.* 2016;222(6):1251–1257.

10. National Academies of Sciences, Engineering, Medicine. *A National Trauma Care System: Integrating Military and Civilian Trauma Systems to Achieve Zero Preventable Deaths After Injury.* Washington, DC: National Academies Press; 2016: xiv, xv. http://www.nationalacademies.org/hmd/Reports/2016/A-National-Trauma-Care-System-Integrating-Military-and-Civilian-Trauma-Systems.aspx. Accessed July 11, 2016.

11. Remick KN. Leveraging trauma lessons from war to win in a complex global environment. *US Army Med Dep J.* 2016;Apr-Sep:106–113.

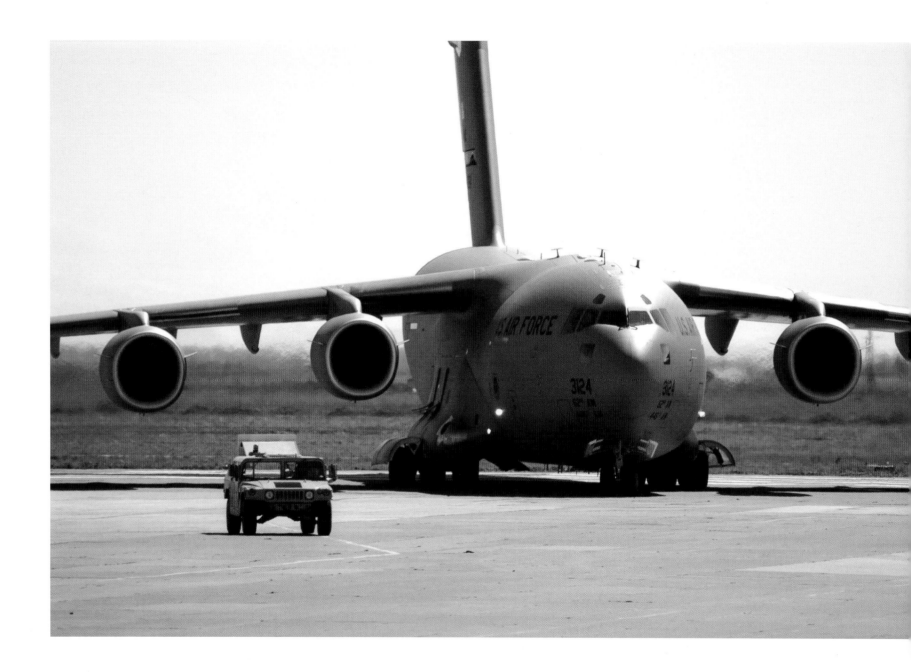

CHAPTER forty-four

Homecoming

LIEUTENANT GENERAL (RETIRED) THOMAS W. TRAVIS, MD, MPH

D URING THE LONG WARS IN IRAQ AND AFGHANISTAN, three times a week, C-17s (Figure 44.1) from Germany would land at Andrews Air Force Base in Maryland, usually packed with patients—some ambulatory, some on litters, and some who required Critical Care Air Transport Teams (CCATTs). On final approach to Andrews, the aircraft flew over the Capital Beltway, filled with commuters who had no idea that just above their heads was a plane full of wounded, ill, and injured young Americans coming home.

In the spring of 2013, during my first year as Air Force surgeon general, I received a call one Sunday morning that an air-evac flight was coming into Andrews that afternoon with a critically wounded Air Force medic on board. This 23-year-old medic had been deployed to Afghanistan for a year and was on her final mission before coming home. She was riding in a mine-resistant ambush-protected vehicle (MRAP) with three battle buddies when they were struck by a 400- to 700-pound improvised explosive device (IED). The massive blast killed one of her Army buddies and severely wounded her and the other two Soldiers. She sustained a punctured lung, three broken ribs, seven spinal compression fractures, two severely broken ankles, six fractures to her pelvis, and shrapnel wounds to her face.

After fellow medics in a trailing vehicle extracted her and rendered lifesaving care, she was taken to a nearby forward operating base (FOB) for additional resuscitative care and prep for evacuation to Craig Joint Theater Hospital at Bagram Airfield. A nurse at the FOB was able to make contact with the medic's mother to let her know how she was, and kissed the medic on the forehead at her mother's request.

FIGURE 44.1. [*Opposite*] A C-17 Globemaster III follows a high-mobility multipurpose wheeled vehicle during airfield operations at Karshi-Khanabad Air Base, Uzbekistan, March 20, 2005, during Operation Enduring Freedom. Photo by Master Sergeant Scott Sturkol, Headquarters, Air Mobility Command. Reproduced from: https://www.dvidshub.net/image/345068/c-17-globemaster-iii-amcs-workhorse-meeting-airlift-needs-across-globe.

Shortly thereafter, a MEDEVAC (medical evacuation) helicopter flew her to Bagram, where she received more treatment. Then she was placed on an air-evac flight in the care of a CCATT and flown to the jointly staffed hospital at Landstuhl, Germany.

The patient's first sergeant at her home base knew some of the nurses and medics at Landstuhl and asked them to wash and braid her hair and put some nail polish on her toes. And again, at her mother's request, a nurse kissed her before she went into surgery. After a brief stay at Landstuhl, she came home on the flight I met at Andrews. This was just three days after the attack that changed her and her family's lives forever.

When she landed at Andrews, she was still intubated[1] and somewhat sedated. I was allowed on board the C-17 to briefly greet the patients before they were taken by ambulance to Walter Reed National Military Medical Center in Bethesda. After speaking to some of the other patients (two of whom were victims of the same IED attack), I approached the young medic.

Her eyes were closed, and she was mildly sedated, but I could tell she was signing. I happen to know sign language because I have a deaf family member. So I held her hand, told her who I was, and let the nurses know that she was asking for the tube[1] to be removed and that she did not want any more [sedating] meds.

Anxious to allow the crew to off-load the plane, I told her I would visit her in the hospital in a few days when she was more awake. As I left the flight, I spent a brief moment with the other two critical care patients, shook the hand of every litter and ambulatory patient to welcome them home, and got out of the crew's way. Because the medic's family had been given regular information about her whereabouts and condition during her journey back from Afghanistan, they were at Walter Reed to meet her when she arrived from the Andrews flight line.

A few days later, I kept my promise and visited the medic at Walter Reed. By then, she was awake and her mom was there. We had a wonderful visit. Her mother told me about all of the touch points of care mentioned above. She called it an unbroken chain of love and care, from the kiss on the forehead at the FOB, to the fingernail polish in Germany, and then my interpreting her daughter's sign language on the plane when she landed.

A few weeks later, I was proud to be asked by the injured medic to present her Purple Heart and Combat Action medals with her family present and her commanders and peers participating via live video stream from her home base.

Since that day, this young lady has required many more surgeries and rehabilitation. It has been a tough road, but at last report, three years after the attack, she is making great progress.

This medic's experience, and that of thousands of casualties like her, represents the care our military health team strives to provide every wounded, ill, or injured service member from the point of injury overseas to definitive care and eventual rehabilitation here at home. Every one of these young Americans is precious to us. Their moms and dads, husbands and wives, sons and daughters, and all who love them rightfully expect us to provide them the best possible care. The leadership of the Army, Navy, and Air Force medical departments and the personnel they lead are committed to this goal. So are the line leaders of our respective services. We understand how important expert medical care is to our nation's military strength. Based on the lessons we've learned over the past 14 years of war, we are absolutely determined, regardless of the obstacles, to be as good at the beginning of the next conflict as we were at the end of this one. Our nation expects no less.

Note

1. Intubated: when a patient is unable to adequately breathe on their own, doctors carefully pass a clear plastic tube, known as an endotracheal tube, through the patient's mouth, between the vocal cords, and into the patient's windpipe, or trachea. The tube is then connected to a ventilator (breathing machine). Healthcare providers often shorten the term "endotracheal tube" to "tube."

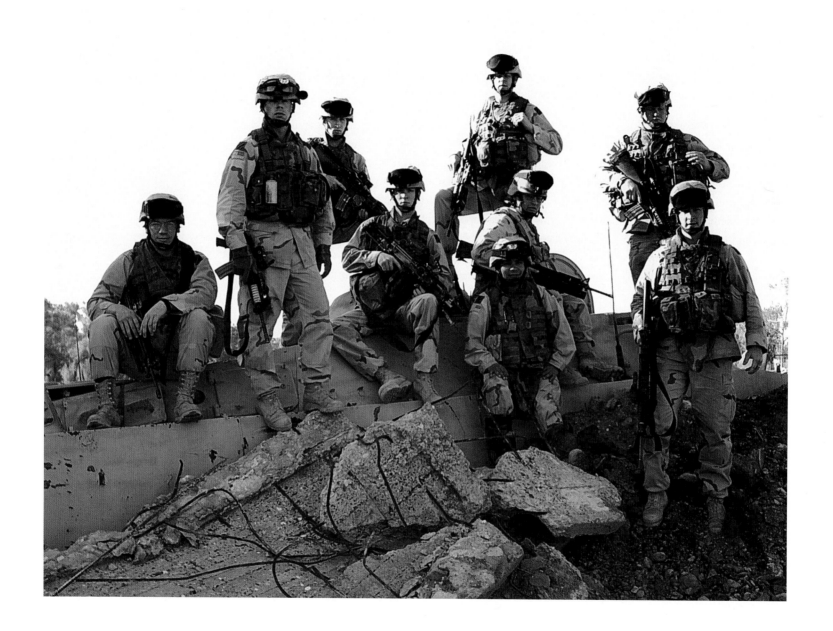

H IPPOCRATES, THE "FATHER OF WESTERN MEDICINE," reportedly said, "He who wishes to be a surgeon should go to war." Hippocrates was voicing a sad truth: the battlefield has long served as the classroom for medical advances. For centuries, under the pressure of delivering care in wartime, medical personnel have used their creativity and powers of observation to develop better methods to treat the ill and injured. Over time, the broader medical community adopted these techniques, to the benefit of us all.

The pace of discovery and knowledge-sharing accelerated during the American Civil War, and more recently, during the two world wars and the conflicts that followed. Today, we take many of these advances for granted: use of helicopters for aeromedical evacuation; use of morphine and other drugs to treat agonizing pain; safe approaches to cross-matching and transfusing blood and plasma; surgical techniques to treat damaged blood vessels and other forms of life-threatening trauma; and rehabilitation to help trauma victims recover from invisible as well as visible wounds.

This tradition continued in the wars in Iraq and Afghanistan. In little more than a decade, the US military transformed its approach to combat casualty care from the point of injury on the battlefield through successful reintegration of wounded warriors into their communities. In the process, the military took a combat care system that was already considered the best in the world and made it better—*much* better.

The results speak for themselves. Despite simultaneously fighting two far distant regional wars, the US military achieved the highest rate of combat casualty survival in the history of warfare. This achievement is even more remarkable because, over the course of the wars, the average severity of combat injuries increased due to the growing power and sophistication of improvised explosive devices, the dominant mechanism of injury in these conflicts.

FIGURE A1. [*Opposite*] Retired Army Staff Sergeant Mitch Court (second from left) stands among his squad in Afghanistan in 2009, the day before he was severely injured in combat. Court's recovery included major surgeries to his legs, face, lung, and ribs. He is now a quality assurance specialist with the Defense Contract Management Agency, Cleveland. Photo courtesy of the Defense Contract Management Agency. Reproduced from: https://www.dvidshub.net/image/1862656/wounded-warrior-comes-home-quality-life.

FIGURE A2. [*Opposite*] May 19,
2007. A UH-60A Black Hawk with
the 45th Medical Company (Air
Ambulance) taxies down the runway at Al Asad Air Base, Iraq. Photograph reproduced from: https://
www.dvidshub.net/image/46478/
air-ambulance-run-ups.

Thanks to the determination, ingenuity, and courage of the medical services of the United States and
our allies, hundreds (if not thousands) of wounded, ill, and injured warriors who would have died in
prior wars came home alive. Furthermore, thanks to equally dramatic improvements in rehabilitation,
prosthetics, behavioral healthcare, and family support, many returned to productive service in their unit
or their community. A surprising number returned to serve on the battlefield.

Several factors contributed to this remarkable success:

1. **The physical condition of those who deployed was the best in our nation's history**. Rigorous
   screening and physical fitness training ensured that those we sent in harm's way were as physically,
   mentally, and emotionally prepared as possible. This not only made them more adaptable in combat,
   it also made them more resilient to injury and adversity (Figure A.1).

2. **The training provided to Army medics, Navy corpsmen, and Air Force med techs was thorough
   and evidence-based**. Long revered for their courage in battle, these front-line providers were taught
   skills that greatly enhanced their effectiveness. Once learned, these techniques were repeatedly
   rehearsed in simulation centers and field exercises that imparted as much realism as possible. This
   assured that when these providers went down range, they were prepared.

3. **The importance of bleeding control was swiftly recognized**. For decades, the optimal sequence
   for resuscitation was "A, B, C." Airway first, followed by breathing, then circulation. However, initial
   data from Afghanistan and Iraq revealed that uncontrolled bleeding was the most common cause
   of preventable battlefield deaths. This made prompt control of life-threatening hemorrhage the top
   priority, and drove rapid improvements in the design and use of tourniquets, topical hemostatics,
   and balanced blood resuscitation. These techniques have already reached the civilian world and are
   incorporated into Advanced Trauma Life Support instruction.

4. **Air supremacy enabled prompt evacuation of the wounded**. Widespread use of MEDEVAC helicopters, soon staffed by paramedics and critical care nurses, minimized the risk of ambush and attacks with roadside bombs during ground travel through hostile terrain (Figure A.2). It also enabled
   wounded service members to reach a forward surgical team or combat support hospital within the
   "golden hour" required for optimal trauma care. Air supremacy also enabled intercontinental air

evacuations to Germany, and from there to the United States, on C-17 flights staffed by Critical Care Air Transport Teams. This allowed the military health system to shrink the medical footprint in combat zones and dramatically shorten time from injury to definitive care (and reunion with loved ones).

5. **Information technology accelerated the sharing of knowledge and expertise.** Telehealth and intercontinental teleconferences enabled teams spread across the world to review and discuss wounded service members' care. Weekly videoconferences linked combat medics, nurses, and trauma surgeons in Balad and Bagram with their colleagues at Landstühl, Walter Reed National Military Medical Center, San Antonio Military Medical Center, and the Institute for Surgical Research. As these medical professionals reviewed each case, they applied the insights gained to subsequent warriors' care. This capability, along with the systematic collection of data through the Joint Trauma Registry, transformed military trauma care into a "learning healthcare system."

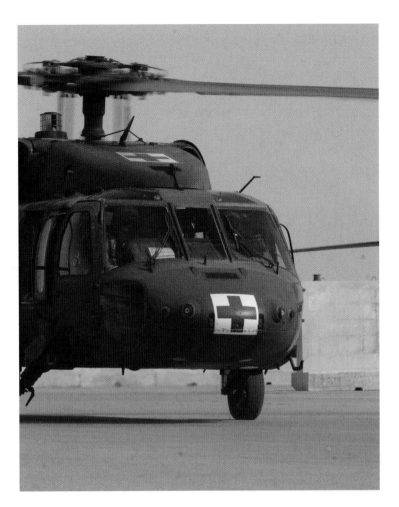

These advances did not happen by chance. They emerged from a clinical culture that values problem-solving, initiative, and leadership. In addition to having excellent people, equipment, and facilities, the military health system benefitted from its inventive and adaptive research infrastructure. Underlying all was American ingenuity, moral courage, and a relentless drive to do better.

When the pace of war recedes, military medical leaders often struggle to ensure that their personnel retain their combat-relevant skills. Failure to do so can result in a costly and painful period of "re-learning" when another war begins. This is a primary reason the US Congress established the Uniformed Services University of the Health Sciences

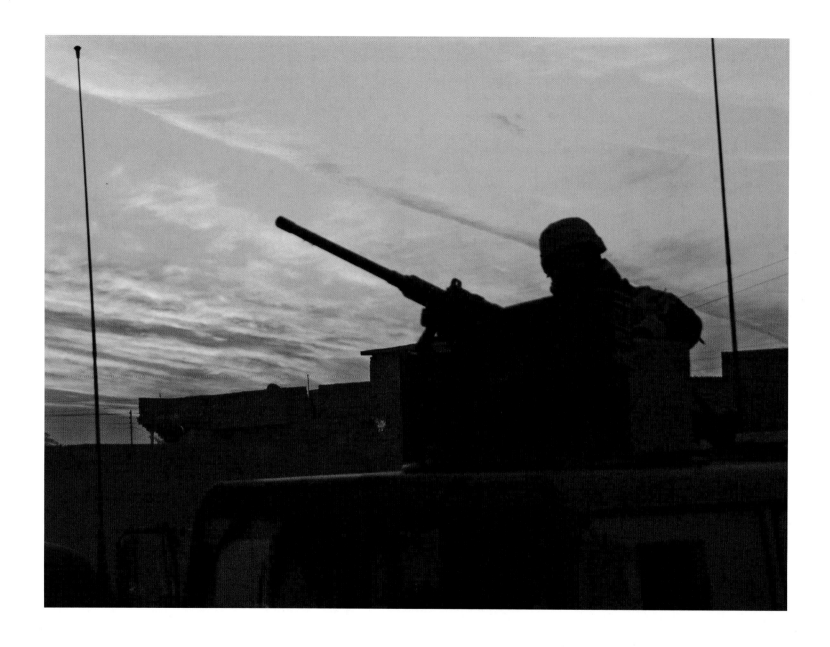

(USU). USU was never intended to supply all the physicians, nurses, and other healthcare professionals needed to support military healthcare operations. Rather, like the military service academies, it produces leaders with the ethos and core values the enterprise can rely on, and serves as a repository of lessons learned from prior conflicts (Chapter 3). USU graduates and faculty members (current and former) played critical roles in Iraq and Afghanistan. Many contributed to this book.

America's military health system has a long and mutually beneficial partnership with civilian medicine. Knowledge sharing is a two-way street. Military medicine works with civilian specialty societies (such as the American College of Surgeons and the American Board of Preventive Medicine) to ensure that its personnel are up-to-date on the latest research and techniques. The visiting surgeon program at Landstuhl is a powerful example of this steadfast and enduring partnership (Chapter 43).

Civilian medicine also benefits from the partnership. As quickly as military doctors develop new innovations on the battlefield, they share their findings with civilian colleagues through conferences, symposia, journal articles, and professional dialog. Many of the innovators who championed achievements documented in this book have transitioned to civilian life as teachers and clinical leaders in our nation's top academic medical centers.

Generals are often accused of "fighting the last war." Military medicine cannot make the same mistake. The next time our nation goes to war, the challenges may be vastly different from those encountered in Iraq and Afghanistan (Figure A.3). For this reason, it is not only vital that our military health system sustain its current capabilities, but we must also ensure that it retains its remarkable capacity to *innovate* in order to defeat emerging health threats. Although America's civilian research agencies are very capable, they focus on different priorities and work at a slower pace than that required to meet military needs.

In "Homecoming," this book's final chapter, the mother of a wounded Air Force medic speaks appreciatively of the "unbroken chain of love and care" that brought her daughter home. The chain she describes was forged in the crucible of war, but it is held together by love. The men and women who make up our nation's military health system love the mission they've been given, those they leave behind when they go into harm's way, the patients they serve at home and overseas, and the nation they are sworn to defend.

JONATHAN WOODSON, MD, and CHARLES L. RICE, MD

FIGURE A3. [*Opposite*] In the early morning of January 15, 2005, Sergeant Bonneau keeps an eye out for any suspicious activity on a street in the city of As Siniyah, Iraq, as his fellow Soldiers perform a sweep for any materials for making improvised explosive devices. Photograph courtesy of the Multi-National Corps Iraq Public Affairs Office. Reproduced from: https://www.dvidshub.net/image/3690/sgt-bonneau-keeps-eye-out-any-suspicious-activity.

abbreviations and acronyms

AAS	All Soldier Study		CAREN	computer-assisted rehabilitation environment
ACME	Advanced Combat Medical Experience		CASF	contingency aeromedical staging facility
ACS	American College of Surgeons		CAT	cognitive assistive technology
ACS-COT	American College of Surgeons Committee on Trauma		CAT	Combat Application Tourniquet
AD	advanced development		CCATT	Critical Care Air Transport Team
ADAPT	After Deployment Adaptive Parenting Tools		CCC	concussion care center
AFIRM	Armed Forces Institute of Regenerative Medicine		CCCRP	Combat Casualty Care Research Program
AFSOC	Air Force Special Operations Command		CDST	clinical decision support tool
AKO	Army Knowledge Online		CHAMP	Consortium for Health and Military Performance
AMBUS	ambulance bus		CI	clinical investigation
AMSUS	Association of Military Surgeons of the United States		CJCS	chairman of the Joint Chiefs of Staff
APACHE	Acute Physiology and Chronic Health Evaluation		CJOA-A	Combined Joint Operating Area–Afghanistan
APS	acute pain service		CME	continuing medical education
ARC	Advanced Rehabilitation Center		CNE	continuing nursing education
ASSET	Advanced Surgical Skills for Exposure in Trauma		CNRM	Center for Neuroscience and Regenerative Medicine
ATLS	Advanced Trauma Life Support		CoTCCC	Committee on Tactical Combat Casualty Care
			CPNB	continuous peripheral nerve block
BAMC	Brooke Army Medical Center		CPPs	cryopreserved platelets
BRAC	Base Realignment and Closure Act		CRCC	concussion restorative care center
			CSC	combat stress control
C4	Combat Casualty Care Course		CSCC	concussion specialty care center
CAM	complementary and alternative medicine		CSH	combat surgical hospital

CSI	congressional special interest	HIV	human immunodeficiency virus
CT	computed tomography	HPM	human performance modification
CTE	chronic traumatic encephalopathy	HPO	human performance optimization
		HPRC	Human Performance Resource Center
DCBI	dismounted complex blast injury	HPSP	Health Professions Scholarship Program
DCoE	Defense Center of Excellence	HRSA	Health Resources and Services Administration
DCR	damage control resuscitation		
DNBI	disease or non-battle injury	ICU	intensive care unit
DoD	Department of Defense	IDE	individual device exemption
DoDTR	Department of Defense Trauma Registry	IDEO	Intrepid Dynamic Extraskeletal Orthosis
DTLOMS	Doctrine, Training, Leader Development, Organization, Materiel, and Soldier	IDES	Integrated Disability Evaluation System
		IED	improvised explosive device
DTRS	Deployable Tele-Radiology System	IFAK	individual first aid kit
DVBIC	Defense and Veterans Brain Injury Center	IND	investigational new drug
		IV	intravenous
ECMO	extracorporeal membrane oxygenation		
EMEDS	Expeditionary Medical Support	JC2RT	Joint Combat Casualty Care Research Team
EMS	emergency medical services	JECC	Joint Enroute Care Course
EMT-B	emergency medical technician–basic	JTAPIC	Joint Trauma Analysis and Prevention of Injury in Combat
ESD	expeditionary transfer dock		
		JTS	Joint Trauma System
FDA	Food and Drug Administration	JTTR	Joint Theater Trauma Registry
FOB	forward operating base	JTTS	Joint Theater Trauma System
FOCUS	Families Overcoming Under Stress		
FRSS	Forward Resuscitative Surgical System	LRMC	Landstuhl Regional Medical Center
FST	forward surgical team	LTCOS	Long Term Clinical Outcomes Study
GI	gastrointestinal	MACE	Military Acute Concussion Evaluation
GME	graduate medical education	MAST	Military Assistance to Safety and Traffic
		MATTERS	Military Application of Tranexamic Acid in Trauma Emergency Resuscitation Study

MATV	MRAP all-terrain vehicle		OEF	Operation Enduring Freedom
MDRO	multidrug-resistant organism		OIF	Operation Iraqi Freedom
MEDEVAC	medical evacuation		O&M	operations and maintenance
MEDHOLD	medical holding company		OND	Operation New Dawn
MERT	Medical Emergency Response Team		OSCAR	Operational Stress Control and Readiness
MFLC	military family life consultant		OT	occupational therapy
MFST	mobile field surgical team		PI	performance improvement
MHS	Military Health System		PJ	pararescueman
MHAT	Mental Health Advisory Team		PLA	product license application
MHSS	Military Health Services System		PMMA	polymethyl methacrylate
MMPL	Military Medical Practice and Leadership		PPDS	Pre-Post Deployment Study
MFP	Medical Field Practicum		PPE	personal protective equipment
MOOTW	military operations other than war		PRT	Provincial Reconstruction Team
MPL	modular prosthetic limb		PSC	Polytrauma/TBI System of Care
MRAP	mine-resistant ambush-protected vehicle		PTSD	posttraumatic stress disorder
MRE	meal, ready-to-eat			
MRI	magnetic resonance imaging		RTD&E	research, development, testing, and analysis
MRMC	Medical Research and Material Command		R&D	research and development
MRSA	methicillin-resistant *Staphylococcus aureus*		RC	regional command
MSSA	methicillin-sensitive *Staphylococcus aureus*		REBOA	resuscitative endovascular balloon occlusion of the aorta
NAM	National Academy of Medicine		RFF	request for forces
NCO	noncommissioned officer		RFT	recreational/fitness technology
NHTSA	National Highway Traffic Safety Administration		ROTC	Reserve Officers Training Corps
NICoE	National Intrepid Center of Excellence		RPG	rocket-propelled grenade
NIH	National Institutes of Health			
NIMH	National Institute of Mental Health		SAAP	selective aortic arch perfusion
NSS	New Soldier Study		SHOS	Soldier Health Outcomes Study
			SOF	Special Operation Forces
			SSRI	selective serotonin reuptake inhibitor

S&T	science and technology	UK	United Kingdom
STARRS	Army Study to Assess Risk and Resilience in Servicemembers	UME	undergraduate medical education
		USAF	US Air Force
STARRS-LS	STARRS–Longitudinal Study	USMLE	US Medical Licensing Exam
		USU or USUHS	Uniformed Services University of the Health Sciences
TBH	tele-behavioral health		
TBI	traumatic brain injury	VA	Department of Veterans Affairs
TCCC	Tactical Combat Casualty Care	VBA	Veterans Benefits Administration
TCCET	Tactical Critical Care Evacuation Team	VCA	vascularized composite allograft
TCCET-E	Tactical Critical Care Evacuation Team–Enhanced	VHA	Veterans Health Administration
TFF	total force fitness	VR	virtual reality
TF-MED	Task Force MED		
TIDOS	Trauma Infectious Disease Outcomes Study		
TRACK-TBI	Transforming Research and Clinical Knowledge in TBI	WRAMC	Walter Reed Army Medical Center
TXA	tranexamic acid		